T0235373

Lecture Notes in Artificial Intelligence   9521

Subseries of Lecture Notes in Computer Science

More information about this series at http://www.springer.com/series/1244

Arjen Hommersom · Peter J.F. Lucas (Eds.)

Foundations of Biomedical Knowledge Representation

Methods and Applications

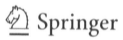 Springer

Editors
Arjen Hommersom
Institute for Computing and Information
  Sciences
Radboud University
Nijmegen
The Netherlands

and

Faculty of Management, Science
  and Technology
Open University
Heerlen, Limburg
The Netherlands

Peter J.F. Lucas
Institute for Computing and Information
  Sciences
Radboud University
Nijmegen
The Netherlands

ISSN 0302-9743   ISSN 1611-3349   (electronic)
Lecture Notes in Artificial Intelligence
ISBN 978-3-319-28006-6   ISBN 978-3-319-28007-3   (eBook)
DOI 10.1007/978-3-319-28007-3

Library of Congress Control Number: 2015958082

LNCS Sublibrary: SL7 – Artificial Intelligence

Printed on acid-free paper

This Springer imprint is published by SpringerNature
The registered company is Springer International Publishing AG Switzerland

Preface

Medicine and health care are currently faced with a significant rise in their complexity. This is partly due to the progress made during the past three decades in the fundamental biological understanding of the causes of health and disease at the molecular, (sub)cellular, and organ level. It is also partly caused by the increased specialization of both biomedical research and clinical practice, and greater involvement of policy makers in health care to control costs. Promises made by biomedical researchers that their research results will have clinical impact, e.g., that cancer can be cured by immune therapy, have also increased expectations from society about what healthcare is able to deliver. However, it is rarely the case that a discovery at the molecular level has immediate consequences for the diagnosis and treatment of patients.

A major problem is that the progress made by the basic sciences increases the quantity of information that one has to deal with when making decisions at the level of the patient or health care in general. An additional problem is that this information arises from research at different levels: from the molecular level, via the subcellular level, at one end of the spectrum, to the patient and health-care level at the other end. How to bridge these different levels is currently unclear although it has given rise to the creation of yet another field: translational medicine.

However, although there are huge differences in the techniques and methods used by biomedical researchers, there is now an increasing tendency to share research results in terms of formal knowledge representation methods, such as ontologies, statistical models, network models, and mathematical models. As there is an urgent need for health-care professionals to make better decisions, computer-based support using this knowledge is now becoming increasingly important. It may also be the only way to integrate research results from the different parts of the spectrum of biomedical and clinical research.

Exploitation of knowledge technologies in biomedicine and health care, ranging from biological ontologies to computerized clinical practice guidelines, has been used as a solution to the aforementioned issues. However, it has been difficult to integrate knowledge from different levels, even when concerning a single disease.

Many different formal representations are being used at the output of biomedical research. Probabilistic methods, such as Bayesian networks, have proved themselves useful for problems where uncertainty is important, such as medical decision making and prognostics, but also in biology. Logic plays a key role as a basis for medical ontologies, but also in the formalization of important medical concepts such as diagnostics. Differential equations are popular for describing the dynamics of biological processes at the molecular level. These methods can be extended with all kinds of semantic concepts, such as space, in the biomedical domain. Space is an important concept when developing probabilistic models of, e.g., the spread of infectious disease, either in the hospital or in the community at large. Reasoning with time is already provided by differential equations, but can also be done in other formalisms, such as probability theory and logic. Temporal reasoning is important in the context of personalized health care.

The aim of the book *Foundations of Biomedical Knowledge Representation* is to shed light on developments in knowledge representation at different levels of biomedical application, ranging from human biology to clinical guidelines, and using different techniques, from probability theory and differential equations to logic. While there is interdisciplinary cooperation between the different fields, there is a clear need for understanding the relationships of representation and reasoning among the different communities.

What the book will certainly make clear is that since the end of the 1970s, when knowledge representation and reasoning in the biomedical field became a separate area of research, huge progress has been made in the development of methods and tools that are finally able to have an impact on the way medicine is being practiced.

We wish to thank all the contributors to this book for their dedication in creating a truly outstanding account of modern methods in biomedical knowledge representation and reasoning.

October 2015

Arjen Hommersom
Peter J.F. Lucas

Contents

Prediction and Prognosis of Health and Disease

Treatment of Disease

Recommendation

List of Contributors

Luca Anselma
Dipartimento di Informatica, Università di Torino, Torino, Italy
e-mail: anselma@di.unito.it

R. Marshall Austin
Magee-Womens Hospital, Department of Pathology, University of Pittsburgh Medical Center, Pittsburgh, USA
e-mail: raustin@magee.edu

Shender María Ávila-Sansores
Instituto Nacional de Astrofísica, Óptica y Electrónica, Puebla, Mexico
e-mail: shender@ccc.inaoep.mx

Alessio Bottrighi
DISIT, Computer Science Institute, University of Piemonte Orientale, Alessandria, Italy
e-mail: alessio.bottrighi@uniupo.it

Stefano Bragaglia
Department of Computer Science and Engineering, University of Bologna, Bologna, Italy
e-mail: stefano.bragaglia@unibo.it

Elizabeth S. Burnside
Department of Radiology, University of Wisconsin School of Medicine and Public Health, Madison, Wisconsin, USA
e-mail: eburnside@uwhealth.org

Michael Caldwell
Marshfield Clinic, Marshfield, Wisconsin, USA
e-mail: caldwell.michael@marshfieldclinic.org

Stefano Ceccon
School of Information Systems Computing and Maths, Brunel University, Uxbridge, UK
e-mail: stefano.ceccon@brunel.ac.uk

Federico Chesani
Department of Computer Science and Engineering, University of Bologna, Bologna, Italy
e-mail: federico.chesani@unibo.it

Jesse Davis
Department of Computer Science, KU Leuven, Heverlee, Belgium
e-mail: jesse.davis@cs.kuleuven.be

Marek J. Druzdzel
Decision Systems Laboratory, School of Information Sciences and Intelligent Systems Programs, University of Pittsburgh, Pittsburgh, USA and Faculty of Computer Science, Białystok University of Technology, Białystok, Poland
e-mail: marek@sis.pitt.edu

Inês Dutra
Departamento de Ciência de Computadores, Faculdade de Ciências, Universidade do Porto, Porto, Portugal
e-mail: ines@dcc.fc.up.pt

Catherine G. Enright
National University of Ireland, Galway, Ireland
e-mail: Catherine.Enright@nuigalway.ie

Arjen Hommersom
Institute for Computing and Information Sciences, Radboud University, Nijmegen, The Netherlands and Faculty of Management, Science and Technology, Open University, Heerlen, The Netherlands
e-mail: arjenh@cs.ru.nl

Anthony Hunter
Department of Computer Science, University College London, London, UK
e-mail: anthony.hunter@ucl.ac.uk

Laura Giordano
DISIT, Computer Science Institute, University of Piemonte Orientale, Alessandria, Italy
e-mail: laura.giordano@uniupo.it

Yuanxi Li
School of Information Systems Computing and Maths, Brunel University, Uxbridge, UK
e-mail: yuanxi.li@brunel.ac.uk

Peter J.F. Lucas
Institute for Computing and Information Sciences, Radboud University, Nijmegen, The Netherlands and LIACS, Leiden University, Leiden, The Netherlands
e-mail: peterl@cs.ru.nl

Anna Łupińska-Dubicka
Faculty of Computer Science, Białystok University of Technology, Białystok, Poland
e-mail: a.lupinska@pb.edu.pl

Michael G. Madden
National University of Ireland, Galway, Ireland
e-mail: Michael.Madden@nuigalway.ie

Paola Mello
Department of Computer Science and Engineering, University of Bologna, Bologna, Italy
e-mail: paola.mello@unibo.it

Gianpaolo Molino
Azienda Ospedaliera San Giovanni Battista, Torino, Italy

Marco Montali
KRDB Research Centre, Free University of Bozen-Bolzano, Bolzano, Italy
e-mail: montali@inf.unibz.it

Stefania Montani
DISIT, Computer Science Institute, University of Piemonte Orientale, Alessandria, Italy
e-mail: stefania.montani@uniupo.it

Agnieszka Onisko
Magee-Womens Hospital, Department of Pathology, University of Pittsburgh Medical Center, Pittsburgh, USA and Faculty of Computer Science, Białystok University of Technology, Białystok, Poland
e-mail: oniskoa@upmc.edu

Felipe Orihuela-Espina
Instituto Nacional de Astrofísica, Óptica y Electrónica, Puebla, Mexico
e-mail: f.orihuela-espina@ccc.inaoep.mx

David Page
University of Wisconsin, Madison, Wisconsin, USA
e-mail: page@biostat.wisc.edu

Peggy Peissig
Marshfield Clinic, Marshfield, Wisconsin, USA
e-mail: peissig.peggy@marshfieldclinic.org

Jose M. Peña
Department of Computer and Information Science, Linköping University, Linköping, Sweden
e-mail: jose.m.pena@liu.se

Vítor Santos Costa
CRACS INESC-TEC and FCUP Universidade do Porto, Porto, Portugal
e-mail: vsc@dcc.fc.up.pt

Marco Scutari
Department of Statistics, University of Oxford, Oxford, UK
e-mail: scutari@stats.ox.ac.uk

Dag Sonntag
Department of Computer and Information Science, Linköping University, Linköping, Sweden
e-mail: dag.sonntag@liu.se

Luis Enrique Sucar
Instituto Nacional de Astrofísica, Óptica y Electrónica, Puebla, Mexico
e-mail: esucar@inaoep.mx

Stephen Swift
School of Information Systems Computing and Maths, Brunel University, Uxbridge, UK
e-mail: stephen.swift@brunel.ac.uk

Paolo Terenziani
DISIT, Computer Science Institute, University of Piemonte Orientale, Alessandria, Italy
e-mail: paolo.terenziani@uniupo.it

Mauro Torchio
Azienda Ospedaliera San Giovanni Battista, Torino, Italy

Allan Tucker
School of Information Systems Computing and Maths, Brunel University, Uxbridge, UK
e-mail: allan.tucker@brunel.ac.uk

Marina Velikova
Embedded Systems Innovation by TNO, Eindhoven, The Netherlands
e-mail: marina.velikova@tno.nl

Matthew Williams
Department of Oncology, Charing Cross Hospital, London, UK
e-mail: mhw@doctors.org.uk

Introduction

Chapter 1
How to Read the Book "Foundations of Biomedical Knowledge Representation"

Peter J.F. Lucas and Arjen Hommersom

1.1 On the Nature of Things

Biology and medicine are very rich knowledge domains in which already at an early stage in their scientific development it was realised that without a proper way to organise this knowledge they would inevitably turn into chaos. Early examples of organisation attempts are for example "*De Rerum Natura* (On the Nature of Things)" by Titus Lucretius Carus (99–55 BC), which explains the natural and physical world as known at the time, and of course the work "*Systema Naturae*" by Carl Linnaeus published in 1735. The latter book can be seen as the clear recognition of the need of using *systematic methods*, here principles of taxonomic organisation, to classify nature. As soon as one considers using systematic methods, computer-based representations and algorithms come to mind.

Today, the size and complexity of medical-biological knowledge has risen to such a dazzling height that one cannot even imagine *not* to use computer-based methods. However, so far this has been especially the case for the representation and storage of basic biological knowledge—not the main focus of the present book—rather than for medical and clinical knowledge. The amount of detailed biological knowledge available nowadays is so large that even people specialised in particular biological areas would not be able to remember this specialised part in toto. Thus, the application of formalisms such as description logics to represent knowledge about genetic mechanisms and the proteins involved was in the end unavoidable. Access to these knowledge bases, such as KEGG[1] (Kyoto Encyclopedia of Genes and Genomes), GO[2] (Gene Ontology), and the RCSB PDB[3] (Protein Databank) is essential for the present-day working biologist and biochemist to make scientific progress. These knowledge bases are standard tools and part of the computational environment used in these research areas.

---

[1] www.genome.jp/kegg.

[2] geneontology.org.

[3] www.rcsb.org/pdb.

© Springer International Publishing Switzerland 2015
A. Hommersom and P.J.F. Lucas (eds.), *Biomedical Knowledge Representation*, LNAI 9521, DOI 10.1007/978-3-319-28007-3_1

The characteristics of the medical area, however, are different from those of research in biology, even though the former area is firmly grounded on biological knowledge. First, knowledge is not mainly used as part of research but primarily for the management of disease, such as the establishment of the diagnosis, treatment, and prognosis in patients. Second, medical doctors are trained to memorise quite a lot of the knowledge involved in decision making, and this knowledge is often simplified to make the memorisation feasible. As a consequence, the need for computer-based methods is not felt as strongly as in biology, where there is not such a clear rationale for simplifying knowledge.

Simplification of knowledge with the aim of keeping the complexity of the decision-making process manageable to humans has a long tradition in medicine. This is, for example, reflected by the frequent use of acronyms, even for procedures (e.g. CABG, pronounced as 'cabbage', i.e. the Coronary Artery Bypass Graft procedure). Yet, with the substantial progress made in biomedical, i.e. both human-biological and clinical, research there are good reasons to consider the biomedical area afresh and wonder whether there may be better, more scientific ways to manage disease in patients. This in itself is not a new idea, and similar ambitions were expressed before in the 1980s by the medical decision making movement [7]. At the same time, there was great belief in the potential of artificial intelligence in medicine with programs such as MYCIN, INTERNIST-I, and CASNET [2, 4]. Reality in biomedicine appeared to be more resistant to change than thought by many people at the time and not much happened.

However, the current circumstances are not the same as those in the 1980s. There is now a stronger tendency to take errors and mistakes in clinical medicine seriously and researchers are identifying ways to prevent them [3]. One also realises that computer-based methods may contribute to a reduction in the avoidable clinical errors and mistakes. At the same time, developments in computing-science methods and tools have continued, which has made it easier to cross the boundary between informal biomedicine and computer-based formalisation.

1.2   Towards Biomedical Knowledge Representation

We have now definitely arrived in the digital age and even healthcare workers have entered this era, mainly because they just followed the rest of society. There is some irony in this part of the evolution in healthcare, since complex information systems have been in use in healthcare at least since the 1970s, and so healthcare was in a perfect position to take the lead in digitisation. Despite several attempts, this never happened at the time, at least not on a global scale, mainly because healthcare workers were not convinced that it would contribute to better and more convenient patient care. Nevertheless, the current situation of almost full digitisation has created new opportunities for using computer-based methods for the representation and reasoning with medical knowledge, and this is where this book is about.

Partly because of the growth in basic biological knowledge and partly because of new clinical insights obtained by clinical and epidemiological research, biomedicine remains one of the most knowledge-intensive areas. Even though basic biological, in particular genetic, knowledge is an important ingredient in clinical decision making nowadays, which is likely to increase more in the near future because of the trends towards personal medicine, there still is this typical practical tendency of medical doctors to control the complexity of the knowledge using its clinical relevancy as the main guiding principle. This is for example reflected in the increasing importance of clinical guidelines and protocols in medical decision making, because clinical guidelines are the result of a process that results in documents that only include what is clinically relevant. Even in this area it is recognised that the impact of the evidence-based medicine movement that is associated with clinical guidelines will have its limitations, because many medical doctors believe that medicine cannot be practised in a systematic way (they call it "cookbook medicine").

The modern research in biomedical computing takes these developments into account, and this explains for example the work on computer-based guideline representation and execution [5]. Rather than starting with new ways to formalise medical knowledge, researchers take existing 'representations', although informal, as a starting point. As researchers working in the computer-based guideline area can only acknowledge, transforming an informal clinical guideline into an executable representation that integrates well with clinical workflow is already a sufficiently big challenge.

There are similar developments in other areas. For example, in the clinical setting of diagnosis most of the work is now focussing on assisting medical doctors in a particular diagnostic task, for example to help in the interpretation of radiological images. There are still people who pursue the old idea, initially investigated with the development of the INTERNIST-I system, of a diagnostic computer-based system that covers the whole area of medicine, but now they do this using modern methods offered by Bayesian networks[4].

Similar developments in techniques has made it possible to assist and give insight to clinicians in treating diseases in patients and in making predictions of the outcome of treatment. Finally, the book also covers modern developments in representation techniques for personal medicine, recommender systems and monitoring of disease, where time is an important aspect of the representation formalism. Disease monitoring is an important topic in the context of eHealth [6].

1.3 Organisation of the Book

Knowledge representation methods [1] have been used for many different types of knowledge-intensive tasks in biomedicine. The concept of 'task' has been used as a way to capture the generic aspects of particular procedures, such as diagnostic problem solving. The same ideas can also be applied to other domains; in that sense only part of the tasks described in this book are domain specific. Nevertheless, in

---

[4]www.symptomate.com.

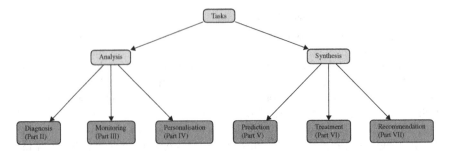

Fig. 1.1 Overview of the book.

this book we distinguish particular tasks and give them the names that they have in medicine even though there may be similar tasks in other domains. The fact that we deal with the domain of biomedicine often has implications for the way we represent the domain, for example, often we use causality as a way to structure the domain knowledge; *abduction*, i.e. explaining observations in terms of active causes is then one possible *method* to implement the task of diagnosis. Many of these issues will hopefully have become clear after reading the introductory chapter (Chap. 2) of the book.

We have made a distinction between tasks that can be seen as a form of *analysis*, and other tasks that put more emphasis on *synthesis*, as summarised in Fig. 1.1. The book consists of 7 parts, where the first part introduces the book and the various techniques used in the book; the other 6 parts are concerned with individual tasks. Each part is started with an introductory chapter that is followed by one or more specialised chapters. The following parts are distinguished:

Part I Introduction. A general description of knowledge representation methods that are relevant for the different chapters included in this book.

Part II Diagnosis of Disease includes a general overview of diagnostic methods and a chapter that describes the use of these methods for medical image interpretation.

Part III Monitoring of Health and Disease and Conformance concerns a description of general characteristics of the monitoring task and applications in the context of clinical guidelines and the individual patient.

Part IV Assessment of Health and Personalisation puts a focus on the use of graphical knowledge-representation formalisms, such as Bayesian networks and chain graphs, to capture the features of disease at the level of the individual. Genetic information and the modelling of the relationship between genetic information and disease is key here.

Part V Prediction and Prognosis of Health and Disease is concerned with statements of what is going to happen in the future, and uncertainty is something one has to take into account. This explains the use of probabilistic methods in this context.

Part VI Treatment of Disease. Treatment is concerned with following a sequence of actions, taking into account the uncertainty in the diagnosis and the uncertainty in the expected outcome of the treatment. Both general principles of knowledge representation of the treatment task and actual applications are described in three chapters.

Part VII Recommendation. This last part of the book deals with supporting physicians through recommendations based on the best available evidence. Knowledge representation techniques have been used to develop computer-interpretable clinical guidelines that can be used for various reasoning tasks. Furthermore, this part also presents an alternative to guidelines by aggregation of clinical evidence through argumentation theory.

With the early work as briefly summarised at the beginning of this chapter in mind it becomes clear that modern knowledge representation and reasoning methods cover a much broader area of biomedicine than the earlier methods, which often only dealt with a specific clinical diagnostic problem. The modern methods now also have a sound mathematical foundation in terms of logic, probability theory and decision theory. This explains the title of the present book "Foundations of Biomedical Knowledge Representation". As the applications described in the book already make clear, we are now finally on the edge that principles of knowledge representation are creating impact in the biomedical field.

References

1. van Harmelen, F., Lifschitz, V., Porter, B. (eds.): Handbook of Knowledge Representation. Elsevier, Amsterdam (2008)
2. Lucas, P.J.F., van der Gaag, L.C.: Principles of Expert Systems. Addison-Wesley, Wokingham (1991)
3. Rylander, M., Guerrasio, J.: Heuristic errors in clinical reasoning. In: Clinical Teaching (2015). doi:10.1111/tct.12444
4. Szolovits, P.: Artificial intelligence in medicine. In: AAAS Selected Symposium, vol. 51. Westview Press, Boulder, Colorado (1982)
5. ten Teije, A., Miksch, S., Lucas, P.J.F. (eds.): Computer-Based Clinical Guidelines and Protocols: a Primer and Current Trends. IOS Press, Amsterdam (2008)
6. Velikova, M., Lucas, P.J.F., van der Heijden, M.: Intelligent disease self-management with mobile technology. IEEE Comput. **48**(2), 32–39 (2015)
7. Weinstein, M.C., Fineberg, H.: Clinical Decision Analysis. Saunders, Philadelphia (1980)

Chapter 2
An Introduction to Knowledge Representation and Reasoning in Healthcare

Arjen Hommersom and Peter J.F. Lucas

2.1 Development of the Field

Healthcare and medicine are, and have always been, very knowledge-intensive fields. Healthcare professionals use knowledge of the structure (molecular biology, cell biology, histology, gross anatomy) and functioning of the human body as well as knowledge of methods and means, some of them described by clinical guidelines, to diagnose and manage disorders. In addition, knowledge of how healthcare is organised is essential for the management of a patient's disease.

Already in the early days of research in artificial intelligence, researchers realised that healthcare and medicine would be suitably challenging fields to drive the development of knowledge representation and reasoning techniques. Quite a large number of different systems were developed in those early days (cf. [23] for a description of the most important early ideas and systems). Typically, researchers developed their own representation methods guided by thoughts on how to handle a particular medical problem. An example of how thoughts on clinical problem solving and computer-based knowledge representation can interact is the work by Pople [21] on heuristic methods for medical diagnostic problem solving. The key idea here is that one needs a kind of structure of the hypothesis space to guide the problem-solving process. In a medical context this means that one needs taxonomic knowledge, i.e. medical knowledge organised according to the principles of a subsumption taxonomy, and causal knowledge, i.e. knowledge that describes the world according to cause-effect relationships. Pople also realised that disease manifestations and the diseases themselves are linked to each other by a, possibly abstract, model of the pathophysiology, and those play a different role in the problem-solving process. Even in that early work it already clear that medicine is a semantically rich field, not only concerned with different type of knowledge of different kind, coming from different sources, but also used for different purposes.

The development of these early systems gave rise to the phrase *knowledge-based system*, or *knowledge system*, which is generally employed to denote information systems in which some symbolic representation of human knowledge of a domain

© Springer International Publishing Switzerland 2015
A. Hommersom and P.J.F. Lucas (eds.), *Biomedical Knowledge Representation*, LNAI 9521, DOI 10.1007/978-3-319-28007-3_2

is applied, usually in a way resembling human reasoning, to solve actual problems in the domain. As this knowledge is often derived from experts in a particular field, and early knowledge-based systems were actually developed in close collaboration with experts, the term *expert system* was the term used in the early days to refer to these systems. Knowledge, however, can also be extracted from literature, or from a datasets by using machine-learning methods. At the time of writing, the terminology of systems that employ formalised knowledge to solve problems is even less clear than it was in the past. For this book this is of little concern, as the focus is on knowledge representation and reasoning for different medical purposes.

Present generation knowledge-based systems are capable of dealing with significant (medical) problem domains. Gathering, maintaining and updating the incorporated knowledge taking into account its associated context, such as working environment, organisation and field of expertise belongs to an area referred to as *knowledge management*. The art of developing a knowledge-based system is called *knowledge engineering*, when there is emphasis on the pragmatic engineering aspects, or *knowledge modelling*, when development of domain models is emphasises. The latter is strictly speaking part of the former. The process of collecting and analysing knowledge in a problem domain is called *knowledge acquisition*, or *knowledge elicitation* when the knowledge is gathered from interviews with experts, normally using interview techniques as developed by psychologists.

Although the early papers on knowledge representation for biomedical problems are still worth reading, there has been significant progress in the techniques, i.e. languages and tools, that act as the basis for knowledge representation. In contrast to the early work, there is now a solid understanding of the importance of logical language to act as a basis for knowledge representation. At the same time, specialised logical languages, such as decoration logics, have been developed to deal with specific knowledge representation and reasoning problems. There has also been a lot of progress in the development of reasoning with uncertainty. Probabilistic graphical models, and in particular Bayesian networks, have come into play since the 1990s as a natural formalism to represent uncertain biomedical knowledge. Specific types of non-monotonic reasoning have also emerged and proven their use in the biomedical context. The theory of argumentation is a typical example. For specific biomedical problems, such as problems that can be handled by clinical guidelines, there are now languages and tools available to represent and to reason with the relevant knowledge.

In general, the significant progress in techniques for knowledge representation and reasoning render it possible to develop knowledge systems of which the foundations are well understood in such way that certainty (computational) properties are guaranteed to be satisfied. Of course, capturing and modelling biomedical knowledge is still a significant challenge. However, with the techniques available nowadays, the modelling is at least supported by sound methods and techniques.

In this chapter, we will review common knowledge representation formalisms in artificial intelligence and link these to the healthcare field.

2.2 Techniques for Knowledge Representation and Reasoning

The knowledge-representation formalism and the types of reasoning supported are of major importance for the development of knowledge-based systems. Logic, probability theory and decision theory are sufficiently general to permit describing the nature of knowledge representation, inference and problem solving without having to resort to special-purpose languages. In the next section, some of the general ideas underlying knowledge representation are summarised and illustrated by means of simple examples.

2.2.1 Horn-clause Logic

Knowledge-based systems usually offer a number of different ways to represent knowledge in a domain, and to reason with this knowledge automatically to derive conclusions. Although the languages offered by actual systems and tools may differ in a number of ways, there are also many similarities. The aspects that the languages have in common can be best understood in terms of a logical representation, as accomplished below.

A *Horn clause* or *rule* is a logical implication of the following form

$$\forall x_1 \cdots \forall x_m ((A_1 \wedge \cdots \wedge A_n) \rightarrow B) \tag{2.1}$$

where A_i, B are literals of the form $P(t_1, \ldots, t_q)$, i.e. without a negation sign, representing a relationship P between terms t_k, which may involve one or more universally quantified variables x_j, constants and terms involving function symbols. As all variables in rules are assumed to universally quantified, the universal quantifiers are often omitted if this does not give rise to confusion. If $n = 0$, then the clause consists only of a conclusion, which may be taken as a *fact*. If, on the other hand, the conclusion B is empty, indicated by $\perp$, the rule is also called a *query*. If the conditions of a query are satisfied, this will give rise to a contradiction or inconsistency, denoted by $\perp$, as the conclusion is empty. So, an empty clause means actually inconsistency.

A popular method to reason with clauses, and Horn clauses in particular, is *resolution*. Let $\mathcal{R}$ be a set of rules not containing queries, and let $Q \equiv (A_1 \wedge \cdots \wedge A_n) \rightarrow \perp$ be a query, then

$$\mathcal{R} \cup \{Q\} \vdash \perp$$

where $\vdash$ means the application of resolution, implies that the conditions

$$\forall x_1 \cdots \forall x_m (A_1 \wedge \cdots \wedge A_n)$$

are not all satisfied. Since resolution is a sound inference rule, meaning that it respects the logical meaning of clauses, it also holds that $\mathcal{R} \cup \{Q\} \models \perp$, or equivalently

$$\mathcal{R} \models \exists x_1 \cdots \exists x_m (A_1 \wedge \cdots \wedge A_n)$$

if $\mathcal{R}$ only consists of Horn clauses. This last interpretation explains why deriving inconsistency is normally not really the goal of using resolution; rather, the purpose is to derive certain facts. Since resolution is only complete for deriving inconsistency, called *refutation completeness*, it is only safe to 'derive' knowledge in this indirect manner. There exist other reasoning methods which do not have this limitation. However, resolution is a simple method that is understood in considerable depth. As a consequence, state-of-the-art resolution-based reasoners are very efficient. Resolution can also be used with clauses in general, which are logical expressions of the form

$$(A_1 \wedge \cdots \wedge A_n) \rightarrow (B_1 \vee \cdots \vee B_m)$$

usually represented as:

$$\neg A_1 \vee \cdots \vee \neg A_n \vee B_1 \vee \cdots \vee B_m$$

Rules of the form (2.1) are particularly popular as the reasoning with propositional Horn clauses is known to be possible in linear time, whereas reasoning with propositions or clauses in general (where the right-hand side consists of disjunctions of literals) is known to be NP-complete, i.e. may require time exponential in the size of the clauses. Note that allowing negative literals at the left-hand side of a rule is equivalent to having disjunctions at the right-hand side. Using a logical language that is more expressive than Horn-clause logic is sometimes unavoidable, and special techniques have been introduced to deal with their additional power.

Using logic to represent (medical) knowledge gives rise to a knowledge base that is sometimes called *object knowledge*.

Let KB be a knowledge base consisting of a set (conjunction) of rules, and let F be a *set of facts* observed for a particular problem $\mathcal{P}$, then there are generally three ways in which a problem can be solved, yielding different types of solutions. The formalisation of problem solving gives rise to knowledge that is sometimes called *meta knowledge*. Let $\mathcal{P}$ be a problem, then there are different classes of solutions to this problem:

- **Deductive solution:** S is a *deductive solution* of a problem $\mathcal{P}$ with associated set of observed findings F iff

$$\text{KB} \cup F \models S \tag{2.2}$$

  and $\text{KB} \cup F \not\models \perp$, where S is a set of solution formulae.
- **Abductive/inductive solution:** S is an *abductive solution* of a problem $\mathcal{P}$ with associated set of observed findings F iff the following *covering condition*

$$KB \cup S \cup K \models F \tag{2.3}$$

is satisfied, where K stands for *contextual knowledge*. In addition, it must hold that $KB \cup S \cup C \nvDash \bot$ (consistency condition), where C is a set of logical constraints on solutions. For the abductive case, it is assumed that the knowledge base KB contains a logical representation of *causal knowledge* and S consists of facts; for the inductive case, KB consists of background facts and S, called an *inductive solution*, consists of rules.

- **Consistency-based solution:** S is a *consistency-based solution* of a problem $\mathscr{P}$ with associated set of observed findings F iff

$$KB \cup S \cup F \nvDash \bot \tag{2.4}$$

Note that a deductive solution is a consistent conclusion that follows from a knowledge base KB and a set of facts, whereas an abductive solution acts as a hypothesis that *explains* observed facts in terms of causal knowledge, i.e. cause-effect relationships. An inductive solution also explains observed facts, but in terms of any other type of knowledge. A consistency-based solution is the weakest kind of solution, as it is neither required to be concluded nor is it required to explain observed findings.

2.2.2   Objects, Attributes and Values

Even though facts or observed findings can be represented in many different ways, in many systems facts are represented in an object-oriented fashion. This means that facts are described as properties, or *attributes*, of objects in the real world. Attributes of objects can be either multivalued, meaning that an object may have more than one of those properties at the same time, or singlevalued, meaning that values of attributes are mutually exclusive.

In logic, multivalued attributes are represented by predicate symbols, e.g.:

$$Parent(John, Ann) \land Parent(John, Derek)$$

indicates that the 'object' John, represented as a constant, has two parents (the attribute 'Parent'): Ann and Derek, both represented by constants. Furthermore, singlevalued attributes are represented as function symbols, e.g.

$$gender(John) = male$$

Here, '*gender*' is taken as a singlevalued attribute, 'John' is again a constant object, and '*male*' is the value, also represented as a constant.

It is, of course, also possible to state general properties of objects. For example, the following bi-implication:

$$\forall x \forall y \forall z ((\text{Parent}(x, y) \land \text{Parent}(y, z)) \leftrightarrow \text{Grandparent}(x, z))$$

defines the attribute 'Grandparent' in terms of the 'Parent' attribute.

Another typical example of reasoning about properties of objects is *inheritance* [2]. Here one wishes to associate properties of objects with the classes the objects belong to, mainly because this yields a compact representation offering in addition insight into the general structure of a problem domain. Consider, for example, the following knowledge base KB:

$$\forall x (\text{Mammal}(x) \rightarrow \text{Endotherm}(x))$$
$$\forall x (\text{Human}(x) \rightarrow \text{Mammal}(x))$$
$$\forall x (\text{Human}(x) \rightarrow \textit{number-of-chromosomes(x)} = 46)$$

Clearly, it holds that

$$\text{KB} \cup \{\text{Human}(\text{John})\} \models \textit{number-of-chromosomes}(\text{John}) = 46$$

as the third rule expresses that as a typical property of humans. However, the knowledge base also incorporates more general properties of humans, such as:

$$\text{KB} \cup \{\text{Human}(\text{John})\} \models \text{Mammal}(\text{John})$$

Now, given the fact that a human is a mammal, we can now also conclude

$$\text{KB} \cup \{\text{Human}(\text{John})\} \models \text{Endotherm}(\text{John})$$

The example knowledge base discussed above can also be represented as a graph, called an object *taxonomy*, and is shown in Fig. 2.1. Here ellipses indicate either classes of objects (Human and Mammal) or specific objects (John). Solid arcs in the graph indicate that a class of objects is a subclass of another class of objects; a dashed arc indicates that the parent object is an element – often the term 'instance' is used instead – of the associated class of objects. The term 'inheritance' that is associated with this type of logical reasoning derives from the fact that the reasoning goes from the children to the parents in order to derive properties.

2.2.3 Description Logics

Describing the objects in a domain, usually but not always in a way resembling a taxonomy, usually with the intention to obtain a formal description of the terminology in a domain, is known as an *ontology*. Instead of describing these properties in standard first-order logic, it is common nowadays to use specialised description logics for that purpose and in particular OWL, the Web Ontology Language [13, 16], is being used for that purpose.

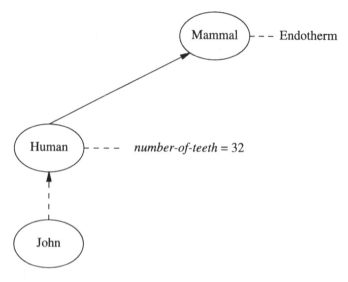

Fig. 2.1 An object taxonomy.

There are two primary ways in which knowledge is being described using OWL:

1. by *combining concepts* using Boolean operators, such as ⊓ (conjunction), and ⊔ (disjunction);
2. by *defining relationships* between concepts (whether primitive or obtained by combining primitive concepts) using the *subsumption* relation ⊑ (also called *general concept inclusion* – GCI).

Thus, a concept description is constructed from

- *primitive concepts C*, e.g., Disease, ⊤ (most general), ⊥ (empty);
- *primitive roles r*, e.g., hasSymptom;
- *conjunctions* ⊓, e.g., Cardiac_Disease ⊓ Cerebral_Disease;
- *disjunctions* ⊔, e.g., Hepatitis ⊔ Cirrhosis;
- a *complement* ¬, e.g., ¬Hepatitis;
- a *value restriction* ∀r.C, e.g., ∀causes.Fever;
- an *existential restriction* ∃r.C, e.g., ∃likelyFatal.Metastasis.

All understood in terms of (groups of) individuals and properties of individuals.
For example, by

$$\text{Hepatitis} \sqcup \text{Cirrhosis}$$

we have combined two concepts, but we have not established how they are related to each other. By writing:

$$\text{Hepatitis} \sqsubseteq \text{LiverDisease}$$

we have established a relationship between the concepts 'Hepatitis' and 'LiverDisease', where the first is less or equally general than the latter. By combining two subsumption relations, it is possible to *define* a new concept:

$$\text{Metastatic\_Cancer} \sqsubseteq \text{Cancer} \sqcap \exists \text{hasMetastasis.Tumour\_Tissue}$$

and

$$\text{Cancer} \sqcap \exists \text{hasMetastasis.Tumour\_Tissue} \sqsubseteq \text{Metastatic\_Cancer}$$

is abbreviated to

$$\text{Metastatic\_Cancer} \equiv \text{Cancer} \sqcap \exists \text{hasMetastasis.Tumour\_Tissue}$$

Note that an expression such as $\exists$hasMetastasis.Tumour_Tissue is also a concept: the role hasMetastasis establishes a relationship between an instance of the concept Tumour_Tissue (the tumour discovered at a distance from the original cancer) and all concepts that participate in the role, which are then intersected with the concept 'Cancer', yielding a definition of 'Metastatic_Cancer'.

General descriptions of a domain form, what is called, the TBox (Terminology Box). In a sense, the TBox restricts the terminology we are allowed to use when describing a domain. The actual domain is described by means of *assertions*, which together form the ABox (Assertion Box).

2.2.4 Temporal Logics

As soon we wish to model the execution of actions in biomedicine, we need to incorporate time into our knowledge-representation formalism, and thus also when it is based on logic.

Several temporal logics have been developed, in particular tense logics since the 1960s. Differences between logics result from different models of time and expressiveness. In linear temporal logics (e.g., Linear Temporal Logic (LTL) [19]), models form a linear trace, while in branching logics models typically (e.g., Computation Tree Logic (CTL) [1, 5, 10]) form a tree.

In LTL, propositional logic is extended with several temporal operators. The temporal operators used are $\mathbf{X}$, $\mathbf{G}$, $\mathbf{F}$, and $\mathbf{U}$. With $\mathbf{X}\varphi$ being true if φ holds in the next state, $\mathbf{G}\varphi$ if φ holds in the current state and all future states, $\mathbf{F}\varphi$ if φ holds in the current state or some state in the future, and $\varphi\mathbf{U}\psi$ if φ holds until eventually ψ holds.

For example:

$$\mathbf{G}(\text{Human} \rightarrow \text{Mammal})$$

expresses that it is always the case that humans are mammals. To specify the mortality of humans, one could model this with a rule such as:

$$\mathbf{G}(\text{Human} \rightarrow \mathbf{F}\,\text{Death})$$

Note the subtle difference with a logical rule such as the following:

$$\text{Human} \rightarrow \mathbf{F}\,\text{Death}$$

which states that only the humans existing at this moment are mortal; this does not specify that those born in the future are mortal. One could even be slightly more precise and specify that humans remain human at least until they die:

$$\mathbf{G}(\text{Human U Death})$$

Of course, reasoning with temporal knowledge is supported as well. One can derive for example that:

$$\mathbf{G}(\text{Human U Death}),\ \text{Human} \models \mathbf{F}\,\text{Death}$$

In contrast to LTL, CTL provides operators for describing events along a multiple computation paths (possible futures), and is therefore sometimes referred to as a 'branching' temporal logic. The path quantifiers $\mathbf{A}$ and $\mathbf{E}$, which are always combined with one of the LTL operators, are used to specify that all or some of the paths starting at a specific state have some property. While LTL formulas describe all possible futures, in CTL we may describe what happens in some or all of the possible futures.

For example, the specify that cancer may lead to metastatic cancer, but at the same time be optimistic that there is a possibility that does not does not occur, one could write the following rules:

$$\mathbf{AG}(\text{Cancer} \rightarrow \mathbf{EF}\,\text{Metastatic\_Cancer})$$
$$\mathbf{AG}(\text{Cancer} \rightarrow \mathbf{EG}\,\neg\text{Metastatic\_Cancer})$$

Automatic reasoning methods for temporal logics have been developed, although reasoning with temporal logic is a hard problem (for example, checking satisfiability and entailment for LTL is PSPACE-complete). One practical method is to look upon temporal logics as first-order formula with a quantification over the temporal states, i.e., each predicates has an additional argument that models the state (and path for CTL) in which the predicate holds. Temporal quantification can then be mapped to ordinary first-order quantification. For example:

$$\mathbf{G}p \equiv \forall t\ p(t)$$

Reasoning methods for first-order logic can then directly be applied to reason about temporal logics, for example, resolution.

2.3   Problem-Solving Methods

Using formalisations of medical knowledge to solve problems can be seen as a form
of meta-level reasoning, as discussed in Sect. 2.2.1. In the section on probabilistic
logic, we already saw a form of meta-level reasoning with uncertain knowledge.
Just to illustrate the idea, we discuss various examples of diagnostic reasoning. In
addition, treatment planning — one of the aspects of guideline execution — is briefly
sketched.

2.3.1   Diagnostic Problem Solving

Above, the general features of knowledge representation and inference were sketched.
Most of the insight that has been gained in the field, however, concerns particular
methods with associated knowledge to handle classes of problems. As said above,
inference or reasoning methods can be used to implement problem-solving methods.
A typical example is the diagnosis of disorders in patients or faults in equipment by
diagnostic methods. Many different methods have been developed for that purpose.
Three well-known diagnostic methods with their associated types of knowledge will
be discussed in the following.

2.3.1.1   Deductive Diagnosis

Most of the early knowledge-based systems, including MYCIN [3], were based on
expert knowledge concerning the relationships among classes expressed by rules.
In the reasoning process these rules were subsequently used to classify cases into
categories. This problem-solving method is known as *heuristic classification*, as most
of the knowledge encoded in the rules is empirical or heuristic in nature rather than
based on first principles [4]. The form of the rules is:

$$(c_1 \wedge \cdots \wedge c_k \wedge \sim c_{k+1} \wedge \cdots \wedge \sim c_n) \rightarrow c$$

where c_i is either a condition on input data or on a subclass. The rules are *generalised*
rules, as conditions may be prefixed by a special negation sign $\sim$, called *negation
by absence*. It represents a special case of the closed-world assumption (CWA); a
condition $\sim c_i$ only succeeds if there is at least one finding concerning the associated
attribute. Formally:

$$\sim A(o, v) \equiv \exists x (A(o, x) \wedge x \neq v)$$

for object o and value v, where o and v are constants. If the attribute A represents
a measurement or test, then negation by absence checks whether the test has been
carried out, yielding a result different from the one specified.

Consider the following toy medical knowledge base KB:

$\forall x ((\text{Symptom}(x, coughing) \wedge \sim \text{Symptom}(x, chest\text{-}pain) \wedge \text{Sign}(x, fever))$
    $\rightarrow \text{Disorder}(x, flu))$
$\forall x ((temp(x) > 38) \rightarrow \text{Sign}(x, fever))$

Then it holds that:

$\text{KB} \cup \{temp(\text{John}) = 39, \text{Symptom}(\text{John}, coughing)\} \models_{\text{NA}} \text{Disorder}(\text{John}, coughing)$

using negation by absence (NA). Note that Sign(John, *fever*) is true, and may be viewed as a classification of the finding *temp*(John) $= 39$; $\sim$ Symptom(John, *chest-pain*) holds due to negation by absence. Both rules in the knowledge base KB above are examples of heuristic classification rules.

2.3.1.2   Abductive Diagnosis

In abductive diagnosis, use is made of causal knowledge to diagnose a disorder in medicine or to determine faults in a malfunctioning device [6, 18, 20]. Causal knowledge can be represented in many ways, but a rather convenient and straight-forward way to represent causal knowledge is by taking logical implication as standing for the causal relationship. Thus, rules of the form:

$$d_1 \wedge \cdots \wedge d_n \rightarrow f \qquad (2.5)$$
$$d_1 \wedge \cdots \wedge d_n \rightarrow d \qquad (2.6)$$

are obtained, where d_i stands for a condition concerning a defective component or disorder; the conjunctions in (2.5) and (2.6) indicate that these conditions interact to either cause observable finding f or another abnormal condition d as effect. Sometimes uncertainty is added, usually represented in a non-numerical way as an assumption α:

$$d_1 \wedge \cdots \wedge d_n \wedge \alpha_f \rightarrow f \qquad (2.7)$$
$$d_1 \wedge \cdots \wedge d_n \wedge \alpha_d \rightarrow d \qquad (2.8)$$

The literals α may be either assumed to be true or false, meaning that f and d are a possible, but not necessary, consequences of the simultaneous occurrence of $d_1, \ldots, d_n$.

An *abductive diagnosis* S is now simply an abductive solution, where literals in S are restricted to d_i's and α's. The contextual knowledge may be extra conditions on rules which cannot be derived, but must be assumed and may act to model conditional causality. For simplicity's sake it is assumed here that K is empty. The set of constraints C may for instance consist of those findings f which have not been observed, and are assumed to be absent, i.e. $\neg f$ is assumed to hold.

Consider, for example, the causal model with set of defects and assumptions:

$$\Delta = \{fever, influenza, sport, \alpha_1, \alpha_2\}$$

and observable findings

$$\Phi = \{chills, thirst, myalgia, \neg chills, \neg thirst, \neg myalgia\}$$

'Myalgia' means painful muscles. The following knowledge base KB contains medical knowledge concerning influenza and sport, both 'disorders' with frequent occurrence:

$$fever \wedge \alpha_1 \to chills$$
$$influenza \twoheadrightarrow fever$$
$$fever \to thirst$$
$$influenza \wedge \alpha_2 \to myalgia$$
$$sport \twoheadrightarrow myalgia$$

For example, $influenza \wedge \alpha_2 \to myalgia$ means that influenza *may cause* myalgia; $influenza \twoheadrightarrow fever$ means that influenza *always causes* fever. For illustrative purposes, a causal knowledge base as given above is often depicted as a labelled, directed graph G, which is called a *causal net*, as shown in Fig. 2.2. Suppose that the abductive diagnostic problem with set of facts

$$F = \{thirst, myalgia\}$$

must be solved. As constraints we take $C = \{\neg chills\}$. There are several solutions to this abductive diagnostic problem (for which the consistency and covering conditions are fulfilled):

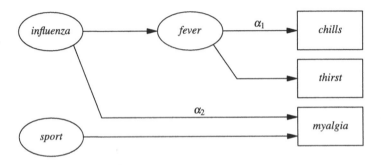

Fig. 2.2 A knowledge base with causal relations.

$$S_1 = \{influenza, \alpha_2\}$$
$$S_2 = \{influenza, sport\}$$
$$S_3 = \{fever, sport\}$$
$$S_4 = \{fever, influenza, \alpha_2\}$$
$$S_5 = \{influenza, \alpha_2, sport\}$$
$$S_6 = \{fever, influenza, sport\}$$
$$S_7 = \{fever, influenza, \alpha_2, sport\}$$

Note that $S = \{\alpha_1, \alpha_2, fever, influenza\}$ is incompatible with the constraints C.

2.3.1.3 Consistency-Based Diagnosis

In consistency-based diagnosis, in contrast to abductive diagnosis, the malfunctioning of a system is diagnosed by using mainly knowledge of the normal structure and normal behaviour of its components [8, 11, 22]. For each component $COMP_j$ its normal behaviour is described by logical implications of the following form:

$$\forall x((COMP_j(x) \wedge \neg Ab(x)) \rightarrow Behaviour_j(x))$$

The literal $\neg Ab(x)$ expresses that the behaviour associated with the component only holds when the assumption that the component is not abnormal, i.e. $\neg Ab(c)$, is true for component c. Sometimes knowledge of abnormal behaviour is added to implications of the form above, having the form:

$$\forall x((COMP_j(x) \wedge Ab(x)) \rightarrow Behaviour_j(x))$$

These may result in a reduction in the number of possible diagnoses to be considered. Logical behaviour descriptions of the form discussed above are part of a *system description*. In addition to the generic descriptions of the expected behaviour of components, a system description also includes logical specifications of how the components are connected to each other (the structure of the system), and the names of the components constituting the system. The system description is now taken as the knowledge base KB of a system. Problem solving basically amounts to adopting particular assumptions about every $COMP_j(c)$, either whether $Ab(c)$ is true or false. This sort of reasoning is called *assumption-based* or *hypothetical reasoning*.

In medicine, a component may be one of the organs or structures that are part of a physiological system. For example, for the cardiovascular system the 'blood' might be one of the components. As for the cardiovascular system it is the blood volume that affects its physiology, we will take 'blood volume' as a component in the medical example below. We will describe how a description of cardiovascular physiology can be employed in diagnosis (cf. [9] for details).

The following logical implications give the steady-state equations of the cardiovascular system, i.e. when the system is stable:

$$\neg Ab(C_{R_{sys}}) \rightarrow \Delta P_{sys} = CO \cdot R_{sys}$$
$$\neg Ab(C_{BV}) \rightarrow P_v = BV/VC$$
$$\neg Ab(C_{VC}) \rightarrow P_v = BV/VC$$
$$\neg Ab(C_{P_v}) \rightarrow \Delta P_v = VR \cdot R_v$$

Here, the following abbreviations are used:

- R_{sys}: the systemic resistance of the cardiovascular system;
- ΔP_{sys}: the difference between arterial and venous pressure;
- CO: the cardiac output (volume of blood per minute pumped out of the heart);
- P_v: the venous pressure;
- BV: blood volume;
- VC: venous compliance (the elastic force of the vessel wall against increased internal volume);
- VR: venous return (volume of blood per minute returned to the heart); it is equal to CO;
- R_v: venous resistance.

With C_X is indicated the corresponding component X that can be malfunctioning, $Ab(C_X)$. Any disturbance of the steady state may violate any of the equations in the right-hand sides of the implications above. In this case, the set of potential 'faulty' components is:

$$COMPS = \{C_{R_{sys}}, C_{BV}, C_{VC}, C_{P_v}\}$$

The cardiovascular system is controlled in such way that changes in its parameters are compensated automatically by changes in other parameters, leading to homeostatis. The following equation describes, for example, how the blood-pressure regulator (baroreceptor system) reacts to a change in arterial blood pressure (P_a) by changing the systemic resistance:

$$R_{sys} = -0.17 P_a + 34 \tag{2.9}$$

Now, assume that a patient gets kidney damage. This will lead to water retention, and thus the blood volume increases. In turn increased blood volume will lead to increase of arterial pressure P_a. The barorecepter system will through Eq. (2.9) compensate for the increased arterial pressure through decrease in systemic resistance R_{sys}.

Let us assume that the following measurements are made in a patient:

$$F = \{P_a = 160 \, mmHg, P_v = 15 \, mmHg, CO = 7 \, l/min\},$$

thus, $\Delta P_{sys} = 160 - 15 = 145 \, mmHg$. $R_{sys} = 6.8 \, mmHG \, min/l$ is the predicted effect of the regulatory baroreceptor mechanism using Eq. (2.9). Clearly, the steady-state equation for the systemic resistance is violated:

$$\Delta P_{sys} = 145 \neq CO \cdot R_{sys} = 7 \cdot 6.8 = 47.6$$

This indicates that the system is malfunctioning. This can also be verified by noting that when assuming all components to behave normally, i.e. $S = \{\neg Ab(c)|c \in$ COMPS$\}$, it follows that

$$KB \cup S \cup F$$

is inconsistent.

Diagnosing the problem simply consists of assuming particular components to be abnormal ($Ab(c)$ is true for those components), and checking whether the result is still inconsistent. If it is not, a diagnosis has been found. So, a *consistency-based diagnosis* is a consistency-based solution S consisting of a conjunction of Ab literals, one for every component.

Consider again the example above. Here,

$$S = \{Ab(C_{R_{sys}}), Ab(C_{BV}), \neg Ab(C_{VC}), \neg Ab(C_{P_v})\}$$

is a consistency-based diagnosis as

$$KB \cup S \cup F \nvDash \bot$$

Note that R_{sys} and BV are, thus, possibly faulty, as assuming them to be abnormal yield no output for this components. There are other solutions as well, such as

$$S' = \{Ab(C_{R_{sys}}), \neg Ab(C_{BV}), Ab(C_{VC}), \neg Ab(C_{P_v})\}$$

2.3.2 Treatment Planning

As medical management is a time-oriented process, diagnostic and treatment actions described in guidelines are performed in a temporal setting. It is assumed that two types of knowledge are involved in detecting the violation of good medical practice:

- Knowledge concerning the (patho)physiological mechanisms underlying the disease, and the way treatment influences these mechanisms. The knowledge involved could be causal in nature, and is an example of *object-knowledge*.
- Knowledge concerning good practice in treatment selection; this is *meta-knowledge*.

Below we present some ideas on how such knowledge may be formalised using temporal logic (cf. [15] for early work).

We are interested in the prescription of drugs, taking into account their mode of action. Abstracting from the dynamics of their pharmacokinetics, this can be formalised in logic as follows:

$$(Gd \wedge r) \rightarrow G(m_1 \wedge \cdots \wedge m_n)$$

where d is the name of a drug or possibly of a group of drugs indicated by a predicate symbol (e.g. $SU(x)$, where x is universally quantified and 'SU' stands for sulfony-lurea drugs, such as Tolbutamid, which are prescribed in diabetes mellitus type 2), r is a (possibly negative or empty) *requirement* for the drug to take effect, and m_k is a mode of action, such as decrease of release of glucose from the liver, which holds at all future times.

The modes of action m_k can be combined, together with an *intention n* (achieving normoglycaemia, i.e. normal blood glucose levels, for example), a particular patient *condition c*, and *requirements* r_j for the modes of action to be effective:

$$(Gm_{i_1} \wedge \cdots \wedge Gm_{i_m} \wedge r_1 \wedge \cdots \wedge r_p \wedge Hc) \rightarrow Gn$$

Good practice medicine can then be formalised as follows. Let $\mathscr{B}$ be background knowledge, $T \subseteq \{d_1, \ldots, d_p\}$ be a set of drugs, C a collection of patient conditions, R a collection of requirements, and N a collection of intentions which the physician has to achieve. A set of drugs T is a *treatment* according to the theory of abductive reasoning if [20]:

(1) $\mathscr{B} \cup GT \cup C \cup R \nvDash \bot$ (the drugs do not have contradictory effects), and
(2) $\mathscr{B} \cup GT \cup C \cup R \vDash N$ (the drugs handle all the patient problems intended to be managed)

If in addition to (1) and (2) condition

(3) $O_\varphi(T)$ holds, where O_φ is a meta-predicate standing for an optimality criterion or combination of optimality criteria φ, then the treatment is said to be *in accordance with good-practice medicine*.

A typical example of this is subset minimality $O_\subset$:

$$O_\subset(T) \equiv \forall T' \subset T : T' \text{ is not a treatment according to (1) and (2)}$$

i.e. the minimum number of effective drugs are being prescribed. For example, if $\{d_1, d_2, d_3\}$ is a treatment that satisfies condition (3) in addition to (1) and (2), then the subsets $\{d_1, d_2\}$, $\{d_2, d_3\}$, $\{d_1\}$, and so on, do not satisfy conditions (1) and (2). In the context of abductive reasoning, subset minimality is often used in order to distinguish between various solutions; it is also referred to in literature as *Occam's razor*. Another definition of the meta-predicate O_φ is in terms of minimal cost O_c:

$$O_c(T) \equiv \forall T', \text{ with } T' \text{ a treatment: } c(T') \geq c(T)$$

where $c(T) = \sum_{d \in T} cost(d)$; combining the two definitions also makes sense. For example, one could come up with a definition of $O_{\subset,c}$ that among two subset-minimal treatments selects the one that is the cheapest in financial or ethical sense.

2.4   Reasoning with Uncertainty

Uncertainty is another essential aspects of much medical knowledge and data. Here again, there has been a lot of research in artificial intelligence.

2.4.1   Bayesian Networks

Up until now, it has been assumed that in representing and solving a problem in a domain dealing with uncertainty is not of major importance. As this does not hold for many problems, the possibility to represent and reason with the uncertainty associated with a problem is clearly of significance. There have been a number of early attempts where researchers have augmented rule-based, logical methods with uncertainty methods, usually different from probability theory, although sometimes also related. However, those methods are now outdated, and have been replaced by methods which take probability theory as a starting point. In the context of knowledge-based systems, in particular the formalism of Bayesian (belief) networks has been successful [7, 12, 14, 17].

A *Bayesian belief network* $\mathcal{B} = (G, \text{Pr})$, also called *causal probabilistic network*, is a directed acyclic graph $G = (V(G), A(G))$, consisting of a set of nodes $V(G) = \{V_1, \ldots, V_n\}$, called *probabilistic nodes*, representing discrete random variables, and a set of arcs $A(G) \subseteq V(G) \times V(G)$, representing causal relationships or correlations among random variables. Consider Fig. 2.3, which shows a simplified version of a Bayesian belief network modelling some of the relevant variables in the diagnosis of two causes of fever. The presence of an arc between two nodes denotes the existence of a direct causal relationship or other influences; absence of an arc means that the variables do not influence each other directly. The following knowledge is represented in Fig. 2.3: variable 'FL' is expressed to influence 'MY' and 'FE', as it is known that flu causes myalgia (muscle pain) and fever. In turn, fever causes a change in body temperature, represented by the random variable TEMP. Finally, pneumonia (PN) is another cause of fever.

Associated with a Bayesian belief network is a joint probability distribution Pr, defined in terms of conditional probability tables according to the structure of the graph. For example, for Fig. 2.3, the conditional probability table

$$\text{Pr}(\text{FE} \mid \text{FL}, \text{PN})$$

has been assessed with respect to all possible values of the variables FE, FL and PN. In general, the graph associated with a Bayesian belief network mirrors the (in) dependences that are assumed to hold among variables in a domain. For example, given knowledge about presence or absence of fever, neither additional knowledge of flu nor of pneumonia is able to influence the knowledge about body temperature, since it holds that TEMP is conditionally independent of both PN and FL given FE.

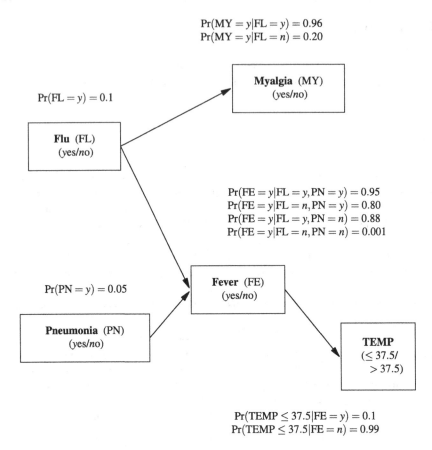

$$\Pr(MY = y | FL = y) = 0.96$$
$$\Pr(MY = y | FL = n) = 0.20$$

$$\Pr(FL = y) = 0.1$$

Myalgia (MY)
(yes/no)

Flu (FL)
(yes/no)

$$\Pr(FE = y | FL = y, PN = y) = 0.95$$
$$\Pr(FE = y | FL = n, PN = y) = 0.80$$
$$\Pr(FE = y | FL = y, PN = n) = 0.88$$
$$\Pr(FE = y | FL = n, PN = n) = 0.001$$

$$\Pr(PN = y) = 0.05$$

Fever (FE)
(yes/no)

Pneumonia (PN)
(yes/no)

TEMP
($\leq 37.5/$
> 37.5)

$$\Pr(TEMP \leq 37.5 | FE = y) = 0.1$$
$$\Pr(TEMP \leq 37.5 | FE = n) = 0.99$$

Fig. 2.3 Bayesian network $\mathscr{B} = (G, \Pr)$ with associated joint probability distribution Pr (only probabilities $\Pr(X = y \mid \pi(X))$ are shown, as $\Pr(X = n \mid \pi(X)) = 1 - \Pr(X = y \mid \pi(X))$).

For a joint probability distribution defined in accordance with the structure of a Bayesian network, it, therefore, holds that:

$$\Pr(V_1, \ldots, V_n) = \prod_{i=1}^{n} \Pr(V_i \mid \pi(V_i))$$

where V_i denotes a random variable associated with an identically named node, and $\pi(V_i)$ denotes the parents of that node. As a consequence, the amount of probabilistic information that must be specified, exponential in the number of variables in general when ignoring the independencies represented in the graph, is greatly reduced.

By means of special algorithms for probabilistic reasoning – well-known are the algorithms by Pearl [17] and by Lauritzen and Spiegelhalter [14] – the marginal probability distribution $\Pr(V_i)$ for every variable in the network can be computed; this is shown for the fever network in Fig. 2.4. In addition, a once constructed Bayesian belief network can be employed to enter and process data of a specific case, i.e. specific values for certain variables, like TEMP, yielding an updated network. Figure 2.5 shows the updated Bayesian network after entering evidence about a patient's body temperature into the network shown in Fig. 2.3. Entering evidence in a network is also referred to as *instantiating* the network. The resulting probability distribution of the updated network, $\Pr^E(V_i)$, which is a marginal probability distribution of the probability distribution $\Pr^E$, is equal to the posterior of the original probability distribution of the same variable, conditioned on the evidence E entered into the network:

$$\Pr^E(V_i) = \Pr(V_i \mid E)$$

Bayesian belief networks have also been related to logic by so called *probabilistic Horn clauses*. This formalism offers basically nothing else then a recipe to obtain a logical specification of a Bayesian belief network. Reasoning with probabilistic Horn clauses is accomplished by logical abduction; the axioms of probability theory are used to compute an updated probability distribution.

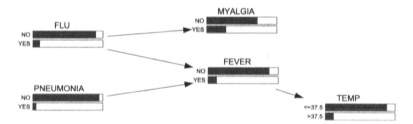

Fig. 2.4 Prior marginal probability distributions for the Bayesian belief network shown in Fig. 2.3.

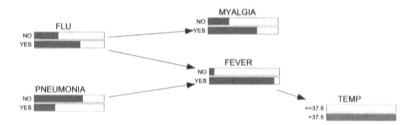

Fig. 2.5 Posterior marginal probability distributions for the Bayesian belief network after entering evidence concerning body temperature. Note the increase in probabilities of the presence of both flu and pneumonia compared to Fig. 2.4. It is also predicted that it is likely for the patient to have myalgia.

2.4.2 Probabilistic Logic

There have been different recent proposals in the AI literature to combine logic and probability theory, where usually predicate logic is combined with probabilistic graphical models. David Poole has developed so-called *independent choice logic* (which later was integrated into AIlog). It combined Prolog-like logic with Bayesian networks. Another approach, developed by Williamson et al. makes use of *credal networks*, which are similar to Bayesian networks but reason over probability intervals instead of probabilities. The last few years *Markov logic* has had an enormous impact on the research area. The idea is to use predicate logic to *generate* Markov networks, i.e., joint probability distributions that have an associated *undirected* graph. Formalisms such as independent choice logic and Markov logic are examples of what is called *probabilistic logic*.

Various probabilistic logics, such as the independent choice logic, are based on logical abduction. The basic idea of these kind of logics is to define the probability of a query in terms of the probability of its *explanations* (sometimes called a *prediction* in theory of logical abduction) of a certain query (cf. Sect. 4.5) given a logic program. Probability of the explanations are defined by a very simple distribution, namely by a set of independent random variables, which makes it possible to (relatively) efficiently compute a probability. The nice thing about this approach is that it truly combines logical reasoning (finding the explanations) with probabilistic reasoning (computing the probability of the set of explanations).

Defining the probability distributions over the explanations is done by associating probabilities to hypotheses in a set Δ. In order to make sure that we end up with a valid probability distribution, we require a partitioning of this set into subsets $\Delta_1, \ldots, \Delta_n$, i.e., such that it holds that:

$$\bigcup_{i=1}^{n} \Delta_i = \Delta$$

and $\Delta_i \cap \Delta_j = \emptyset$ for all $i \neq j$. Each possible grounding of Δ_i, i.e. $\Delta_i \sigma$ with σ a substitution, is associated to a random variable $X_{i,\sigma}$, i.e., $dom(X_{i,\sigma}) = \Delta_i \sigma$. While you could imagine that every random variable is different, here we will assume that every grounding of $h \in \Delta$ has to have the same probability, i.e., for all substitutions σ, σ':

$$P(X_{i,\sigma} = h\sigma) = P(X_{i,\sigma'} = h\sigma')$$

whereas each pair of random variables as we have just defined is assumed to be independent, the hypotheses *in the same partition* are dependent. Suppose for example, we have a random variable X with three possible hypotheses:

$$dom(X) = \{influenza, sport, not\_sport\_or\_influenza\}$$

In each possible state (element of the sample space), each random variable is exactly in one state at the time, i.e., in this case, we assume that we either have influenza, or we sport, or neither, but we do not sport while we have influenza. In other words: sport and influenza are considered to be inconsistent.

To understand the space of explanations that we may consider is by picking a possible value for each random variable. In the language of the *independent choice logic*, this is called a *choice* (hence, the name). In order to make this work probabilistically, we need some slight restrictions on our logic program. First, it is not allowed to have two hypotheses in Δ that unify. Further, it is not allowed that an element from Δ unifies with a head of one of the clauses. Finally, mostly for convenience here, we will restrict ourselves to acyclic logic programs consisting of Horn clauses and substitutions that can be made using the constants in the program.

The probability distribution over Δ is now used to define a probability for arbitrary atoms. As mentioned earlier, this will be defined in terms of explanations, which are slightly different than we have seen before due to the probabilistic semantics. Given a causal specification $\Sigma = (\Delta, \Phi, \mathcal{R})$, a (probabilistic) explanation $E \subseteq \Delta\sigma$ for some formula $F \in \Phi$ is:

$$\mathcal{R} \cup E \models F$$
$$\mathcal{R} \cup C \cup E \not\models \perp$$

where

$$C = \{\perp \leftarrow h_1, h_2 \mid \Delta_i \text{ is one of the partitions of } \Delta, h_1, h_2 \in \Delta_i\}$$

and $\Delta\sigma$ grounded. Note that the consistency condition entails that we only pick at most one value for each random variable. The intuitive assumption that is now being made is that an atom is true if and only if at least one of its (grounded) explanations is true. Suppose $\mathscr{E}(F)$ is the set of all explanations for F, then we define:

$$F = \bigvee_{E_i \in \mathscr{E}(F)} E_i$$

Notice that this definition is equivalent to assuming Clarke's completion of the given theory (cf. Sect. 4.3.1).

Recall that an explanation E is called minimal if there does not exist an explanation E' such that $E' \subset E$. It is not difficult to see that we can restrict our attention to the set of *minimal explanations* $\mathscr{E}_m(F)$: by logical reasoning it holds that, if $E' \subset E$ then $E' \vee E = E'$, so it can be shown that $\mathscr{E}(F) = \mathscr{E}_m(F)$. We then have:

$$F = \bigvee_{E_i \in \mathscr{E}_m(F)} E_i$$

Again, there is a close connection to the semantics of abduction, as $\bigvee_{E_i \in \mathscr{E}_m(F)} E_i$ is sometimes referred to as the *solution formula*. Of course, if two things are equal, then their probability must be equal:

$$P(F) = P\left(\bigvee_{E_i \in \mathscr{E}_m(F)} E_i \right)$$

It is now clear how we can solve the problem of computing the probability of F: first we find the (minimal) explanations of F and then we use the probability distribution defined over the hypotheses to compute the disjunction of the explanations.

Consider the causal specification $\Sigma = (\Delta, \Phi, \mathscr{R})$, with

$$\Delta = \{influenza, sport, not\_sport\_or\_influenza, \alpha_1, not\_\alpha_1, \alpha_2, not\_\alpha_2\}$$

and

$$\Phi = \{chills, thirst, myalgia\}$$

and the set of logical formulae $\mathscr{R}$ as presented in Fig. 2.2.

First we need to define a probability distribution over Δ. For example, we may assume to have three independent random variables X, Y, Z, such that:

$$P(X = sport) = 0.3$$
$$P(X = influenza) = 0.1$$
$$P(X = not\_sport\_or\_influenza) = 0.6$$
$$P(Y = \alpha_1) = 0.9$$
$$P(Y = not\_\alpha_1) = 0.1$$
$$P(Z = \alpha_2) = 0.7$$
$$P(Z = not\_\alpha_2) = 0.3$$

Note that explanations containing e.g., *sport* and *influenza* are inconsistent with this probability distribution, as X can only take the value of one of them (they are mutually exclusive).

Suppose we have interested in the probability of myalgia, i.e., $P(myalgia)$. The set of all minimal explanations for myalgia, i.e., $\mathscr{E}_m(myalgia)$ is $\{E_1, E_2\}$, where:

$$E_1 = \{influenza, \alpha_2\}$$
$$E_2 = \{sport\}$$

Clearly, there are many more explanations, e.g.,

$$E_3 = \{influenza, sport, \alpha_2\}$$
$$E_4 = \{influenza, \alpha_1, \alpha_2\}$$
$$E_5 = \{influenza, not\_\alpha_1, \alpha_2\}$$
$$\vdots \qquad \vdots$$

Note that for example, the set:

$$E' = \{influenza, \alpha_1, not\_\alpha_1, \alpha_2\}$$

is inconsistent, because α_1 and not_α_1 cannot both be true. Therefore, it is not an explanation.

Since we assumed that a formula is true if only if at least one of its explanations is true, the probability of myalgia is defined it terms of influenza and sport:

$$P(myalgia) = P((influenza \wedge \alpha_2) \vee sport)$$

Since $influenza \wedge \alpha_2$ and $sport$ are mutually exclusive, the probability of the disjunction is the sum of the disjuncts, i.e.:

$$\begin{aligned} P(myalgia) &= P(influenza \wedge \alpha_2) + P(sport) \\ &= P(influenza)P(\alpha_2) + P(sport) \\ &= 0.1 \cdot 0.7 + 0.3 = 0.37 \end{aligned}$$

2.5 Conclusions

In this introductory chapter we have briefly reviewed the most important languages for knowledge representation as using in medicine. It is not possible given the scope of this chapter to be complete, but since logic and probability theory act as the core of the majority of the modern work on knowledge representation, this introduction will at least pinpoint the most important ideas.

References

1. Ben-Ari, M., Manna, Z., Pnueli, A.: The temporal logic of branching time. Acta Inform. **20**, 207–226 (1983)
2. Brachman, R.J.: What IS-A is and isn't: an analysis of taxonomic links in semantic networks. IEEE Comput. **16**(10), 30–36 (1983)
3. Buchanan, B.G., Shortliffe, E.H.: Rule-Based Expert Systems: The MYCIN Experiments of the Stanford Heuristic Programming Project. Addison-Wesley, Reading (1984)
4. Clancey, W.J.: Heuristic classification. Artif. Intell. **27**, 289–350 (1985)
5. Clarke, E.M., Emerson, E.A.: Design and synthesis of synchronization skeletons using branching time temporal logic. In: Kozen, D. (ed.) Logic of Programs. LNCS, vol. 131, pp. 52–71. Springer, Heidelberg (1981)
6. Console, L., Theseider Dupré, D., Torasso, P.: A theory of diagnosis for incomplete causal models. In: Proceedings of the 10th International Joint Conference on Artificial Intelligence, pp. 1311–1317 (1989)
7. Cooper, G.F.: A method for using belief networks as influence diagrams. In: Proceedings of the 4th Workshop on Uncertainty in Artificial Intelligence, pp. 55–63 (1988)
8. de Kleer, J., Williams, B.C.: Diagnosing multiple faults. Artif. Intell. **32**, 97–130 (1987)
9. Downing, K.: Physiological applications of consistency-based diagnosis. Artif. Intell. Med. **5**(1), 9–30 (1993)

10. Emerson, E.A., Clarke, E.M.: Characterizing correctness properties of parallel programs using fixpoints. In: de Bakker, J., van Leeuwen, J. (eds.) Automata, Languages and Programming. LNCS, vol. 85, pp. 169–181. Springer, Heidelberg (1980)
11. Forbus, K.D., De Kleer, J.: Building Problem Solvers. The MIT Press, Cambridge (1993)
12. Glymour, C., Cooper, G.F.: Computation. Causation & Discovery. MIT Press, Menlo Park (1999)
13. Hitzler, P., et al. (eds.): OWL 2 Web Ontology Language: Primer. W3C Recommendation, 27 October 2009. http://www.w3.org/TR/owl2-primer/
14. Lauritzen, S.L., Spiegelhalter, D.J.: Local computations with probabilities on graphical structures and their application to expert systems. J. R. Stat. Soc. (Ser. B) 50, 157–224 (1987)
15. Lucas, P.J.F.: The representation of medical reasoning models in resolution-based theorem provers. Artif. Intell. Med. **5**(5), 395–414 (1993)
16. W3C OWL Working Group. OWL 2 Web Ontology Language: Document Overview. W3C Recommendation, 27 October 2009. http://www.w3.org/TR/owl2-overview/
17. Pearl, J.: Probabilistic Reasoning in Intelligent Systems: Networks of Plausible Inference. Morgan Kaufmann, Palo Alto (1988)
18. Peng, Y., Reggia, J.A.: Abductive Inference Models for Diagnostic Problem Solving. Springer, New York (1990)
19. Pnuelli, A.: A temporal logic of concurrent programs. Theor. Comput. Sci. **13**, 45–60 (1981)
20. Poole, D.: Explanation and prediction: an architecture for default and abductive reasoning. Comput. Intell. **5**(2), 97–110 (1989)
21. Pople, H.E.: Heuristic methods for imposing structure on ill-structured problems: the structure of medical diagnostics. In: Szolovits, P. (ed.) Artificial Intelligence in Medicine. AAAS Selected Symposium, vol. 51, pp. 119–190. Westview Press, Boulder (1982)
22. Reiter, R.: A theory of diagnosis from first principles. Artif. Intell. **32**, 57–95 (1987)
23. Szolovits, P.: Artificial Intelligence in Medicine. AAAS Selected Symposium, vol. 51. Westview Press, Boulder (1982)

Diagnosis of Disease

Chapter 3
Representing Knowledge for Clinical Diagnostic Reasoning

Peter J.F. Lucas and Felipe Orihuela-Espina

3.1 A Bit of History: From Rule-based to Model-based

The early medical diagnostic applications often had the form of rule-based expert systems and started to appear around the mid 1970s. Soon, it became apparent that developing reliable diagnostic systems required an understanding of the principles underlying diagnosis, which at the time were poorly understood. Thus, during the 1980s, a research effort was made on developing the conceptual and formal aspects of diagnosis. In the early systems, knowledge from human experts was encoded as empirical classification rules, probably best seen as Horn clauses with limited expressive power [16]. Later, a model-based paradigm started to gain popularity, where the idea was to use a formal language with sufficient expressive power, such as predicate logic and timed automata, to model the part of reality that was relevant for the diagnostic problem at hand [11]. Under the new model-based paradigm, knowledge of a system's structure and function were captured using those formal languages. Notwithstanding the efforts and progress, still in the late 1980s the understanding of the diagnostic problem principles and the characterization of diagnostic systems remained challenging. At that time, diagnostic reasoning was increasingly seen as a method to reduce uncertainty and probabilistic methods, such as offered by Bayesian networks, were investigated in the hope that they would offer a model-based method of sufficient strength and generality to handle most diagnostic problems [18]. Whereas probabilistic methods have left their mark on diagnostic problem solving, at the moment there are still many different methods being used for diagnostic applications although probabilistic methods are now dominant.

3.2 Elements of Diagnostic Reasoning

Making a diagnosis is normally seen as the first step towards the clinical management of illness in people; it is not possible to treat a person without having a sufficiently

© Springer International Publishing Switzerland 2015
A. Hommersom and P.J.F. Lucas (eds.), *Biomedical Knowledge Representation*, LNAI 9521, DOI 10.1007/978-3-319-28007-3_3

accurate diagnosis. Whereas the *diagnosis* is the outcome, the steps that are taken in obtaining this outcome constitute what is called the *diagnostic process*. Thus, the outcome of the diagnostic process is either the absence of illness or the presence of one or more disorders at the same time. In clinical medicine, the diagnostic process takes a particular form, consisting of taking the *medical history*, followed by a *physical examination* and supplemented by *laboratory investigations* (biochemistry and radiology). Taking the medical history involves recording subjective findings, called *'symptoms'*, whereas the physical examination and lab tests will yield objective results, called *'signs'*. The diagnostic process tries to obtain an explanation for the symptoms and signs in terms of disease processes, and this not only involves making observations, but also to actively collect findings, often called *information gathering*. This way of looking at the diagnostic process is often called *diagnostic reasoning*.

The diagnostic conclusions drawn by the clinical professional are based on expertise, obtained after many years of training, and clinical intuition about which diagnostic test should be performed and how to interpret the test results in the context of the patient's characteristics. From a more abstract point of view, the medical knowledge involved has a particular structure and meaning. In addition, in interpreting diagnostic test results uncertainty is explicitly taken into account. Although most researchers will probably agree that making a diagnosis is a process that inevitably involves uncertainty, there is no consensus about how important this uncertainty is and about whether this uncertainty should always be made explicit.

Diagnostic reasoning always involves at least two different aspects. First, one needs to represent in what way a conclusion is taken as being a 'diagnosis'. This concerns the representation of what is seen as the definition of a diagnosis. It will become clear later in this chapter that there are many different definitions of the notion of diagnosis possible. Second, a diagnosis is always based on the interpretation of specific domain knowledge. Clearly, the representation of this knowledge is also an important issue. A third aspect of diagnostic reasoning, that is not always taken into account when describing diagnostic reasoning, is a strategy involving the dynamic collection of information to rule-in and rule-out particular diagnoses.

This chapter provides an overview of the first two aspects to give the reader an entrance point to this section on knowledge-based diagnosis.

3.3 Conceptual Basis of Diagnosis

Several formal theories have been proposed to capture the concept of diagnosis more precisely. Most of these theories have been developed with fault diagnosis and trouble shooting of technical devices, such as photo-copiers, in mind. Despite the different nature of the objects of study, technical and medical diagnostic reasoning have much in common, both in their terminology and diagnostic methods. This similarity explains why we start with ideas that mostly come from the diagnosis of technical devices. However, all of these methods have also been applied to the clinical domain.

Researchers have become aware that there are actually various *conceptual models* of diagnosis that underly the formal theories, determined by the kind of knowledge involved. Diagnosis always concerns the interpretation of observed findings in the context of knowledge from a problem domain. A good starting point for describing diagnosis at a conceptual level are the various types of knowledge that play a role in diagnostic applications.

The knowledge embodied in a diagnostic system may be based on one or more of the following descriptions:

(1) A description of the *normal* structure and behaviour.
(2) A description of *abnormal* behaviour of a system, possibly augmented with a description of abnormal structure.
(3) An enumeration of disorders and collections of observable findings for every possible disorder concerned, without the availability of explicit knowledge concerning the (abnormal) functional behaviour of the system.

These types of knowledge may coexist in real-life diagnostic systems, but it is customary to emphasise their distinction in conceptual and formal theories of diagnosis. Similar classifications of types of knowledge appear in the literature on diagnosis, although often no clear distinction is made between the conceptual, formal and implementation aspects of diagnostic systems. For example, [6, 19] distinguish diagnostic rule-based systems, by which they mean diagnostic systems based on knowledge of the third type mentioned above, from diagnostic systems incorporating knowledge of structure and behaviour, i.e. knowledge of the first and second type mentioned above. However, rule-based systems with a sufficiently expressive rule formalism, e.g. based on predicate logic, can be used to implement any diagnostic system, including those based on knowledge of structure and behaviour.

An observed finding that has been gathered in diagnosing a problem is often said to be either a 'normal finding', i.e. a finding that matches the normal situation, or an 'abnormal finding', i.e. a finding that does not match the normal situation. Based on the three types of knowledge mentioned above, and the two sorts of findings, three different conceptual models of diagnosis are usually distinguished; they will be called:

- *Deviation-from-Normal-Structure-and-Behaviour diagnosis*, abbreviated to *DNSB diagnosis*,
- *Matching-Abnormal-Behaviour diagnosis*, abbreviated to *MAB diagnosis*, and
- *Abnormality-Classification diagnosis*, abbreviated to *AC diagnosis*.

Below, we shall discuss the relationship between these three conceptual models of diagnosis and the three types of knowledge mentioned above. A formal theory of diagnosis has been proposed for each of these conceptual models of diagnosis. In the remainder of this section, each of the three conceptual models of diagnosis will be discussed, and the corresponding formal theory of diagnosis is mentioned.

DNSB diagnosis. For diagnosis based on knowledge concerning normal structure and behaviour, little or no explicit knowledge is available about the relationships between disorders, on the one hand, and findings to be observed when certain disorders are present, on the other hand. Hence, DNSB diagnosis typically employs knowledge of the first type mentioned above. From a practical point of view, the primary motivation for investigating this approach to diagnosis is that in many domains little knowledge concerning abnormality is available, which is certainly true for new human-created artifacts. For example, for a new device that has just been released from the factory, experience with respect to the faults that may occur when the device is in operation is lacking. Thus, the only conceivable way in which initially such faults can be handled is by looking at the normal structure and functional behaviour of the device. In clinical medicine, this will normally happen when one is encountering a new disease. Here, as with the technical disciplines, the only thing one can do is make use of knowledge of normal physiology and compare predicted behaviours with those observed.

For the purpose of diagnosis, the actual behaviour of an actual system, called *observed behaviour*, is compared with the results of a model of normal structure and behaviour of the system, which may be taken as *predicted behaviour*. Both types of behaviour can be characterised by findings. If there is a *discrepancy* between the observed and the predicted behaviour, diagnostic problem solving amounts to isolating the parts of the system that are not properly functioning, using the model of the normal structure and behaviour. In doing so, it is assumed that the model of normal structure and behaviour is sufficiently accurate and correct. Figure 3.1 depicts DNSB diagnosis in a schematic way. DNSB diagnosis is frequently erroneously called model-based diagnosis in the literature, as if it were the only instance of model-based diagnosis. It is also called consistency-based diagnosis, but here this term is reserved for the corresponding formal theory of diagnosis. DNSB diagnosis has been developed in the context of troubleshooting in electronic circuits [6]. A well-known program that supports DNSB diagnosis, and includes various strategies to do so efficiently, is the *General Diagnostic Engine* (GDE) [7].

The formal counterpart of DNSB diagnosis, called *consistency-based diagnosis*, originates from work by R. Reiter, [24]. DNSB diagnosis-like approaches have been used in medical applications on a limited scale (cf. for example [9]); there is more work in which DNSB diagnosis has been applied to solve technical problems (cf. [2]).

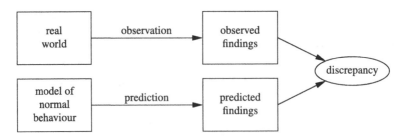

Fig. 3.1 Deviation-from-normal-structure-and-behaviour (DNSB) diagnosis.

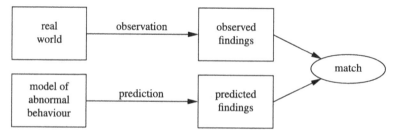

Fig. 3.2 Matching-abnormal-behaviour (MAB) diagnosis.

MAB diagnosis. For diagnosis based on knowledge of abnormal behaviour, diagnostic problem solving amounts to simulating the abnormal behaviour using an explicit model of that behaviour. Hence, in MAB diagnosis the use of knowledge of abnormal behaviour (the second type of knowledge mentioned above) is emphasised. By assuming the presence of certain defects, some observable abnormal findings can be predicted. It can be investigated which of these assumed defects account for the observed findings by *matching* the predicted abnormal findings with those observed. In Fig. 3.2, MAB diagnosis is depicted schematically. In most applications of MAB diagnosis, the domain knowledge that is used for diagnosis consists of causal relationships. Two, strongly related, formal counterparts of MAB diagnosis have been proposed in the literature. The first formal theory, referred to as the *set-covering theory of diagnosis*, is based on set theory: causal knowledge is expressed as mathematical relations, used for diagnosis. This theory originates from work by J.A. Reggia and others [23]. The second theory is based on logic. Early work in this area has been done by Poole [19, 20], and Console and Torasso [5, 28]. Based on the type of reasoning employed to formalise MAB diagnosis, i.e. reasoning from effects to causes instead of from causes to effects, this theory of diagnosis is also referred to as *abductive diagnosis*. Theorist [20] and its successor AILog [21] are two systems supporting MAB diagnosis.

AC diagnosis. Whereas DNSB and MAB diagnosis employ a model of normal or abnormal structure and behaviour for the purpose of diagnosis, the third conceptual model of diagnosis uses neither. The knowledge employed in this conceptual model of diagnosis consists of the enumeration of more or less typical evidence that can be observed, i.e. observable findings, when a particular defect or defect category is present (the third type of knowledge mentioned above). For example, sneezing is a finding that may be typically observed in a disorder like common cold. This form of knowledge has been referred to as *empirical associations* (the phrase '*compiled knowledge*' is also employed) [3].

Diagnostic problem solving amounts to establishing which of the elements in a finite set of defects have associated findings that account for as many of the findings observed as possible, as is shown in Fig. 3.3. The enumeration of findings for the normal situation (knowledge of the fourth type mentioned above) is sometimes also used in AC diagnosis, together with knowledge of the third type; then, observed findings

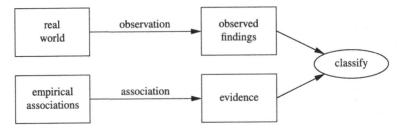

Fig. 3.3 Abnormality-classification (AC) diagnosis.

are classified in terms of present and absent defects. The main goal of AC diagnosis, however, remains the classification of observed findings in terms of abnormality. AC diagnosis is often referred to in the literature as *heuristic classification* [4], although this term is broader, since it also includes a reasoning strategy. AC diagnosis can be characterised in terms of logical deduction in a straightforward way. We shall refer to this formalisation of AC diagnosis as *hypothetico-deductive diagnosis*.

3.4 Formalisation and Implementation

Any formal system aiming to determine a valid (and perhaps most likely) diagnosis establishes a projection to hidden event sources (diseases, conditions or syndromes) and observable findings, that is symptoms and signs. However, the form of this mapping differs depending on the formalisation theory supporting the knowledge representation. A diagnostic system can be described as in Chap. 2 in terms of *object knowledge*, the domain knowledge that is used to determine a diagnosis, and *meta knowledge*, here the actual definition of what a diagnosis is.

3.4.1 Diagnostic Object Knowledge

The most common object knowledge representations in diagnostic systems are:

- A *causal specification* of relationships between (the interaction of) causes and effects. Formally a causal specification can be represented by logical implications of the form

$$C \rightarrow E$$

  or by means of functions or relations $E = f(C)$, and by a family of probability distributions $P(E \mid C)$ if in addition uncertainty is represented in the specification. Causality is as central to science as it has proved elusive to define. There is no single nor agreed definition of causality, with many attempts demanding two critical elements: (i) some kind of temporal precedence or ordering, e.g. Granger's [10] or Lamport's [14], and (ii) context, e.g. Pearl's [17] or Rubin-Holland's [25]. The first demand maybe implicit, ergo the model still might be static. The second demand is perhaps even more difficult to comply and thus it is too very often neglected abusing the causal sufficiency assumption or alleviated under the close-world assumption. Here, in the context of diagnosis it just refers to a particular way to model the reality (without pretending it captures the physics of causality). Consequently throughout this chapter, we will use the words cause, effects and causality without necessarily entailing formal causality. Moreover, causal relations are not necessarily strict [22].

- A model of *structure and behaviour*, often referred to as functional model or *first principles*, represented in logical or in algebraic form, whereas timed automata are used when temporal behaviour is being modelled, and temporal or dynamic Bayesian networks are used if the model includes uncertainty.
- An *associational specification* (non-causal) incorporating empirical relations as logical rules determined from human expertise, or statistical intuition.

3.4.2   Diagnostic Meta Knowledge

In order to define a diagnosis for a problem, using object representations of relevant knowledge, we need diagnostic meta knowledge, as introduced in Chap. 2. Basically, for causal knowledge the meta knowledge has the form of the covering condition, i.e. abductive diagnosis:

$$KB \cup D \models F$$

where KB is a set of causal, local rules, F is a set of observed findings and D is the diagnostic, abductive solution.

From the above statement it may be inferred that there is a one-to-one mapping joining a formalization theory with a particular knowledge representation. While this is not a universal truth, there remains a strong benefit from using a particular type of object knowledge with a particular type of meta knowledge under a particular framework. Chapter 2 gives details about the most popular symbolic diagnostic approaches. See [15] for a detailed analysis of the relationship between object and meta knowledge in diagnostic systems.

3.4.3   Probabilistic Diagnosis

As mentioned at the beginning of this chapter, many people see uncertainty as an essential ingredient of a diagnostic problem [27]. Bayesian networks are a popular formalism to represent object knowledge, and often arcs in a Bayesian networks are given a causal reading. As symptoms, signs and test results in Bayesian networks are often sink nodes, i.e. have no outgoing arcs, whereas diseases act as source nodes, i.e. have no incoming arcs, reasoning with such a Bayesian network can be looked upon as abductive reasoning, very similar to purely symbolic or logical forms of diagnostic reasoning.

In probabilistic diagnostic reasoning systems the diagnostic value of specific symptoms, signs and tests are used to rule in or rule out a diagnosis [1, 8]. Probabilistic reasoning requires knowing (i) the pre-test or prior probability of the diagnosis being considered, and (ii) the degree to which a positive or negative result from a specific test adjusts the probability of that diagnosis. The pre-test probability of a sease is known as the *prevalence* of the disease. Interpretation of the post-test or a posteriori probability strongly depends on the prevalence (i.e. pre-test probability). The most likely diagnosis is computed by Bayes' rule:

$$P(d \mid t) = \frac{P(t \mid d)P(d)}{P(t)}$$

where $P(t) = P(t \mid d)P(d) + P(t \mid \bar{d})P(\bar{d})$. The probability $P(t \mid d)$ is the likelihood that the test t is positive given that the disease d is present, i.e. the true positive rate (also called sensitivity in the medical literature), and the probability $P(\bar{t} \mid \bar{d})$ is the likelihood that the test result is negative given that that the disease is absent. It is also known as the true negative rate (specificity in the medical literature). Both rates are usually in the range [0.90, 0.99].

As an example, consider the the diagnosis of flu f based on measuring the body temperature t (equal or above 38 °C) and $\bar{t}$ (below 38 °C) on two different occasions. The first is under conditions of a severe flu epidemic and the second is in the middle of the summer. Now, the prevalence of flu under epidemic conditions is assumed to be $P(f) = 0.5$, whereas in midsummer it is $P(f) = 0.05$. Using Bayes' rule and assuming that $P(t \mid f) = P(\bar{t} \mid \bar{f}) = 0.95$, we compute the post-test probability for those two possibilities:

- $P(f \mid t) = P(t \mid f)P(f)/P(t) = 0.95 \cdot 0.5/0.5 = 0.95$.
- $P(f \mid t) = P(t \mid f)P(f)/P(t) = 0.95 \cdot 0.05/0.095 = 0.5$

Since the true positive and negative rates do not change, the prevalences have a major effect on how likely a diagnosis is. We also have the following observations:

- Under low prevalence: A negative test is enough to rule out a diagnosis, but a positive test is likely to be a false positive.
- Under medium prevalence: Tests work often at their best. With a positive test it is reasonable to assume the condition is present, and with a negative test it is reasonable to assume this is not the case.
- Under high prevalence: A positive test is enough to confirm a diagnosis, but a negative test is likely to be a false negative.

As patient often have two or more diseases at the same time, known as multimorbidity, one actually has to compute the maximum a posteriori probability (MAP) assignment [13]

$$D^\star = \mathrm{argmax}_D P(D \mid E)$$

Table 3.1 Comparison conceptual and formal theories of diagnosis and their implementation.

	DNSB	MAB	AC
Object knowledge	Normal structure and behaviour	Causal model of (ab)normality	Empirical associations
Formalisation of diagnosis	Consistency-based	Bayesian network abductive and diagnosis set-covering diagnosis maximum a postiori probability assignment	Hypothetico-deductive diagnosis
Examples of software systems	GDE	Theorist/AILog Bayesian network package	Rule-based systems

where D is a set of instantiated disease variables and E the evidence (symptoms, signs, and lab test results). Since the computations are NP-hard, one usually resorts to computing the marginal probability $p(d \mid E)$ for individual diseases d.

3.4.4   From Conceptual to Formalisation and Implementation

A comparison of the three conceptual and formal models of diagnosis is given in Table 3.1. Obviously, the various models of diagnosis discussed above can also be combined. To solve real-life diagnostic problems in a domain, it is likely that a mixture of conceptual models of diagnosis as distinguished above will be required. Since the resulting systems use various types of knowledge, e.g. both knowledge of structure and behaviour, and empirical associations, the result is known as diagnosis with *multiple models*.

Although in the literature it is emphasised that the conceptual models of diagnosis discussed embody different forms of diagnosis, they have much in common. For example, the type of knowledge used in DNSB diagnosis can be viewed as an implicit, or intensional, version of the type of knowledge used in AC diagnosis (if restricted to normality classification), which is an explicit or extensional type of knowledge; the associations between normal observable findings and the absence of defects are hidden in the specified normal behaviour in DNSB diagnosis. DNSB and MAB diagnostic problem solving are based on some kind of simulation of behaviour; such simulation of behaviour is absent in AC diagnosis. In all cases, the diagnostic problem is seen as an ordered pair $\mathscr{P} = (K, O)$, with $K = (C, R, E)$ in turn a tuple of causes C, association rules R, and effects or possible observations E corresponding to the description of the causal model, and O a set of actual findings or observations such that $O \subseteq E$. The particular form, as well as the semantic, of the elements and subelements of the diagnostic problem depends on the chosen formalisation paradigm. For instance in consistency based diagnosis the system description is a finite set of first-order logic formulae R implicitly encoding the projection from system components C to observed findings E, whereas in the case of set covering diagnoses R is explicitly a subset of the Cartesian product between disorders C and manifestations E.

Finally, several programs have been developed that offer limited possibility to carry out diagnostic problem solving using multiple models; examples of such programs are GDE [12]. These programs use DNSB diagnosis as their core approach.

3.5 Conclusions

This chapter introduces the book section on the use of knowledge representation to solve the diagnostic problem. The chapter has briefly overviewed important formalisation theories which arise from the two reasoning frameworks dominating formal medicine; namely deductive and probabilistic. Each of these ways to explaining events are archetypical of two attitudes towards clinical diagnosis; deterministic and evidence-based diagnosis [26]. Whatever the reasoning chosen to address the diagnosis, it seems clear that our GP has now a wealth of formal approaches at her hand to reason the most solid diagnosis on the light of the signs. The different options available have different expressive capabilities and their choice depends on the type of knowledge base available to the system designer. Notwithstanding, *uncertainty* and *meaning* can be combined in a unified framework such as offered by probabilistic logics, such as AILog [21].

The rest of this book section presents two specific examples of formal diagnostic systems, each of them addressing different clinical problems and founded on different knowledge representation paradigms.

References

1. Arroll, B., Allan, G.M., Elley, C.R., Kenealy, T., McCormack, J., Hudson, B., Hoare, K.: Diagnosis in primary care: probabilistic reasoning. J. Prim. Health Care **4**(2), 166–173 (2012)
2. Beschta, A., Dressler, O., Freitag, H., Montag, M., Struss, P.: DPNet – a second generation expert system for localizing faults in power transmission networks. In: Proceedings of the International Conference on Fault Diagnosis (Tooldiag93), pp. 1019–1027. Toulouse (1993)
3. Buchanan, B.G., Shortliffe, E.H.: Rule-based Expert Systems: the MYCIN Experiments of the Stanford Heuristic Programming Project. Addison-Wesley, Reading (1984)
4. Clancey, W.J.: Heuristic classification. Artif. Intell. **27**, 289–350 (1985)

5. Console, L., Theseider Dupré, D., Torasso, P.: A theory of diagnosis for incomplete causal models. In: International Joint Conference on Artificial Intelligence (IJCAI 1989), pp. 1311–1317. AAAI Press (1989)
6. Davis, R., Hamscher, W.: Model-based reasoning: troubleshooting. In: Shrobe, H.E. (ed.) Exploring Artificial Intelligence: Survey Talks from the National Conference on Artificial Intelligence, pp. 297–346. Morgan Kaufmann, San Mateo (1988)
7. de Kleer, J., Williams, B.C.: Diagnosing multiple faults. Artif. Intell. **32**, 97–130 (1987)
8. Doust, J.: Diagnosis in general practice: using probabilistic reasoning. Br. Med. J. **339**(b3823), 1080–1082 (2009)
9. Downing, K.L.: Physiological applications of consistency-based diagnosis. Artif. Intell. Med. **5**, 9–30 (1993)
10. Ganger, C.W.J.: Investigating causal relations by econometric models and cross-spectral methods. Econometrica **37**, 424–438 (1969)
11. Hamscher, W., Console, L., De Kleer, J.: Readings in Model-based Diagnosis. Morgan Kaufmann, San Mateo (1992)
12. de Kleer, J., Williams, B.C.: Diagnosis with behavioural modes. In: Proceedings of the 11th International Joint Conference on Artificial Intelligence, pp. 1324–1330. AAAI Press (1989)
13. Kwisthout, J.: Most probable explanations in Bayesian networks: complexity and tracability. Int. J. Approximate reasoning **52**, 1452–1469 (2011)
14. Lamport, L.: Time, clocks and the ordering of events in a distributed system. Commun. ACM **21**(7), 558–565 (1978)
15. Lucas, P.J.F.: Analysis of notions of diagnosis. Artif. Intell. **105**(1–2), 293–341 (1998)
16. Lucas, P.J.F., van der Gaag, L.C.: Principles of Expert Systems. Addison-Wesley, Wokingham (1991)
17. Pearl, J.: Causality: Models, Reasoning and Inference, 2nd edn. Cambridge University Press, Cambridge (2009)
18. Pearl, J.: Probabilistic Reasoning in Intelligent Systems: Networks of Plausible Inference. Morgan Kaufmann, San Mateo (1988)
19. Poole, D.: Representing knowledge for logic-based diagnosis. In: Proceedings of the International Conference on Fifth Generation Computer Systems 1988, pp. 1282–1290. ICOT (1988)
20. Poole, D., Goebel, R., Aleliunas, R.: Theorist: a logical reasoning system for defaults and diagnosis. In: Cercone, N., Mc Calla, G. (eds.) The Knowledge Frontier, pp. 331–352. Springer, Berlin (1987)
21. Poole, D., Mackworth, A.: Artificial Intelligence: Foundations of Computational Agents. Cambridge University Press, Cambridge (2010)
22. Poole, D.: Representing diagnosis knowledge. Ann. Math. Artif. Intell. **11**, 33–50 (1994)
23. Reggia, J.A., Nau, D.S., Wang, Y.: Diagnostic expert systems based on a set-covering model. Int. J. Man Mach. Stud. **19**, 437–460 (1983)
24. Reiter, R.: A theory of diagnosis from first principles. Artif. Intell. **32**, 57–95 (1987)
25. Rubin, D.: Causal inference using potential outcomes. J. Am. Stat. Assoc. **100**(469), 322–331 (2005)
26. Soltani, A., Moayyeri, A.: Deterministic versus evidence-based attitude towards clinical diagnosis. J. Eval. Clin. Pract. **13**, 533–537 (2007)
27. Sox, H., Higgens, M.C., Owens, D.K.: Clinical Decision Making, 2nd edn. Wiley, Hoboken (2013)
28. Torasso, P., Console, L.: Diagnostic Problem Solving. North Oxford Academic Publishers, London (1989)

Chapter 4
Automated Diagnosis of Breast Cancer on Medical Images

Marina Velikova, Inês Dutra and Elizabeth S. Burnside

Abstract The development and use of computerized decision-support systems in the domain of breast cancer has the potential to facilitate the early detection of disease as well as spare healthy women unnecessary interventions. Despite encouraging trends, there is much room for improvement in the capabilities of such systems to further alleviate the burden of breast cancer. One of the main challenges that current systems face is integrating and translating multi-scale variables like patient risk factors and imaging features into complex management recommendations that would supplement and/or generalize similar activities provided by subspecialty-trained clinicians currently. In this chapter, we discuss the main types of knowledge—object-attribute, spatial, temporal and hierarchical—present in the domain of breast image analysis and their formal representation using two popular techniques from artificial intelligence—Bayesian networks and first-order logic. In particular, we demonstrate (i) the explicit representation of uncertain relationships between low-level image features and high-level image findings (e.g., mass, microcalcifications) by probability distributions in Bayesian networks, and (ii) the expressive power of logic to generally represent the dynamic number of objects in the domain. By concrete examples with patient data we show the practical application of both formalisms and their potential for use in decision-support systems.

4.1 Introduction

According to the American Cancer Society (ACS), breast cancer is the second leading cause of cancer death in women, exceeded only by lung cancer. The chance that breast cancer will be responsible for a woman's death is about 3 %. Death rates from breast cancer have been declining since about 1990, with larger decreases in women younger than 50. These decreases are believed to be the result of earlier detection through screening and increased awareness, as well as improved treatment, changes in clinical procedures, for example, genetic testing, and innovation in technologies like digital mammography and tomosynthesis [7, 11]. The increased use of computerized

© Springer International Publishing Switzerland 2015
A. Hommersom and P.J.F. Lucas (eds.), *Biomedical Knowledge Representation*, LNAI 9521, DOI 10.1007/978-3-319-28007-3_4

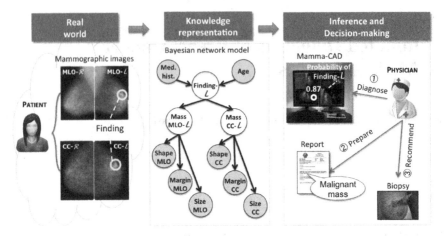

Fig. 4.1 Knowledge representation for decision-support in breast cancer diagnosis.

decision support systems that can detect breast cancer based on breast images or on the patient's history and clinical information, has the potential to contribute to improved outcomes [3, 5]. The severe consequences of breast cancer for many patients' health and life, and for their families well-being are still present and much room for improvement in the management of the disease is needed.

In this respect, a number of major challenges for clinical practicioners can be outlined, such as processing of huge amounts of data (e.g., interpretation of medical images) in short time, uncertainty in establishing a diagnosis or a treatment due to the variety of breast cancer pathologies. Another important problem is the lack of standardization and organization of what information to collect, which may be confusing and create delay in the diagnosis of diseases. This mostly concerns recording results in free text dictations, use of different terms for the same concepts and use of different metrics for the same values. Fortunately, and unique as compared to other medical fields, breast imaging has its own lexicon created by the American College of Radiology, the Breast Imaging Reporting and Data System (BI-RADS) [1], to facilitate the organization and standardization of information gathered. While this lexicon provides a good basis, it is not sufficient to support fully the management process of breast cancer.

Computer-based systems mitigate these problems by (1) efficiently organizing patient information, (2) preventing and eliminating errors and data inconsistencies; (3) extracting reliable statistics and non-trivial knowledge from the data, and (4) supporting clinical decision. Figure 4.1 presents a general scheme for such computerized support for the detection and diagnosis of breast cancer, where the knowledge about the parallel interpretation of two breast image views is represented once and in a consistent manner by means of a Bayesian network (probabilistic graphical model), and it is embedded into a computer-aided system for multiple use by a clinician.

In this work we assume that the data was entered correctly, is consistent, and is stored in some structured format. Our goal is to represent the "knowledge" attached to those data, which implies encoding not only primitive data (objects, attributes and their values), but also their relationships (causal, uncertain) that can convey useful information about the patient health conditions. In order to have knowledge with a good quality it is important to choose a good representation. In this chapter we will focus on logical and probabilistic knowledge representations.

4.2   The Domain of Breast Cancer

Breast cancer is a type of cancer originating from breast tissue, most commonly from the inner lining of milk ducts (ductal carcinomas) or the lobules (lobular carcinomas) that supply the ducts with milk. Any lump, abnormality, or alteration in the breast tissue's integrity that may represent a breast cancer can be designated as a *finding*.

Figure 4.2 depicts the main tasks related to the identification and management of a finding, and the common methods used to perform them. The first task is called detection, which includes the identification of a finding as a physical object and its characterization (e.g., size, shape, density, and location). This is mostly done by a physical examination (e.g., palpation either by a woman herself or by a doctor) or by means of breast cancer (usually imaging) screening. The latter is performed regularly in asymptomatic women above certain age (usually between 40–50) to detect cancer at early stages and it is currently based on mammographic examinations. Such examination involves an X-ray of each breast—a *mammogram*—which is taken while carefully compressing the breast. On a mammogram, small changes in the breast tissue can be detected, which may indicate cancer that is too small to be felt. Mammograms are usually taken in two views: (1) mediolateral oblique (MLO), taken under 45° angle and showing part of the pectoral muscles, and (2) craniocaudal (CC), taken head to toe. Two main types of mammographic findings are distinguished: microcalcifications and masses. *Microcalcifications* are tiny deposits of calcium and are associated with extra cell activity in breast tissue. Microcalcifications that are scattered throughout the mammary gland are usually a non-cancerous sign, while their occurence in clusters might indicate early stage breast cancer. According to the BI-RADS definition, "a *mass* is a space occupying lesion seen in two different projections." When visible in only one projection, it is referred as a mammographic "asymmetry". However, asymmetry may be a mass, perhaps obscured by overlying glandular tissue on the other view, and if it is characterised by enough suspicious features then it may indicate breast cancer.

Based on the detection results of a finding, the physician may or may not request additional exams, for example, fine needle aspiration (FNA) or core needle biopsy (CNB) in order to perform the second task—diagnosis. It concerns the identification of a finding either as *benign (non-cancerous)* or as *malignant (cancerous)*. In benign tumors, the cells will not invade surrounding tissues or spread to distant organs. In most

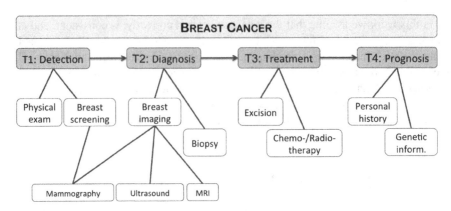

Fig. 4.2 Tasks (T#) and common methods involved in the management of breast cancer.

cases, a benign tumor can be removed. In a malignant tumor, the cells have the potential to behave aggressively, invading adjacent tissue and spreading to distant organs.

If the diagnosis is a malignant finding, the next task is to recommend and perform a treatment such as chemo-/radiotherapy or an excision surgery. Finally, the physician can study the effects of the treatment, and perform a prognostic analysis for cancer recurrence and chances for survival of the patient, by using, for example, genetic information or the patient's history.

Therefore, in this domain, we can count on information about the patient (demographics, personal history, family history, social information, and environmental exposures), about mammography images and reports, descriptors of abnormalities associated with a mamography, pathology information (details of histological analysis such as kind of breast cancer or cells associated with calcifications), and details about surgeries (kind of biopsy procedure, kind of needle, number of specimens collected etc.).

4.3   Knowledge Representation for Breast Cancer Diagnosis

4.3.1   Motivation

The information concerning the breast cancer diagnosis can come from various sources, e.g., image modalities, laboratory tests, and different medical experts, e.g., radiologists, surgeons, pathologists. As a result, we end up with heterogeneous type of information about the same patient that need to be represented and processed in a relational form as opposite to the traditional propositional approach that uses a single table to collect all information about a patient. One of the forms of representing relational data is to store it in relational databases. These databases allow only for querying the primitive (basic) data itself, and do not support queries about more

Human-defined knowledge

Probability of upgrade increases for stereotactic biopsy if the finding is microcalcifications
and biopsy results reveal atypical ductal hyperplasia (ADH).

First-order logic   Bayesian network

```
upgrade(A): IF
    biopsyResults(A,ADH) AND
    calcifications(A,a,f) AND
    biopsyProcedure(A,stereo).
```

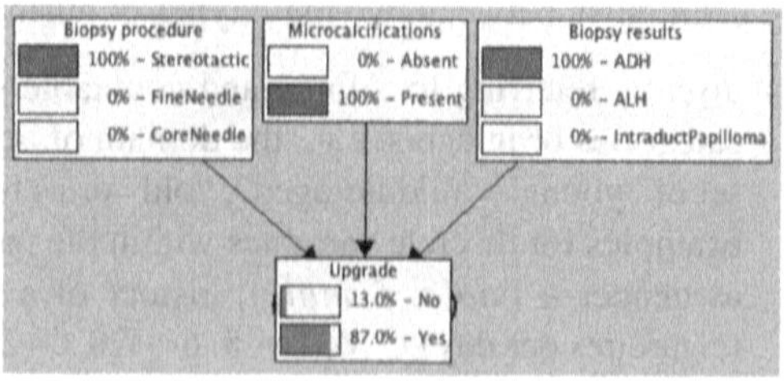

Fig. 4.3 Human-defined knowledge and its representation by FOL and a BN.

complex relationships such as "What is the relation between a malignant diagnosis
and a combination of some patient attributes", "What is the disease evolution along
the time and what is the prognosis of a given patient?", or even "What is the pattern of
a discordant biopsy (the one that gave a result that is not agreeable by all physicians
in a medical conference)?" From a clinical point of view, giving answers to these
questions means to save patients from the inconvenience of undergoing invasive procedures and save other patients of being sent home without an adequate treatment,
while reducing costs to patients and to hospitals.

To be able to answer such questions, more advanced approaches need to be used
to represent relational knowledge. In this chapter we will focus on first order logic
and graphical probabilistic models. To illustrate the basic knowledge representation
principles of these methods, Fig. 4.3 presents an example in the domain of breast cancer. In the left-hand side, we have a first order logic (FOL) definition for an upgraded
biopsy (an upgraded biopsy is the one that gave a negative result for malignancy, but
proved to be malignant after recommended surgery). In the right-hand side we have a
graphical probabilistic representation in the form of a Bayesian network (BN). Both
representations make use of the attributes A related to an object $Biopsy$ to build
a relation among attributes. The first-order logic relates atypical ductal hyperplasia (ADH), microcalcifications (amorphous and fine-linear), and biopsy procedure
to infer cases when the biopsy is an upgrade. The same information is represented
in the Bayesian network, but in another format and uses additional probabilistic
information.

To design a knowledge representation system, we need to identify the types of
knowledge that exists in the domain of interest—the diagnosis of breast cancer. We
distinguish between two categories of knowledge: (i) knowledge about primitive data,
which are objects and attributes and (ii) knowledge about relationships between the
primitive data.

4.3.2 Object-Attribute Knowledge

Table 4.1 presents examples of physical objects O relevant for our domain of interest, their attributes (features) A with the respective range of values $dom(A)$.

We distinguish between two main types of attribute domains:

(i) *discrete* referring to a finite and countable set of values. It can be defined by categories or integers, e.g., the domain of age can be defined as the categorical set of "young", "middle-aged", "old" or as the integer set $\{1, \ldots, 120\}$. Typical examples for discrete variables within the medical domain are risk factors such as gender $\in \{male, female\}$, history of a disease $\in \{no, yes\}$, and smoking (cigarettes per day) $\in \{0, 1-5, 6-20, >20\}$.

(ii) *continuous* referring to an infinite set of values between two points. Thus the domain is real-valued and values follow a distribution, e.g., Gaussian or Gamma. Typical examples of continuous attributes are the image features extracted by a computer-aided system or the size of a finding. From a knowledge representation point of view, continuous attributes are often *discretized*, i.e., their range is divided into a finite set of values that may or may not have a semantical meaning, but allow for an easier interpretation for human experts. For example, the size of a finding can be discretized into $\{<1\,cm, 1–3\,cm, >3\,cm\}$ or $\{small, medium, large\}$. A recent work on discretization of mammographic features has shown the advantages of this data pre-processing method for improving the detection performance of a CAD system [8].

More than one value can be assigned to some of the variables in breast cancer. For example, both values "fine" and "linear" can be assigned to the calcifications variable, or more than one pathology may be associated with a tumour. In that case, physicians may use a precedence list that indicates orders like Fine > Linear > ...

Table 4.1 Examples of objects, attributes, and their values in the domain of breast cancer

Object O	Attribute $A \in dom(A)$
Patient	age $\in$ {"young", "middle-aged", "old"}
	gender $\in$ {"male","female"}
Exam	time $\in$ {"prior", "current"}
	type $\in$ {"physical", "screening"}
Image	quality $\in$ {"low", "medium", "high"}
	modality $\in$ {"MRI", "mammography", "CT"}
	breast-view $\in$ {"MLO", "CC"}
Finding	location-in-breast (quadrant) $\in$ {"upper-outer", "upper-inner", ...}
	location (side) $\in$ {"left", "right"}
Mass	shape $\in$ {"oval", "round", "irregular"}
	margin $\in$ {"circumscribed", "indistinct", "spiculated"}

or ALH < LCIS < ADH < DCIS. This information can be used to give preferences to certain attribute values ranking their relevance.

Coding medical object-attribute knowledge is straightforward once there is an established convention for naming variables and terms, such as the BI-RADS lexicon for mammographic features and findings. For example, the shape (attribute) of a mass (object) using first-order logic (FOL) can be represented by the two-valued predicate $massShape(F, Value)$, where F is a variable referring to a mass object and $Value$ is a variable referring to one of the attribute values (see Table 4.1). In terms of probabilistic graphical models, such as Bayesian networks (BNs), the same knowledge is to be represented by a node called "massShape" whose domain will contain the three exclusive values describing shape.

Another way of coding the same attribute "massShape" is to use a boolean representation where a new attribute is created for each possible value of the original "massShape". Therefore, if "massShape" could assume values "oval," "round," or "irregular," the new representation would be done through three new variables, say, "massShapeOval," "massShapeRound," and "massShapeIrregular" with boolean values (for example, value 1 indicating presence and value 0 indicating absence). This kind of representation can be very useful when one attribute can assume several possible values or if the data is to be used for classification, as some classifiers work better with binary feature vectors. It is also helpful to improve the quality of data as each possible value of the variable will be properly discriminated. For example, assume the variable we have is "massShape." If this variable is left blank for any reason, we can not conclude anything about "oval," "round," or "irregular." On the other hand, if we represent this same variable by three new variables, chances are that at least one of them will not be left blank.

4.3.3   Relational Knowledge

Relational representations can be conceptualised as a binding between a relation symbol and a set of ordered tuples of elements. For example, the relation-symbol *larger* is bound to the set of ordered pairs: {(5, 2), (3, 1)...}. The symbol represents the "intension" of a relation and specifies which relation is intended; for example, elements are ordered by size. The ordered tuples represent the "extension" of a relation. They can include knowledge learned by experience, and can provide statistical knowledge of the world [4].

4.3.3.1   Causality

While object-attribute relationships are relatively straightforward to represent given a standardized naming, the relationships between the objects in the domain of interest may be more complex to formally express. One type of relationship concerns

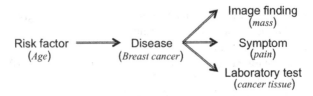

Fig. 4.4 Example of causal dependencies

causal dependencies. A typical example of such dependencies in a medical domain, including the breast cancer diagnosis, is presented in Fig. 4.4:

The concept on the left-hand side of each arc represents the cause whereas the concept on the right-hand side is the effect. While these causal arcs reflect the direction of influence, they do not necessarily express a deterministic dependence. In other words, the presence of a risk factor (elderly woman) increases the *chance* that a disease (breast cancer) may occur, but it does not imply that it will occur for sure. The same holds for the presence of a disease and its appearance on an image— breast cancer may or may not appear as a mammographic mass, for example. Clearly such relationships are inherent with uncertainty and they can be represented by probabilistic approaches such as Bayesian networks, where the network structure reflects exactly the direction of causality, and the probability distributions represent its strength. Certain causal relationships such as "Disease" ⟶ "Laboratory tests" may be more probable and even in some cases deterministic, as in the example shown in Fig. 4.4, which can be expressed by the FOL rules.

Another type of relational knowledge that is more challenging to represent, especially in image interpretation, concerns aggregations such as the "part-whole" relations. A common assumption in this case is that given evidence about parts, the goal is to hypothesise and try to draw conclusions about the whole. In particular, evidence for certain characteristics in one or more parts increases the likelihood that the same characteristics are present in the whole. This type of relationship is illustrated in Fig. 4.5 where various levels of object image analysis are given, namely an image is "part-of" an exam, and the exam is "part-of" a patient case. Detecting cancer on the image will imply that the respective exam and patient case are also assigned a label of "cancerous". The problem of this type of reasoning is, however, that the errors in the low(part)-level image analysis will be propagated to the higher(whole)-level analysis. An alternative is to represent and reason about additional knowledge such as spatial, temporal, and hierarchical relationships to better analyse the part-whole dependencies.

4.3.3.2 Spatial Knowledge

Another key knowledge used in breast cancer diagnosis on medical images are spatial relationships that indicate the context dependency to the objects locations. There are two general forms of spatial knowledge: (i) absolute position of the objects on the

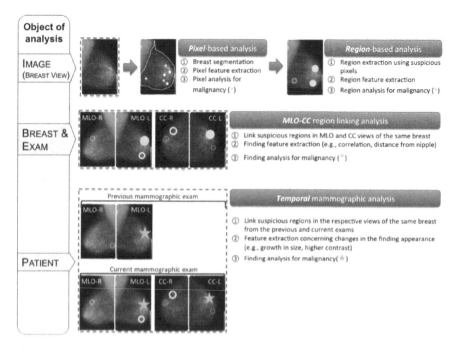

Fig. 4.5 Various levels of object image analysis by computer-aided detection systems.

image, usually in XY-coordinate system for 2D images, and (ii) relative positions of the objects to each other.

The first type of spatial knowledge in image interpretation for breast cancer diagnosis is relatively straightforward to represent. Let us consider a finding detected by a CAD system or a human reader in the MLO view of the left breast. The location of this finding will be represented by a node for each coordinate, e.g., "LocX-MLO" in BNs, and by a binary predicate, e.g., $locX\_MLO(F, Value)$ in FOL with F referring to the finding and $Value$ to the X-location value. Depending on the available data, the range of values that location can take will be (i) continuous: obtained from the automated processing of the MLO image or (ii) discrete: based on a manual annotation (e.g., breast quadrant) or discretization of the continuous values.

The relation of objects in terms of space requires a more complex, and not necessary unique, representation. In mammographic analysis, it is well-known that two regions of interest (or findings) on MLO and CC views of the same breast that are approximately at the same distance from the nipple and exhibit similar features (e.g., mass shape is the same) are *very likely* to refer to one finding. In FOL, this knowledge concerning the findings F_1 and F_2 can be expressed as follows:

Fig. 4.6 A BN representing the linking between two findings on the MLO and CC views of the same breast. The grey circles represent the observed features of the findings on both views.

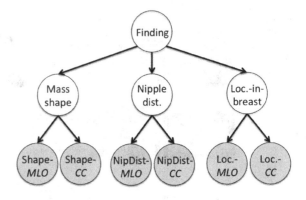

$$same\_finding(F_1, F_2) \longleftarrow MLOView(F_1) \wedge CCView(F_2) \wedge$$
$$nipple\_distance(F_1, D_1) \wedge nipple\_distance(F_2, D_2) \wedge$$
$$(abs(D_1 - D_2) < \epsilon) \wedge$$
$$side(F_1, left) \wedge side(F_2, left) \wedge$$
$$quadrant(F_1, upper\_outer) \wedge quadrant(F_2, upper\_outer) \wedge$$
$$massShape(F_1, oval) \wedge massShape(F_2, oval).$$

The problem with the representation above is that it is deterministic and it does not reflect a likelihood that F_1 and F_2 are the same finding. To do so, we can use a BN with probabilistic information as shown in Fig. 4.6.

The lowest network level captures the observed features O_i of an image finding on each breast view, modeled as effects of the unobserved finding features X_j (white circles). The top level node corresponds to finding F with values "no", "benign," and "malignant". The conditional probability tables $P(O_i|X_j)$ and $P(X_j|F)$ can be obtained based on expert knowledge or statistics derived from image data. These can be expressed as qualitative or quantitative constraints as shown in Table 4.2.

Table 4.2 Probabilistic qualitative constraints and quantities

Probabilistic qualitative constraints
$P(MassShape =' oval'|Finding =' benign') >$
$P(MassShape =' oval'|Finding =' malignant') >$
$P(MassShape =' oval'|Finding =' no')$
$P(nipple\_distance =' 0 - 2cm'|Finding =' benign') >$
$P(nipple\_distance =' 0 - 2cm'|Finding =' malignant')$
Probabilities
$P(MassShape =' oval'|Finding =' benign') = 0.73$
$P(nipple\_distance =' 0 - 2cm'|Finding =' malignant') = 0.24$

4.3.3.3 Temporal Knowledge

Temporal knowledge implies a dependence to time and may lead to different inferences in different temporal contexts. In medical domain, including breast cancer diagnosis, modelling and reasoning about such knowledge is of particular importance due to a progressive nature of a disease. In breast screening programs, for example, it is typical that images of the same breast are taken over regular intervals of time. Detecting interesting changes amounts to recognising corresponding objects, if present, in these images.

We used the examples of mammographic patient data from Table 4.3 to illustrate knowledge representation principles of temporal knowledge using graphical models and logic. Table 4.3 contains observational data such as the column "Calc F/L" reporting if a radiologist saw fine or linear calcifications in the mammogram image, and the column "Location" reporting the quadrant in the breast image related to the finding.

Table 4.3 includes two interesting relations for patient P1, who has three mammographic exams. The first and the second exams seem to reveal the same finding, given the common location in the breast, and observed at different periods of time (5/02 and 5/04). This finding refers to a tumor that appears on the mammogram as a mass that has grown in size in the second examination and as newly observed microcalcifications—clearly signs for malignancy. At the same time, another tumor was found in patient P1 during the examination made in 5/04, which appears to be benign.

In terms of probabilistic graphical models, a common representation method of temporal knowledge are *dynamic Bayesian networks*—temporal models where the same variables of interest, describing both the state of the system, observables, conditions, and actions that may change the state at different points of time [6]. A usual assumption underlying these models is that: (i) the future state is conditionally independent of the past state given the present state (first-order Markov property), and (ii) the probabilistic temporal relations between adjacent states do not change over time (time invariance or stationarity condition). This way, a dynamic Bayesian network becomes a compact process representation that can be employed in forecasting.

Figure 4.7 presents a dynamic Bayesian network in the context of patient data shown in Table 4.3. We have two time slices representing, for example, mammographic exams taken over two years. Within each slice static causal relationships are represented by solid arcs whereas the temporal relationship between both slices is represented by the dashed line. The former expresses, for example, that the

Table 4.3 Examples with mammographic patient data

Patient	Month/Year	Finding	Calc F/L	Mass size	Location	Diagnosis
P1	5/02	1	No	0.03	RU4	Benign
P1	5/04	2	Yes	0.05	RU4	Malignant
P1	5/04	3	No	0.04	LL3	Benign
P2	6/00	4	No	0.02	RL2	Benign

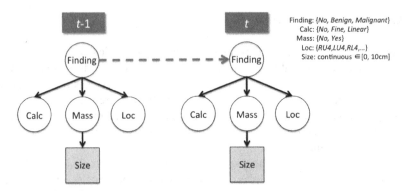

Fig. 4.7 A structure of a dynamic Bayesian network representing the relations in Table 4.3. The dashed arc represents a temporal relationship *between* two time slices whereas the solid arcs represent static relationships *within* a time slice.

presence of *Finding* is a causal factor for the presence of calcifications or a mass as well as for a location characteristic. Furthermore, *Mass* has a probabilistic influence on the distribution of the size attribute, which can be expressed, for example, as $P(Size|Mass = yes) = \mathcal{N}(0.03, 0.001)$, with $\mathcal{N}$ denoting a normal distribution with a respective mean and standard deviation. A temporal relationship in the network expresses the fact that a finding detected in a previous time slice $t - 1$ increases the probability for a finding in the current time slice t, which is expressed by the conditional probability distribution $P(Finding_t|Finding_{t-1})$, e.g., $P(Finding_t = benign|Finding_{t-1} = benign) = 0.42$, and $P(Finding_t = malignant|Finding_{t-1} = benign) = 0.25$.

The relations in Table 4.3 can also be easily represented in logic as shown below, where names such as "previous_finding," "mammo," and "date" are regular first order logic predicates and P, F_1, F_2 are logical variables.

$$previous\_finding(F_1, F_2) \longleftarrow mammo(P, F_1) \wedge mammo(P, F_2) \wedge$$
$$date(F_1, D_1) \wedge date(F_2, D_2) \wedge$$
$$(D_1 < D_2 \vee D_2 < D_1)$$

This rule relates two findings F_1 and F_2 for the same patient P, separated in time (date of F_1 is before or after the date of F_2). It can be further used to simulate temporal reasoning in the context of other rules such as:

$$is\_malignant(A) \longleftarrow mass(A, present) \wedge previous\_finding(A, B) \wedge$$
$$\left(massSize(A) < massSize(B)\right) \wedge calc(B, present) \wedge$$
$$previous\_finding(A, C) \wedge calcFineLinear(C, yes)$$

In this rule, we have explicit relations among different rows of Table 4.3 with the use of the predicate *previous_finding* which relates finding A with finding B, each one having its own properties. This rule also relates finding A with a third finding C (not shown in Table 4.3), which has calcification fine-linear.

4.3.3.4 Hierarchies and Concept Aggregation

Up to now we discussed ways for representing mostly low-level image interpretation information, which concerns findings, manual annotations, and their features. Although this forms the basic step for automated decision-support in breast cancer diagnosis, the ultimate goal is that computerized systems should be able to analyze data and provide feedback at a patient level. In particular, as physicians are capable of simultaneous interpretation of various contexts (e.g., spatial and temporal), multiple types of findings (e.g., masses, calcifications, distortions) and modalities (e.g., X-ray, MRI, ultrasound), the systems should represent and reason with various sources and levels of information and knowledge. A useful representation scheme for systematic structuring of such variety of complex relationships and facilitating physician's reasoning is a *concept hierarchy*, where knowledge and information sources are integrated both horizontally and vertically. Such a hierarchical structure in the domain of breast cancer image diagnosis is presented in Fig. 4.8.

The horizontal integration refers to combining various sources at the same level of processing, where each source supports part of an entire task. A typical example in the context of breast cancer image diagnosis is a parallel interpretation of multiple mammographic signs, such as microcalcifications $MCAL$ and masses $MASS$, to provide a complete picture whether or not breast cancer BC (i.e., a malignant finding)

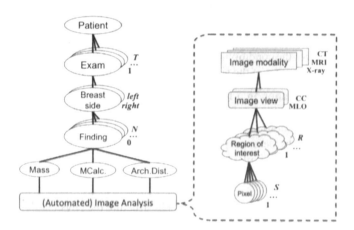

Fig. 4.8 A hierarchical structure of concepts used in breast cancer diagnosis. The left structure presents the semantical concepts as used by physicians whereas the right structure presents the top-down layers in image analysis.

Table 4.4 Aggregated concepts in establishing the risk for breast cancer with a respective example for a representation in FOL

Concepts	Example representation in FOL
Proximity	$highRisk(F) \longleftarrow calcifications(F, yes) \wedge location(F, X) \wedge$ $location\_calcifications(F, Y) \wedge distance(X, Y, E) \wedge E < Error$
Quantity	$lowRisk(F) \longleftarrow numberOfFoci(F, N) \wedge N = 1$
Similarity	$lowRisk(F) \longleftarrow previous\_finding(F, BF) \wedge date(BF, D1) \wedge$ $date(F, D2) \wedge D1 < D2 \wedge pathology(BF, benign), similar(F, BF)$
Timing	$lowRisk(F) \longleftarrow previous\_finding(F, BF) \wedge date(BF, D1) \wedge$ $date(F, D2) \wedge D1 < D2 \wedge pathology(BF, benign)$
Association	$highRisk(F) \vee excise(F) \longleftarrow calcifications(F, yes)$
Priority	$incidental(P) \longleftarrow pathologyPriority(P, low) \wedge pathologyType(P', ARS')$

is present. In terms of probabilistic graphical models, this integration can be expressed in two ways depending on available knowledge and data:

- $MCAL \longleftarrow BC \longrightarrow MASS$: This *descriptive* representation expresses the causal knowledge that microcalcifications and masses are signs (effects) of the disease "breast cancer" (cause) and given that the disease is present then it is expected to appear as a mammographic sign. The uncertainty in this appearance (e.g., obscurity in the image due to high breast density) is provided by the conditional probability tables of $MCAL$ and $MASS$ based on domain knowledge, e.g., $P(MCAL =' malignant'|BC =' present') = 0.86$ and $P(MASS =' malignant'|BC = 'present') = 0.93$. Once a sign is observed, the probability $P(BC|MCAL, MASS)$ can be computed using the Bayes theorem.

- $MCAL \longrightarrow BC \longleftarrow MACC$: This *discriminative* representation aims at predicting the probability for breast cancer given the mammographic observations. When sufficient data from image processing or human annotation reports are available, one can learn the conditional probabilities $P(BC|MCAL, MASS)$, expressing the combined effect of the signs in breast cancer dignosis.

The vertical integration in a hierarchy, on the other hand, is a knowledge representation at different levels of abstraction. An example in the current context is the parallel interpretation of multiple two-dimensional breast projections, such as MLO and CC, to provide a complete picture whether or not a finding is present in the breast B as a whole. Similarly to the horizontal integration, the vertical knowledge representation can be expressed in various forms based on domain knowledge or available data.

Abstract concepts can be represented to help structure the physician's reasoning. Table 4.4 presents a number of typical concepts in establishing the risk for breast cancer.

4.3.4   Observations and Hypotheses

From a knowledge representation point of view, we distinguish between observations and hypotheses. *Observations* are factual information obtained by means of a visual (physical) inspection, reporting, tests, or computer processing. Typical examples include risk factors (age, medical history), image features (location and shape of a finding), image findings (mass, microcalcifications), symptoms (pain, palpable mass) or laboratory results (breast biopsy).

A *hypothesis* is a possible explanation for the phenomenon we observe and it is often related to a variable of interest (output). Examples include the diagnosis of a disease (e.g., breast cancer) or determining the state of organ functioning (e.g., renal dysfunction). In the knowledge representation process, hypotheses may be included as separate entities that establish dependencies between the observations. In this case, we refer to hypotheses as "hidden variables".

Despite this hard distinction between observed and hidden variables, in practice a variable can play the role of both, depending on available information or the problem at hand. For example, in certain situations, an image finding of mass may be reported by a human reader and be used as evidence for determining whether or not breast cancer is present, whereas in another situation the goal might be to predict whether mass is present given a number of observed image features.

4.4   Inference and Decision-Making in the Management of Breast Cancer

4.4.1   Deductive Inference

A deductive system uses the data combined with pre-defined rules to draw conclusions and to support the decision-making process. For example, after the first screening, a medical doctor can lookup the guideline on Breast Screening and Diagnosis produced by the National Comprehensive Cancer Center (NCCN)[1], to assist his/her the decision-making. With the guideline, depending on the symptoms found during a screening, the physician can follow different paths suggesting a possible follow-up to a patient. A guideline implements a limited form of deduction, where, given some knowledge about a patient, the physician infers a decision based on the paths followed in that guideline. This inference of deduction can be done automatically if we use formal languages such as mathematical logic that, for example, uses complete and sound proof procedures such as resolution [9]. In fact, there are several works in the literature that represent guidelines (or parts of) by means of logics [10, 13]. The knowledge represented in Sect. 4.3, using the logic formalism, can be used to automatically answer questions such as "what are the findings that are malignant?"

---

[1] http://www.nccn.org/professionals/physician_gls/pdf/breast.pdf, available after registration.

(in logic: $\exists\, F malignant\,(F)$) or "Is there a benign finding with a high mass density?"
(in logic: $\exists\, F\; pathologyType(F, benign) \wedge massDensity(F, high)$), using resolution.

4.4.2 Inductive Inference

Inductive systems, on the other hand, support the decision-making by automating
the process of creating models based on available data or expert knowledge. Systems
that fall in this category are usually called machine learning systems. In the case of
creating rules, a machine learning algorithm can automatically produce a guideline
as defined by NCCN or the rule presented in Fig. 4.9, or even complement a guideline
with a newly created rule.

The example rule shown in Fig. 4.9, written with the Prolog syntax, was automatically extracted from a database containing more than 65,000 patients. This rule
suggests that a set of patients may have had a delayed treatment, because they had
obtained a BI-RADS category of 3 (low-risk benign, b3) in past exams, which later
became 5 (high-risk malignant, b5) [2]. In fact, this rule was validated against the
dataset, and this condition held true for seven positive patients and for none of the
negative ones with benign findings.

Inductive learning with logic is very useful to extract readable and interpretable
models from the data. Rather than producing a black-box classifier, logical rules
can explain the classifier itself to the physician. This can further contribute to the
refinement of the expert knowledge in a way that the inductive system learns rules,
the physician can modify or refine them, then the system learns new rules from the
refinements and the process continues.

One good side-effect of inductive learning is that the rules found during this
interactive process can shed some light on the most relevant primitive features that

Human-defined knowledge

If finding A was classified as BI-RADS 5, had a mass present in a patient who was between the
ages of 65 and 70, had two prior mammograms B and C, and prior mammogram B had no mass
shape described, had no punctate calcifications, and prior mammogram C was classified as BI-
RADS 3 then finding A is malignant.

Prolog-based rule

```
is_malignant(A):-
    birads_category(A,b5), massPAO(A,present), age(A,age6570),
    previous_finding(A,B,C), massesShape(B,none),
    calc_Punctate(B,notPresent),
    previous_finding(A,C), birads_category(C,b3).
```

Fig. 4.9 An example of knowledge representation using a Prolog rule.

can suggest a diagnosis. For example, some of the features may consistently appear in every learning step. The health professionals can then concentrate on studying these features and even improving the quality of the data values entered for these features by enforcing better data collection.

4.4.3 Application

In this section we demonstrate the application of knowledge representation formalism for mammographic diagnosis. We show two different formalisms. One is based on a probabilistic graphical model and the second one is based on first order logic. In the first one, features are automatically extracted from image processing. In the second one, features come from multiple tables generated by annotations performed by doctors when preparing medical reports about mammography, pathology analysis and biopsy procedures.

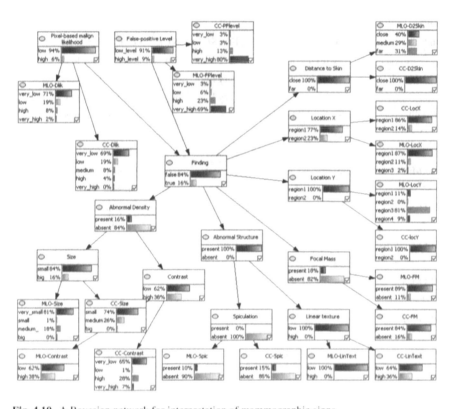

Fig. 4.10 A Bayesian network for interpretation of mammographic signs

4.4.3.1   Probabilistic Graphical Model

Figure 4.10 presents a Bayesian network model whose structure was manually built using domain knowledge and its parameters were learnt from real-world mammographic data. The model aims at detecting a malignant finding on a mammogram based on image features automatically extracted from a CAD system and following the two-view image interpretation as done by radiologists. For a more detailed description of the model, the reader is referred to [8, 12].

Table 4.5 presents the data for three real-world cases obtained from the Dutch mammographic screening program, which contains a number of automatically extracted regions of interest and their respective features on a breast view (image). The ground-truth of each region is provided by pathology reports. The last row in

Table 4.5 A sample of three real-world cases with mammographic regions of interest (ROI) and respective features extracted from a CAD system. Variable Finding is the ground-truth.

Cases (C#)	C1 (right breast)		C2 (left breast)		C3 (right breast)	
ROI#	ROI1	ROI2	ROI1	ROI2	ROI1	ROI2
Finding	FALSE	TRUE	FALSE	TRUE	FALSE	TRUE
MLO-FPlevel	very high	low	very high	high	very high	low
CC-FPlevel	very high	very low	very high	very low	very high	very low
MLO-Dlik	very low	high	very low	very low	very low	low
CC-Dlik	very low	low	very low	high	very low	medium
MLO-Spic	present	present	present	present	absent	absent
CC-Spic	absent	present	present	present	absent	absent
MLO-FM	present	absent	present	present	present	present
CC-FM	present	absent	present	present	present	present
MLO-Size	very small	very small	medium	medium	very small	very small
CC-Size	small	small	small	medium	small	small
MLO-Contrast	low	low	low	low	low	low
CC-Contrast	very low	very low	very low	high	very low	very low
MLO-LinText	low	low	low	low	low	low
CC-LinText	low	low	low	low	low	low
MLO-D2Skin	far	medium	close	medium	medium	medium
CC-D2Skin	close	close	close	close	close	close
MLO-LocX	region1	region1	region1	region1	region1	region1
CC-LocX	region2	region1	region1	region1	region1	region1
MLO-LocY	region3	region3	region4	region3	region1	region3
CC-LocY	region1	region1	region1	region1	region1	region1
$P(Finding = T)$	**0.07**	**0.89**	**0.11**	**0.77**	**0.11**	**0.62**

Table 4.5 shows the Bayesian network (shown in Fig. 4.10) computed probability that a malignant finding is present, given the features in each view.

4.4.3.2 First Order Logic (FOL)

Another example using a logic representation is shown in Fig. 4.11, where each of the rules, automatically learned from data, is true for 30 out of 79 benign findings (with 40 % Recall) while not missing any malignant finding out of 17 (with 100 % precision). In other words, when these rules are used to classify new cases, a true malignant case is never missed and mistakenly sent home. On the other hand, some benign cases will may be misclassified, but not all. The dataset used to train the rules consists of non-definitive biopsies collected from the Medical School of the University of Wisconsin-Madison, USA. The relevance of this result is that the classifier is

$benign(F) \longleftarrow$	
$patientID(F,P) \wedge previousSurgery(P, ps\_no) \wedge$	The patient did not have a previous surgery, imag-
$marginSpiculated(F,no) \wedge$	ing did not present a spiculated mass margin, the
$disappearanceAbn(F,'N')$	abnormality remained in post-biopsy imaging
$benign(F) \longleftarrow$	
$biopsyAbn(F,Abn) \wedge$	Imaging did not present an indistinct mass margin,
$marginIndistinct(Abn, not\_present) \wedge$	imaging did not present a spiculated mass margin,
$marginSpiculated(Abn, not\_present) \wedge$	the abnormality remained in post-biopsy imaging
$disappearanceAbn(F,'N')$	

Fig. 4.11 FOL rules

abnID(bio53,abn24).	abnID(bio76,abn94).
patientID(bio53,patient771964).	patientID(bio76,patient60244).
biopsyDate(bio53,667).	biopsyDate(bio76,747).
age(bio53,68).	age(bio76,63).
biopsySide(bio53,'R').	biopsySide(bio76,'L').
biopsyProcedure(bio53,'UsCore').	biopsyProcedure(bio76,'MriCore').
needleType(bio53,'vacuum-assisted').	needleType(bio76,'vacuum-assisted').
needleGauge(bio53,9).	needleGauge(bio76,9).
samplesNum(bio53,6).	samplesNum(bio76,10).
clipInSiteBX(bio53,0).	clipInSiteBX(bio76,0).
disappearanceAbn(bio53,'Y').	disappearanceAbn(bio76,'N').
outcome(bio53,'Y').	outcome(bio76,'N').
familyHistory(patient771964,fh_none).	familyHistory(patient60244,fh_none).
personalHistory(patient771964,ph_no).	personalHistory(patient60244,ph_yes).
previousSurgery(patient771964,ps_yes).	previousSurgery(patient60244,ps_no).
patientID(bio53,patient771964).	patientID(bio76,patient60244).
marginIndistinct(abn24,not_present).	marginIndistinct(abn94,not_present).
marginMicrolobulated(abn24,not_present).	marginMicrolobulated(abn94,not_present).
marginCircumscribed'(abn24,not_present).	marginCircumscribed'(abn94,not_present).
marginSpiculated(abn24,not_present).	marginSpiculated(abn94,not_present).
marginObscure(abn24,not_present).	marginObscure(abn94,not_present).

Fig. 4.12 Instances represented in FOL

capable of sparing some women from excision while not missing any malignant finding. Currently, when biopsies are inconclusive (non-definitive), the common practice is to excise all women in this situation.

In order for that to work, data instances need also to be represented in FOL. Two examples are shown in Fig. 4.12. These instances are coded from medical mammography reports, and include extra information about the biopsy procedures and about the patient data. They also use the BI-RADS encoding. Applying the rules from Fig. 4.11 to the two instances, classifies correctly the left instance as malignant and the right instance as benign. We only show partial data for the instances, since the rules only describe mass margins (mammographic finding), biopsy features and patient data.

4.5   Discussion and Conclusion

We outlined various types of knowledge available in the domain of image interpretation of breast cancer diagnosis and their representation using two main formalisms from the field of artificial intelligence—Bayesian networks (BNs) and first-order logic (FOL). While both formalisms are capable of explicitly expressing domain knowledge, for example, in terms of causal, spatial and temporal relations, they differ in the form of this expression.

The power of Bayesian networks lies in their capabilities to deal in a probabilistic manner with uncertainty, which is often encountered in medical image intepretation due to, for example, image quality or resemblance in the image appearance between abnormalities and normal body structures. In the current context, we demonstrated how Bayesian networks can be used to model multi-view image interpretation by using a hierachical representation following the human expert's working principles.

As a propositional method, however, Bayesian networks are restricted in the representation of a dynamic number of objects and relationships, which is naturally done by FOL. In the context of breast cancer diagnosis based on medical images, we showed how the latter can be applied in formalizing expert knowledge in a compact manner.

Recent advances in medical imaging have led to a variety of modalities such as MRI, tomosynthesis, and ultrasound, to augment the current tools (primarily mammography) for breast cancer screening. The integrated interpretation of these modalities at a patient level imposes even more challenges for human readers and new modelling techniques are needed to handle both uncertainty and dynamics in findings. Probabilistic logics—the merge of probability theory and logic—is a promising direction for future research in this application domain.

References

1. D'Orsi, C.J., Bassett, L.W., Berg, W.A., et al.: BI-RADS: Mammography, 4th edn. American College of Radiology Inc., Reston (2003)
2. Davis, J., et al.: Knowledge discovery from structured mammography reports using inductive logic programming. In: 2005 Annual Symposium American Medical Informatics Association, pp. 86–100 (2005)
3. Fenton, J.J., et al.: Influence of computer-aided detection on performance of screening mammography. N. Engl. J. Med. **356**(14), 1399–1409 (2007). PMID: 17409321, http://wwwnejm.org/doi/pdf/10.1056/NEJMoa066099
4. Halford, G.S., Wilson, W.H., Phillips, S.: Relational knowledge: the foundation of higher cognition. Trends Cogn. Sci. **14**(11), 497–505 (2010). doi:10.1016/j.tics.2010.08.005
5. Horsch, K., et al.: Classification of breast lesions with multimodality computer-aided diagnosis: observer study results on an independent clinical data set. Radiology **240**(2), 357–368 (2006). doi:10.1148/radiol.2401050208. PMID: 16864666
6. Murphy, K.P.: Dynamic Bayesian networks: representation, inference and learning. PhD thesis, UC Berkeley (July 2002)
7. Pisano, E.D., et al.: Diagnostic performance of digital versus film mammography for breast-cancer screening. N. Engl. J. Med. **353**(17), 1773–1783 (2005). PMID: 16169887, http://wwwnejm.org/doi/pdf/10.1056/NEJMoa052911
8. Robben, S., et al.: Discretisation does affect the performance of Bayesian networks. In: Bramer, M., Petridis, M., Hopgood, A. (eds.) Research and Development in Intelligent Systems XXVII, pp. 237–250. Springer, London (2011)
9. Robinson, J.A.: A machine-oriented logic based on the resolution principle. J. ACM **12**(1), 23–41 (1965)
10. Shiffman, R.N., Greenes, R.A.: Improving clinical guidelines with logic and decision-table techniques: application to hepatitis immunization recommendations. Med. Decis. Making **14**(3), 245–254 (1994)
11. Skaane, P., et al.: Comparison of digital mammography alone and digital mammography plus tomosynthesis in a population-based screening program. Radiology **267**(1), 47–56 (2013)
12. Velikova, M., et al.: On the interplay of machine learning and background knowledge in image interpretation by Bayesian networks. Artif. Intell. Med. **57**(1), 73–86 (2013)
13. Wilk, S., et al.: Clinical practice guidelines and comorbid diseases: a MiniZinc representation of guideline models for mitigating adverse interactions. Stud. Health Technol. Inform. **192**, 352–356 (2013)

Monitoring of Health and Disease and Conformance

Chapter 5
Monitoring in the Healthcare Setting

Federico Chesani, Catherine G. Enright, Marco Montali,
and Michael G. Madden

5.1 Introduction

Monitoring is an activity in which a running system is observed, so as to become aware of its state. The fact that the system is *observed* makes monitoring complementary to approaches like formal verification and validation, which are tailored to assess the quality and trustworthiness of the system before the execution. While verification/validation works on a model of the system, as discussed in Chap. 19 monitoring observes real system executions. The fact that the system is typically observed while *running* makes monitoring complementary to approaches like data/process mining, which are applied post-mortem, i.e., on historical, logged information.

Typically, monitoring does not only work solely on a *stream of data* representing the evolving trace of an *actual* system behavior, but also considers a *model* capturing the *expected* system behavior. In this light, monitoring is concerned with continuously contrasting the actual and expected behavior, so as to correspondingly provide a meaningful feedback to the actors responsible for the system execution, not only to make them aware of its current state and of deviations with the expected state, but also to make them able to promptly react to exceptional situations. This is why it is considered to be one of the main pillars of what is termed *operational decision support* [1, 2].

5.2 Monitoring Tasks

Figure 5.1 depicts a generic monitoring framework, and the typical tasks involved. We briefly describe them.

Calibration involves adapting system parameters so that the model of expected behaviour is attuned to the individual patient being monitored, as opposed to an idealized patient. This is a key component of personalized medicine.

© Springer International Publishing Switzerland 2015

A. Hommersom and P.J.F. Lucas (eds.), *Biomedical Knowledge Representation*, LNAI 9521, DOI 10.1007/978-3-319-28007-3_5

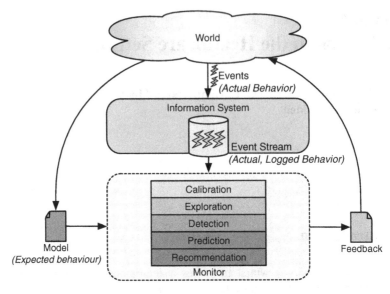

Fig. 5.1 A generic monitoring framework (inspired by [2])

Exploration deals with the proper reconstruction of the current system state (and possibly of the history) by using the events collected so far, and the model of the system. This typically includes a range of visualization techniques, tailored to provide an intuitive, end-user oriented representation of the system current state (and history).

Detection is meant to check the alignment between the actual behavior (reconstructed from the stream of events), and the expected behavior (obtained from the model). When the two behaviors are indeed aligned, we say that the actual behavior is *conformant* or *compliant* with the expected one.[1] If instead a deviation is detected, a warning is issued by the monitor, so as to make the responsible actors aware of the misalignment.

Prediction exploits the model, and typically also historical data about past executions of the system, so as to determine the likely future evolution(s) of the currently monitored behavior. When the resulting predicted behavior has undesired aspects, proper countermeasures can be taken in advance so as to properly redirect the system.

Recommendation refines prediction by automatically providing suggestions on what to do next. Obviously, the generated recommendations have to be continuously reconsidered in the light of new, incoming events.

---

[1]The latter acception is typically employed when the model of the system carries a normative meaning.

5.3   Monitoring Issues and Knowledge Representation

From Fig. 5.1, the main issues involved in a generic monitoring framework can be inferred. We briefly review such issues, highlighting in particular how they relate with Knowledge Representation. This is by no means an exhaustive discussion, and the literature lacks a proper systematization of the field (for a recent attempt along this direction, the reader can refer to [22]).

Fetching the events is the *conditio sine qua non* for monitoring. To make monitoring applicable, the information system on which the monitoring framework is applied must be able to collect (and log) the relevant events occurring in the system, so as to construct a representation of the actual system execution that is as accurate as possible. This is typically difficult for those settings, like healthcare, in which part of the work is carried out by human actors in the physical world, without a direct computerized support. While this means, in general, that the logged trace of the system is only an incomplete representation of the real one, the presence of a model of the system makes it possible to exploit automated reasoning techniques so as to (partially) reconstruct the missing information. An example of the usage of KR techniques in this respect is [5].

Represent and process the events: Orthogonally to how the events are collected by the information system, there is the issue of how these events are represented. In fact, real-worlds events are typically heterogeneous both for what concerns their attached data, and their level of abstraction. As a simple example, consider the problem of monitoring the everyday life of a patient. In this setting, an event type may refer to the measurement of a (continuous) patient's vital parameter (such as the blood pressure), whereas another event type could denote that the patient took some medicine at a given time. This heterogeneity is depicted in Fig. 5.2. How signals/sub-symbolic events, as well as abstract/high-level symbolic events, are represented and related to each other is a central, longstanding problem of KR. It is worth noting that these two types of events could be reduced to each other before being processed by the monitoring system. On the one hand, symbolic events may be *reduced* to signals (e.g., through serialization into a binary stream). On the other hand, sub-symbolic events may be analyzed by an *activity recognition* module, so as to extract symbolic events by suitably correlating subsymbolic information.

Construct and represent the model: Similar to the problem of representing and process-ing the events is the representation and exploitation of the system model. This requires identifying the relevant aspects of the system to be modeled, trying to bal-ance between expressiveness and tractability (which, as KR suggests, cannot be separated from "how" this model is used for reasoning). Since monitoring focuses on the system dynamics, a central aspect is obviously constituted by time. This motivated the extensive research on monitoring and runtime verification using variants of temporal logics (see, e.g., the *Runtime Verification* conference series[2]).

---

[2]http://runtime-verification.org/.

How events are modeled (e.g., atomic vs non-atomic events), whether time must be considered in a qualitative or quantitative fashion, which kind of data must be modeled, how to represent provenance information and event originators, are important questions for the KR community. Finally, beside how to represent the model, it is central to understand how such model is constructed. In particular, in addition to standard, top-down modeling, data/process/specification mining techniques can be exploited to semi-automatically extract model-level information from historical data about the system. An alternative approach is to transform existing models of a different type into a form amenable for use in monitoring [13, 14].

Perform online reasoning: While it is obvious that the reasoning techniques embedded by the monitoring framework depend on how events/models are represented, and on which task(s) are of interest (cf. Sect. 5.2), there are some specific key requirements that monitoring poses, no matter the application domain. First of all, since monitoring is an online, continuous activity, efficiency and *reactivity* are a must: the monitoring feedbacks must be produced in a timely fashion, and continuously revised taking into account newly incoming events. This calls, in turn, for *incremental* reasoning techniques, which exploit the previously computed results instead of recalculating everything from scratch [17]. A second specific aspect of monitoring is that it must provide *continuous support*, In particular, since the monitored system is in general not under the control of the monitor, the monitor must be able to follow the system evolution also in exceptional, unforeseen situations.

Calibrate the feedback: A final important aspect is how the monitoring outcome is represented, communicated to the actors responsible for the system execution, and possibly automatically exploited. This ranges from the extreme case in which the monitor is only able to observe the system and provide "symbolic" feedbacks to humans, to the one in which the monitor can (automatically or semi-automatically) supervise and adapt the real system depending on the monitoring outcome. An example of a system that automatically adapts to the patient is described in Chap. 7.

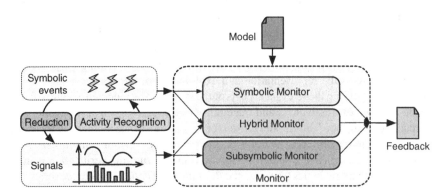

Fig. 5.2 Monitoring heterogeneous events

5.4   Monitoring in Healthcare

5.4.1   Where Monitoring Can Be Applied in Healthcare

The generic monitoring framework described in the previous section can be applied to a wide range on tasks in the healthcare setting.

- Monitoring patient signals
- Monitoring therapeutic interventions
- Monitoring disease progression
- Monitoring recovery
- Monitoring the execution of guidelines
- Monitoring alarms
- Combinations of the above

Traditionally, monitoring in the healthcare setting was carried out locally, but with the advent of telemedicine, remote patient monitoring is growing in popularity, mainly due to its convenience and effectiveness for both patients and clinicians.

It is important to emphasize that monitoring involves the observation of a system over time and reasoning with these observations. Much previous work on prediction and decision support in the healthcare sector was concerned with reasoning a particular point in time with a particular set of inputs. Examples include predicting morbidity, mortality and length of stay on admission [4, 8, 25]. The advantage of a continuous monitoring system is the monitor can learn about the individual patient and adapt to them in real-time.

5.4.2   Artificial Intelligence Techniques for Healthcare Monitoring

Artificial Intelligence techniques have been applied in the medical settings for many years. The ICU is particularly suited to the use of AI tools due to the wealth of available data and the opportunities for increased efficiencies [18]. The purpose of this section is not to present a complete history or ontology of AI applications in the ICU setting but rather to give a flavour of the variety of applications that have been proposed. The 2001 review by Hanson et al. [18] of artificial intelligence tools in the ICU provides a good overview. They conclude that neural networks and fuzzy systems are particularly useful for waveform analysis; fuzzy controllers can be integrated into bedside devices such as fluid and medication infusion devices, mechanical ventilators, and dialysis machines; Bayesian networks and neural networks can be used in the development of smart alarms; case-based reasoning, machine learning algorithms, and visualization tools can be used to analyse information from data warehouses describing the characteristic of an individual ICU.

Tools for predicting morbidity, mortality and length of stay have also been proposed. Barbini et al. [4] and Cevenini et al. [8] compared different models for predicting ICU morbidity following cardiac surgery. They found Bayesian classifiers and logistic regression models to be superior to an artificial neural network and the k-nearest neighbour classifier in terms of generalisation and calibration for this particular task. Ramon et al. [25] consider four different data mining algorithms for predicting 14 different tasks including probability of survival, length of stay in the ICU, probability of developing inflammation and the probability of developing kidney dysfunction. Their results for predicting probability of survival were better than the results obtained using the standard APACHE II score method [19] used by most ICUs. Using the APACHE II score the area under the ROC-curve (AUC) was 75 %. The best results were obtained using a Naive Bayes Classifier (AUC = 88 %). The AUC for Tree-Augmented Nave Bayesian networks was 86 % and for First Order Random Forests was 82 %. (First Order Random Forests are Random Forests in which the tests are first order logic queries [28].) Decision Trees provided the least promising results with AUC = 79 %. It is interesting to note that no one technique proved superior for all 14 tasks.

Other research includes Cismondi et al.'s fuzzy system for predicting the outcome of lab results [12], and the INTCARE system [23, 27] which combines data mining techniques and decision support systems to predict organ failure and suggest therapeutic treatment. The INTCARE research also addresses the need to distribute the application so it is available to doctors via mobile devices as well as in the ICU.

MIMIC II is a project undertaken by MIT, Philips Medical Systems and the Beth Israel Deaconess Medical Centre to develop and evaluate advanced ICU patient monitoring systems that will improve the efficiency, accuracy and timeliness of clinical decision making in intensive care. They aim to develop a research database from more than 30000 ICU patients. Their research includes estimating blood pressure and heart rate derived from the ABP waveform [20], using a Bayesian Network to estimate fluid requirements in the ICU [7], eliminating false alarms using classification trees and neural networks [29] and a decision tree to predict hypoglycaemia in intensive care patients [30].

A 2012 review by Bright et al. [6] shows the widespread interest across all medical fields in clinical decision-support systems. They examined 128 trials. From these they conclude that clinical decision support had a favourable effect on prescribing treatments, facilitating preventive care services, and ordering clinical studies across diverse venues and systems. They also stress the importance of delivering the right information to the right person in a timely manner.

5.4.3 Challenges in Healthcare Monitoring

Monitoring the physiological responses of a patient during recovery or in response to therapeutic interventions presents challenges. Substantial variability exists in the responses of different patients to medical interventions. This can be due to a variety of reasons including genetics, severity of illness and comorbidities. In addition an individual's response to events and interventions can fluctuate as their condition changes. These changes can be sudden or take place over a long time period. For a monitoring system to be truly useful it must be calibrated to the individual patient in real-time and adjust in real-time as the patient condition changes.

As mentioned in Sect. 5.4 human actors carry out events and/or manually record data in the Healthcare environment. These events may not be carried out at precisely the prescribed time, they may not be recorded in a timely manner nor with the precision that a monitoring system may require. Even automatically recorded information can be subject to measurement error. The monitoring system must be designed to deal with these uncertainties.

Healthcare is also an environment where disparate data may need to be integrated to provide the most complete picture. This is one area where monitoring systems can add huge value. A computational model can incorporate a much larger number of variables into its decision support process than a human can when making decisions unaided by a computer-based decision support system.

5.4.4 Probabilistic Monitoring Methods for Healthcare Monitoring

These challenges make healthcare monitoring particularly amenable to probabilistic approaches. Bayesian Networks (BNs) and Dynamic Bayesian Networks (DBNs) are used in the medical setting and here we note a few examples. An excellent introduction to the field is provided by Lucas et al. [21].

Aleks et al. [3] describe an application of DBNs to analysing ICU data. They demonstrated accurate detection and removal of artefacts in the arterial-line blood pressure sensor data. Charitos et al. [9] developed a DBN to successfully diagnose ventilator-associated pneumonia in ICU Patients. Research from the MIMIC II project mentioned in Sect. 5.4.2 includes applying a Kalman Filter to estimate blood pressure and heart rate derived from the ABP waveform in the presence of high levels of persistent noise and artefact [20], using a Bayesian Network to estimate fluid requirements in the ICU [7] and using a Bayesian network to model the cardiovascular system [26].

Techniques have been developed to learn both BN and DBN structure and parameters from data. More recently techniques for combining expert knowledge and automated learning for building BN structure [15, 24] have been published. However most models, including the ones noted here, are manually constructed using knowledge elicited from domain experts [11, 21]. This is a time consuming task [15, 21]. Knowledge elicitation therefore remains a bottleneck; this is clear in the paper of van Gerven et al. [16], for example, which provides an excellent demonstration of the steps required to build a DBN model for prognosis of carcinoid patients. In order to bypass this bottleneck, Enright et al. [13, 14] propose a methodology for automatically constructing DBNs from mathematical models since mathematical models can be considered to embody existing expert knowledge.

5.4.5   *Characteristics of an Effective Monitoring System*

In order for a monitoring system to be accepted and used in a healthcare setting it must be easily understood. A system that is understood by clinicians is more likely to be gain traction. This applies both to the internal workings of the monitoring system as well as the feedback provided to clinicians and patients. Feedback should be clear, concise and easily interpreted.

The monitoring system must be fully validated on realistic data. As mentioned in Sect. 5.4.3, data in healthcare is noisy. The monitoring system must therefore be designed to reason with incomplete and inaccurate data in a principled manner. It must also be thoroughly validated with this data.

The monitoring system must be suited to the task in hand. If monitoring a patient it must be individualised to that patient. That individualisation should be a continual process to adapt to ever changing patient conditions. If monitoring a process the system must be flexible to adapt to the variety of paths and outcomes.

Monitoring systems are of most value when they run in real-time. In order to achieve practical run-time speeds models must often be simplified. However a delicate balance is needed to avoid over-simplification and to preserve a practical model of the underlying system.

This trade-off between complexity and practicality also emerges when deciding what model parameters should be allowed vary. Models with a minimal number of parameters to be individualised work better when dealing with noisy-data [10].

5.5   Conclusion

We have reviewed the role of monitoring in the healthcare setting, delineating the main forms of operational support that monitoring can provide to healthcare professionals, and the main corresponding challenges from the point of view of knowledge representation.

The following two chapters in this book provide two notable, and quite diverse, examples of effective monitoring systems for healthcare, built by taking into consideration all the key characteristics enunciated in Sect. 5.4.5.

Chapter 7 describes a Probabilistic Real-time Intelligent Monitor (PRIM) that can be used for *Exploration, Detection, Prediction* and *Recommendation*. The chapter describes a methodology for *constructing and representing* the monitoring model and an efficient algorithm for *online reasoning*. The framework is designed specifically to address the challenges of the healthcare environment i.e. inaccurate and incomplete data, inter-patient variability and patient instability. The issues described in Sect. 5.3 in relation to a generic monitoring framework are addressed in a principled manner. The probabilistic approach adopted enables a reasoned method to handle incomplete data and represent events. The proposed approach for model construction involves exploiting existing models thus expediting and simplifying the model construction phase. The Adaptive Time Particle Filtering algorithm presented is an efficient mechanism for online Reasoning which in the context of this probabilistic monitoring system meets the requirements for incremental reasoning and continuous support in exceptional and unforeseen circumstances.

Chapter 5 describes a very different application of monitoring in a clinical environment. The chapter deals with monitoring conformance to clinical guidelines. The challenge explored is how to build a generic framework to *Detect* deviations. In this case *knowledge representation* is a huge challenge because, as will be explained, clinical guidelines encompass many different types of knowledge. Human actors execute clinical guidelines and it is this behaviour that is monitored. In this chapter we again see how this leads to inaccurate and incomplete data.

References

1. van der Aalst, W.M.P., et al.: Auditing 2.0: using process mining to support tomorrow's auditor. IEEE Comput. **43**(3), 90–93 (2010)
2. van der Aalst, W.M.P.: Process Mining: Discovery, Conformance and Enhancement. Springer, Heidelberg (2011)
3. Aleks, N., et al.: Probabilistic detection of short events, with application to critical care monitoring. In: Proceedings of NIPS 2008: 22nd Annual Conference on Neural Information Processing Systems. Vancouver, Canada, pp. 49–56 (2008)
4. Barbini, E., et al.: A comparative analysis of predictive models of morbidity in intensive care unit after cardiac surgery part I: model planning. BMC Med. Inf. Decis. Making **7**, 35 (2007)
5. Bertoli, P., Dragoni, M., Ghidini, C., Martufi, E., Nori, M., Pistore, M., Di Francescomarino, C.: Modeling and monitoring business process execution. In: Basu, S., Pautasso, C., Zhang, L., Fu, X. (eds.) ICSOC 2013. LNCS, vol. 8274, pp. 683–687. Springer, Heidelberg (2013)
6. Bright, T.J., et al.: Effect of clinical decision-support systems a systematic review. Ann. Intern. Med. **157**, 29–43 (2012)
7. Celi, L.A., et al.: An artificial intelligence tool to predict fluid requirement in the intensive care unit: a proof-of-concept study. Crit. Care **12**(6), R151 (2008)
8. Cevenini, G., et al.: A comparative analysis of predictive models of morbidity in intensive care unit after cardiac surgery part II: an illustrative example. BMC Med. Inform. Decis. Making **7**, 36 (2007)
9. Charitos, T., et al.: A dynamic bayesian network for diagnosing ventilator-associated pneumonia in ICU patients. Expert Syst. Appl. **36**(2), 1249–1258 (2009)
10. Chase, J.G., et al.: Physiological modeling, tight glycemic control, and the ICU clinician: what are models and how can they affect practice? Ann. Intensive Care **1**, 11 (2011)
11. Chatterjee, S., Russell, S.: Why are DBNs sparse? In: International Conference on Artificial Intelligence and Statistics, Sardinia, pp. 81–88 (2010)
12. Cismondi, F.C., et al.: Reducing ICU blood draws with artificial intelligence. Crit. Care **16**, 436 (2012)
13. Enright, C.G., Madden, M.G., Madden, N.: Bayesian networks for mathematical models: techniques for automatic construction and efficient inference. Int. J. Approximate Reasoning **54**, 323–342 (2013)
14. Enright, C.G., Madden, M.G., Madden, N., Laffey, J.G.: Clinical time series data analysis using mathematical models and DBNs. In: Peleg, M., Lavrač, N., Combi, C. (eds.) AIME 2011. LNCS, vol. 6747, pp. 159–168. Springer, Heidelberg (2011)
15. Flores, J.M., et al.: Incorporating expert knowledge when learning bayesian network structure: a medical case study. Artif. Intell. Med. **53**(3), 181–204 (2011)

16. van Gerven, M.A.J., Taal, B.G., Lucas, P.J.F.: Dynamic bayesian networks as prognostic models for clinical patient management. J. Biomed. Inform. **41**(4), 515–529 (2008)

17. Ghezzi, C.: Evolution, adaptation, and the quest for incrementality. In: Calinescu, R., Garlan, D. (eds.) Monterey Workshop 2012. LNCS, vol. 7539, pp. 369–379. Springer, Heidelberg (2012)

18. Hanson III, C.W., Marshall, B.E.: Artificial intelligence applications in the intensive care unit. Crit. Care Med. **29**, 427 (2001)

19. Knaus, W.A., et al.: APACHE II: a severity of disease classification system. Crit. Care Med. **13**, 818–829 (1985)

20. Li, Q., Mark, R.G., Clifford, G.D.: Artificial arterial blood pressure artifact models and an evaluation of a robust blood pressure and heart rate estimator. BioMed. Eng. Online **8**(1), 13 (2009)

21. Lucas, P.J.F., van der Gaag, L.C., Abu-Hanna, A.: Bayesian networks in biomedicine and health-care. Artif. Intell. Med. **30**(3), 201–214 (2004)

22. Ly, L.T., et al.: A framework for the systematic comparison and evaluation of compliance monitoring approaches. In: Gasevic, D., Hatala, M., Motahari Nezhad, H.R., Reichert, M. (eds.) Proceedings of the 17th IEEE International Enterprise Distributed Object Computing Conference (EDOC 2013), pp. 7–16. IEEE (2013)

23. Portela, F., et al.: Knowledge discovery for pervasive and real-time intelligent decision support in intensive care medicine, 2011. Fundao para a Cincia e a Tecnologia (FCT) - PTDC/EIA/72819/ 2006, SFRH/BD/70156/2010

24. Radstake, N., Lucas, P.J.F., Velikova, M., Samulski, M.: Critiquing knowledge representation in medical image interpretation using structure learning. In: Riaño, D., ten Teije, A., Miksch, S., Peleg, M. (eds.) KR4HC 2010. LNCS, vol. 6512, pp. 56–69. Springer, Heidelberg (2011)

25. Ramon, J., et al.: Mining data from intensive care patients. Adv. Eng. Inform. **21**, 243–256 (2007)

26. Roberts, J.M., et al.: Bayesian networks for cardiovascular monitoring. In: Annual International Conference of the IEEE Engineering in Medicine and Biology Society, pp. 205–209. IEEE Engineering in Medicine and Biology Society (2006)

27. Santos, M.F., Portela, F., Vilas-Boas, M.: INTCARE: multi-agent approach for real-time intelligent decision support in intensive medicine. Fundao para a Cincia e a Tecnologia (FCT) (2011)

28. Vens, C., Van Assche, A., Blockeel, H., Džeroski, S.: First order random forests with complex aggregates. In: Camacho, R., King, R., Srinivasan, A. (eds.) ILP 2004. LNCS (LNAI), vol. 3194, pp. 323–340. Springer, Heidelberg (2004)

29. Zhang, Y., Szolovits, P.: Patient-specific learning in real time for adaptive monitoring in critical care. J. Biomed. Inform. **41**(3), 452–460 (2008)

30. Zhang, Y.: Predicting occurrences of acute hypoglycemia during insulin therapy in the intensive care unit. In: 30th Annual International Conference of the IEEE Engineering in Medicine and Biology Society. EMBS 2008, pp. 3297–3300 (2008)

Chapter 6
Conformance Verification of Clinical Guidelines in Presence of Computerized and Human-Enhanced Processes

Stefano Bragaglia, Federico Chesani, Paola Mello and Marco Montali

Abstract Clinical Guidelines (CGs) capture medical evidence and describe standardized high quality health processes. Their adoption increases the quality of the service offered by health departments, with direct advantage for treated patients. However, their application in real cases is often tempered by a number of factors like the context, the specific case itself, administrative processes, and the involved personnel. In this chapter we analyse the issues related to the problem of representing CGs in a formal way, and to reason about the differences between what is prescribed by CGs, and what is observed during their application/execution. Our approach is based on a general, abstract framework that should be flexible enough to cope with the raised issues. Possible technical solutions are also presented and their limits discussed.

6.1 Introduction

Clinical Practice Guidelines (or simply Clinical Guidelines, CGs), in their original definition, are "systematically developed statements to assist practitioner and patient decisions about appropriate health care for specific clinical circumstances" [14]. Nowadays, the focus of CGs has been broader to any aspect related to the health care processes, from disease diagnosis, to treatment and intervention, up to administrative issues for health-related services.

Based on medical evidence, CGs provide (1) definitions and terminology, (2) workflows, (3) rules, and (4) temporal constraints. They aim to capture evidence-based new findings and to bring advances into daily medical practice. Their adoption ensures an increase of services quality, and promote the standardization of the health processes across different organizations (at the local, regional, or national level). CGs are also closely related to Clinical Pathways (CPs), that differ from CGs "as they are utilised by a multidisciplinary team and have a focus on the quality and co-ordination of care"[1].

---

[1] See http://www.openclinical.org/clinicalpathways.html.

© Springer International Publishing Switzerland 2015
A. Hommersom and P.J.F. Lucas (eds.), *Biomedical Knowledge Representation*, LNAI 9521, DOI 10.1007/978-3-319-28007-3_6

Thanks to the pervasive diffusion of IT systems both the CGs, as well as the log of their application to each specific patient, have become available in an electronic form, thus prospecting the possibility of automatically confront the CGs models with what happened in real cases. Hence, the evaluation of how "things have gone" w.r.t. "how things should have gone", named as *conformance*, has become a required analysis step to revise, update and adapt the CGs.

Evaluating the conformance of a CG execution against the CG model however raises a number of technical problems, ranging from the formal representation of CGs and execution logs, up to the reasoning techniques used to establish if and when a CG has not been respected. The aim of this chapter is to analyse all these issues, and to discuss an abstract framework powerful enough to cover many aspects. We do not provide any technical, complete solution: the "final word" on the CGs conformance is far from being achieved. However, we briefly point out how some techniques that can be successfully exploited to overcome many of the current issues.

6.1.1 What Is "Conformance", and Why?

In the context of business processes *conformance* is a property of an observed execution of a *process* (i.e., an *instance* or a *case* of the process), when confronted with a certain *process model*. Conformance indicates if and how much an instance *adheres* to a process model, where such model (explicitly or implicitly) brings some prescriptive information about allowed and forbidden characteristics of process instances.

Thus, a proper definition of conformance depends on three notions: the *instance* of a process, the *model* of a process, and a *matching function* that computes how much an instance matches the model. Definitions of these concepts can vary greatly, depending on the domain and the context. E.g., in a specific hospital department an instance might be the set of actions and events related to a specific patient within a hospitalization; the process model might be a CG that should be applied to that patient; finally, the evaluation function might be a measure of which activities where envisaged by the CG, that were not applied to the patient. The *conformance verification task*, also named as *conformance checking*, amounts to apply the evaluation function to a given instance and to a given model. Usually, it is applied to a number of instances w.r.t. the same model.

Conformance verification is a fundamental and required step whenever a proper analysis of a process is conducted. Indeed, for a variety of reasons, process executions often deviate from the expected model. The conformance verification task answers to the questions: *"Does a case deviate? Where?"*. Notice that from the process management viewpoint some deviations are indeed desirable, while others are to be avoided: the concept of deviation itself does not have a negative meaning, neither a positive one. For example in [13] the authors introduce the distinction of deviations as (acceptable) *exceptions*, versus (undesirable) *anomalies*. Deciding if a deviation is acceptable or not is up to the process manager, that can decide for example to extend the process model to allow/forbid new (previously unforeseen) cases.

6.1.2 Why Executions of Clinical Guidelines Deviate from the CG Model?

CGs capture medical evidence on the basis of statistical data, thus making (at least) three strong implicit assumptions [6]:

(*i*) *ideal patients*, i.e., patients that have "just the single" disease considered in the CG (thus excluding the concurrent application of more than one CG), and are "statistically relevant" (they model the typical patient affected by the given disease), not presenting rare peculiarities/side-effects;

(*ii*) *ideal physicians* executing the CG, i.e., physicians whose basic medical knowledge always allows them to properly apply the CGs to specific patients;

(*iii*) *ideal context* of execution, so that all necessary resources are available.

Moreover, when adopted within local organizations, CGs are typically subject to an adaptation process, which customizes the CG w.r.t. the peculiarities of the specific organization.

Hence, when concretely applying the CGs, three types of issues might arise:

(a) the implicit assumptions (*i*) − (*iii*) might not hold, for various practical reasons;

(b) depending on specific contexts, peculiar additional rules and workflows might need to be enacted together with the CGs recommendations (e.g., a certain health department might have its own administrative workflows); consequently, the patient could be subjected to practices not envisaged in the original guideline;

(c) when applying a CG to a specific case at hand, the physician (and the other health-related professionals) exploits also her/his general knowledge (Basic Medical Knowledge, BMK from now on). The interplay between these two types of knowledge can be very complex: e.g., actions recommended by a CG could be prohibited by the BMK, or a CG could force some actions despite the BMK discouraging them.

Note that independently of the type ((*a*), (*b*) or (*c*)) of the arising issue, it is always the physician (and other humans actors) that addresses the problems, and has the responsibility of taking decisions. Thus, healthcare processes can be considered an example of a *socio-technical system* [20], where humans interact with devices, manual and automated activities coexist, and human players ultimately need to cope with an unpredictable, highly dynamic environment that requires continuous adaptation.

Summing up, *CGs propose a model, but when dealing with its effective implementation, many factors might deviate the execution course from the model.* In this light, it becomes extremely important to assess what is effectively going on, and relate actual executions with the "ideal" model. Although each case can be considered in its uniqueness, the focus of the conformance task is upon the totality of the CG implementations versus the CG model.

Conformance checking in CG has another important characteristic: it is not an evaluation of the behaviour of the involved personnel. Indeed, the variety and dynamism of the situations does not allow to automatically (algorithmically) evaluate the personnel's course of actions and taken decisions. However when applying the CG to a patient, the conformance checking might be of interest for the physicians himself, as a sort of decision support. E.g., each deviation captures an aspect of the current state of affairs that differ from the expected model, and can consequently be analysed by domain experts to formulate a corresponding explanation (e.g., by relying on the conformance framework described in [23]).

6.1.3 Organization of This Chapter

In Sect. 6.2 we briefly introduce Clinical Guidelines, in particular by highlighting the type of information (or, better say, the type of knowledge) that CGs usually contain. In Sect. 6.3 we present an abstract framework, where conformance is expressed in terms of expectations of what should happen, and matching functions between observed (logged) events and expectations. Section 6.4 is devoted to discuss in deep detail how to conjugate two different aspects usually found in CGs, i.e. the interplay between procedural and declarative CG prescriptions. Section 6.5 presents some technical solutions, while finally in Sect. 6.7 we discuss the limits of our current approach, and future works.

6.2 Clinical Guidelines

Clinical Guidelines usually come as documents addressing many different aspects related to the health-care processes. In particular, they address a specific disease or pathology, suggesting the best practices that should be followed/enacted by health practitioners. The principal aim is to provide the patient with the best treatment possible, and guaranteeing quality standards at the same time. The majority of clinical guidelines are provided by national and international public health institutions, although it is frequent to have guideline specifications provided at local levels such as hospitals or departments.

When approaching the conformance task some common CGs features can have a huge impact on the understanding of the conformance issue itself:

Different knowledge types within a CG.
CGs often comprise many type of knowledge. In particular, it is quite usual to encounter:

- *Definitions and terminology:* each CG provides definitions for the terms adopted within the CG, so as to limit misunderstandings. Moreover, each CG usually specifies the disease and the type of patient for which the CG is applicable: in other words, it defines the criteria for applying the CG to a certain patient with a certain disease.
- *Workflows:* a CG can define the set of actions, and their correct execution order, in terms of workflows. Indeed, a plethora of languages and projects has been developed to create domain-independent computer-assisted tools for managing, acquiring, representing and executing CGs [12, 29], paying particular attention to the *procedural and control-flow dimension*.
- *Rules:* particular cases and exceptions are often tackled by CG by means of rules. Sometimes these rules can be applied only when inside a specific execution context of the CG implementation; sometimes the rules must be considered valid for the whole duration of the CG.
- *Linguistic labels:* conditions, (patient) features, and criteria are often measured by means of linguistic labels such as, for example, "low", "medium" and "high". While linguistic labels fit perfectly with the involved human actors, their translation into algorithms for the conformance task might be not straightforward.
- *Temporal constraints:* usually a workflow already provides (implicitly or explicitly) a set of temporal constraints, in the sense that a workflow clearly establishes a specific order for the actions execution. Moreover, it is quite common to find explicit constraints related to temporal aspects, such as "a certain B action must be executed within X time unit from action A" (relative-time constraints), or "every day at time Y a certain action must be executed" (absolute-time constraints).

Interplay between CGs and BMK.
CGs must not be intended as mandatory: they are "Not prescriptive: don't override clinical judgement"[2]. Indeed, it happens that a CG execution trace could seem conformant to the CG and not conformant to the BMK, or vice-versa. Actually, both the CG knowledge and the BMK can be defeated, while it is the physician's own responsibility to prefer a certain course of actions.

Interplay between workflows and rules.
Both CGs and the BMK contain a mix of procedural (workflows) and declarative knowledge (rules). Procedural knowledge comes into play when there is a set of well-accepted, predefined *sequences of operations* that must be followed by the involved stakeholders. Contrariwise, declarative knowledge typically captures *constraints* and *properties* that must be satisfied during the execution, without explicitly fixing how the stakeholders must behave in order to satisfy them. The majority of the approaches available in the literature have focused either on CGs or BMK in isolation, without

---

[2]http://www.openclinical.org/clinicalpathways.html.

taking into account how they mutually affect each other. Few works have attempted to consider both these aspects at the same time [6, 10].

Human actors are involved.
Indeed, CGs are mostly implemented by human players. This in turn affects the notion of conformance, that must be adapted to the peculiarities of human players. Let us consider, for example, a rule with a temporal deadline such as "every day the patient temperature must be recorded at 3 p.m.". What happens if the temperature is recorded 5 min later? Should we consider it as conformant with the rule, or not? Although only a physician can answer our question, it seems clear that any conformance approach should allow some flexibility: for example, we might expect that if the temperature is taken with a delay of 5 min, then we could consider it as conformant with a *score* of 0.99, while if the delay is above the hour we could lower the score to 0.40. This example points out to the notion of a *grade of conformance*, against the simpler idea of *conformance yes/no*.

6.2.1 A CG Example

Let us consider a real CG, taken from the on-line repository provided by the "National Institute for Health and Clinical Excellence"[3], a public UK organization sponsored by the UK's Department of Health. In particular, let us consider the "Quick Reference Guide" of the Clinical Guideline 56.[4] The guideline address the emergency treatment for head injuries, as well as subject admission to specific care units.

After few generalities about the document itself, the first section of the guideline quick reference is devoted to provide *definitions* of the terms. E.g., exact definitions of concepts like "infants", "children", and "adults", are given on the basis of the subject's age. Another example is the explanation of the "Glasgow Coma Scale", referred as GCS: no exact definition is given this time, possibly because GCS is assumed as being part of the staff's Basic Medical Knowledge.

The document then provides a mix of algorithms and rules for dealing with specific tasks; in Fig. 6.1 we show a simple excerpt from the "Assessment in the emergency department" section. There is a procedural part, that is guided by the evaluation of the GCS score: depending on the value assumed at the start of the assessment, different actions should be followed. In this particular case all the paths lead to assess "the need for CT imaging of head and/or cervical spine": such assessment is defined later in the guideline quick reference as another workflow. Moreover, the small CG excerpt in Fig. 6.1 shows at least two rules: the first one is a general rule about stabilizing airway, breathing and circulation (ABC). Another rule instead is a recommendation about "excluding significant brain injury before ascribing depressed conscious level to intoxication", hence suggesting that prior to formulate intoxication, involved personnel should exclude the hypothesis of brain injury.

---

[3]NICE, http://www.nice.org.uk.

[4]CG56: http://www.nice.org.uk/nicemedia/live/11836/36257/36257.pdf.

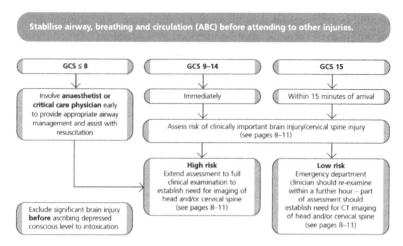

Fig. 6.1 An example of a part of a CG taken from UK NICE CG56.

The workflow specifies only few actions. However, interestingly, specific deadlines are provided depending on the different path: in one case, for example, assessment of brain injury must be performed *immediately*, while in another case it can be performed within *15 min*.

Finally, notice that although it is not explicitly specified, the workflow assumes the existence and availability of a "anaesthetist or critical care physician": i.e., the CG envisages certain roles, and assumes that qualified personnel is available for playing the roles.

6.3   A Generic Conformance Framework

In this section, we outline the main components and features of a generic framework for evaluating conformance, following the abstract schema of Fig. 6.2.

6.3.1   Types of Processes and Their Impact on Conformance

In Sect. 6.1.1, we discussed that conformance is about three elements: a *process model*, a *process instance*, and a *matching function*. In particular, there exist many different types of processes. However, from the conformance viewpoint, some process types have a huge impact on the notion of conformance itself.

Open versus Closed processes.
Closed, structured processes are based on the assumption that the model is completely defined, i.e. it explicitly captures all the possible situations. Therefore, any course

of action that is not mentioned in the model is forbidden. Any slightly difference observed within the execution must be intended as a deviation (non conformance) w.r.t. the model. An example of such type of processes is given by bank transactions, where the only and exactly allowed actions are those envisaged by the model.

On the opposite, open processes explicitly define what is allowed, and what is prohibited. Courses of actions for which no information is given are allowed and not required. Open approaches usually adopt a constraint based solution, where a trace is considered conformant if it satisfies all the imposed constraints. Open process are typical of many human interactions, where the involved players can enact many actions not necessarily envisaged by the model.

Summing up, closed approaches require only to specify the desired/allowed actions or events, while open solutions require (at least) two distinct concepts: one for desired actions and one for prohibited actions.

Open- versus Closed-time-view processes.
In principle, the conformance task can be applied "post-mortem", i.e. to already completed executions of the CG, or at run-time, when the execution is still running. This dichotomy needs to be reflected in the adopted conformance checking technique. In the first case, the course of events characterizing the execution is "closed", expected events can be missing either because they did not happen at all, or because they did happen but they were not properly recorded in the underlying information system. In the open-time-view case instead the course of events is "open", since further events can still occur in the future. In principle, this could make some deviations to be only temporary deviations, i.e., apparent deviations that will be fixed thanks to the suitable, future occurrence of new events. The ability of dealing with this open-time-view is typical of runtime verification and monitoring facilities.

With respect to this dimension, a careful consideration must be taken about the real implementations of CGs. In the majority of the cases it happens that health

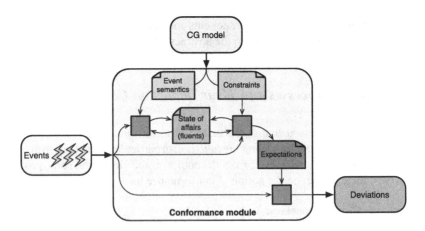

Fig. 6.2 An abstract architecture for conformance

practitioners apply a CG (by executing the foreseen actions), and only at a later moment they record the actions course. This means that two different time instants can be observed: the time instant when an action is executed, and the time instant when the execution of an action is recorded. Such instants are typically referred as *valid time vs. transaction time*. If the difference between these two time instants is relevant, it does not make sense at all to speak about run-time conformance: only a-posteriori, post-mortem analysis can be performed.

6.3.2   An Abstract Architecture for Conformance

Let us first consider a generic matching function as a black-box. It takes as input:

1. a formal model of the clinical guideline, covering the aforementioned different types of knowledge;
2. a set of correlated events describing a single (partial or complete) execution trace of the clinical guideline;

and it computes all the *deviations* between the actual behaviour and the ideal behaviour captured by the guideline model. As for conformance, the CG model can be conceived as constituted by two aspects: one providing the *event semantics*, and the other specifying a set of *constraints* that should be respected by the actual behaviours. Statements about the semantics of an event help in understanding how the occurrences of such an event modify the state of affairs, e.g., by introducing or modifying information about the patient ("measure glucose level has the effect of updating the glucose level of the patient"), or by affecting the state of durative activities ("a complete event marks the termination of an active execution of the corresponding activity").

The term "constraints" is here used as an umbrella term for all those parts of the CG model that specify the intended behaviour foreseen by the evidence-based studies and/or the BMK. Here we find the workflow dimension of the guideline, as well as rules dealing with exceptions or representing a portion of the medical knowledge. The combination of constraints with observed events and state of affairs determines which are the events/actions that are expected to be observed (in the future, as well in the past).

6.3.3   Conformance Based on "Expectations"

Our approach to conformance is inspired by the three elements previously introduced, i.e. the *process case*, the *process model*, and the *matching function*. The first concept we introduce is the *happened event*. Events represent the minimal possible observable information. They are the tiniest bit of information that can be recorded within the system. They are made of a description of *what* happened, together with information about *when* they happened. In our perspective happened events are characterized by having a single time-point duration. Durative actions are given in terms of *start* events and *end* events. Obviously, for each durative action with start time t_s and end time t_e, it must hold $t_s \leq t_e$.

$$\text{Happened Event} \doteq \langle \text{Event Description, When} \rangle$$

Depending on the type of event, the description of the observed event might contain different, structured data fields: in case of the execution of actions, the description might contain the name and the role of the action originator, as well as the name and role of the action destination; in case of observed facts, the description might contain some data that have been observed.

Given the simple notion of event, we introduce in a straightforward manner the notion of a *process instance*, intended as a set of (not necessarily ordered) process events:

$$\text{Process Case} \doteq \{ ev_i | i \in 1 \ldots n \}$$

where n is the number of events belonging to that instance. Although it is possible to have process cases of infinite length, quite often real cases resort to a finite number of events. The choice of closed- vs. open-time-view processes affects the intended meaning of the process trace: respectively, it contains all the happened events, or rather only a subset of a larger process case.

The second fundamental concept is the *expectation*. The desired behaviour, i.e. the ideal model specified by the CGs, can be expressed by means of expectations, that again are made of *what* is expected, and *when* it is expected. With the term "expectations" we want to capture the notion that depending on the current (dynamic) state of the observed CG execution, the CG model indicates what has to be done and possibly observed. The *what* can be only partly specified, thus allowing to capture larger sets of possible future outcomes. E.g., we might want to expect that a patient is served with food, but we might not want to explicitly specify who is going to serve him, since anyone is fine provided the patient is fed. The *when* instead can be an exact time value, or rather as a time interval when any event happening at a time instant belonging to the interval is fine. E.g., we might expect that patient temperature is taken exactly one hour after the last measurement, or we might expect that the temperature is taken within three hours since the last visit.

$$\text{Expected Event} \doteq \langle \text{What, When} \rangle$$

Depending on the adopted process model (open or close), expectations can be only *positive* (i.e., about the happening of something), or they can be also *negative* (about the non-happening of something, or simply prohibition). Moreover, expectations can be about the happening of events, or rather about properties. In the latter case, expectations can be about *achievement properties*, i.e. about a property being true in a certain time instant; or they can be about *maintenance properties*, i.e. about a property being maintained "true" along a temporal interval. Note that negative expectations implicitly introduce universal quantification over time intervals. Indeed, expecting that a certain event (or property) does not happen within a time interval means that *for all* the time instants within the interval, the event does not happen.

Given the concept of expectations, a process model can be thought as a specification of what is expected for any possible process case. The expressivity of the language used for defining such specifications defines the complexity of the processes that can be modelled.

Finally, the third fundamental concept is the *matching function* that is used to determine if an event or a property matches an expectation. The matching function provides the reasoning capabilities needed to fully support the different knowledge types that are found in a CG, as explained in Sect. 6.2. If we want to support definitions and terminology, we might expect the matching function to support ontological reasoning. If we need to support linguistic labels and grades of conformance, then the matching function should support fuzzy reasoning as well as uncertainty. Minimum capabilities of temporal reasoning are required to establish if an event indeed happened within the expected time interval or not. Finally, a sort of a fuzzy temporal reasoning is required to cope with deviations typically introduced when a process (a CG) is enacted by human players.

Roughly speaking, given *events* and *expectations*, conformance can be established by simply looking which expectations are "satisfied", and which not. To this end, a positive expectation is satisfied if there is an event (a property) that *matches* the expectation, while it is violated if there is not such event. On the contrary, a negative expectation is satisfied if there is no event (property) matching the expected *what/when*, while it is violated if a matching one is found.

Given the concepts of events, expectations and matching functions, only one important question is still open: how a CG (plus a BMK and other rules, standards etc.) can be represented so as to support these concepts? Our current answer is given by tackling in the next Sections three different sub-problems, that we believe as the being the principal issues when dealing with CG: (*a*) the integration between procedural and declarative knowledges; (*b*) representing and reasoning on the state of

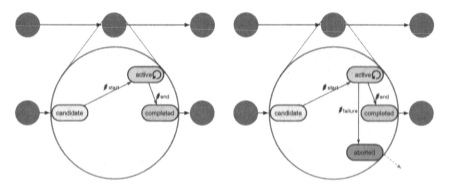

Fig. 6.3 A simple activity life-cycle, and an extension towards exception management

execution of a CG, and how the happening of events affects such states and properties; and (c) how to represent declarative knowledge in terms of rules.

6.4   The Interplay Between Procedural and Declarative Knowledge

Clinical Guidelines typically embrace both a procedural, workflow-like dimension, and a more declarative, rule-based component. The first aspect deals with structured, prescriptive and well-established fragments of the guideline, such as for example administrative processes or laboratory procedures. The second instead focuses on the management of less structured fragments of the guideline, as well as with general rules (such as the ones coming from the BMK) that should be always respected during the CG execution. In this section, we discuss the conformance problem by first considering the procedural knowledge, then the declarative knowledge, and finally their combination.

6.4.1   Conformance with Procedural Knowledge

The procedural knowledge defined within a CG takes often the form of a structured workflow, with simple blocks representing the actions to be executed, and control-blocks such as parallel execution, and/or splits, etc. Several workflow-like CG specification languages have been proposed in the literature, such as Asbru [4], GLARE [30], and PROForma [28]. Independently of the specific features of the language, as for conformance all such approaches comprise *intra-* and *inter-activity dynamic constraints*.

6.4.1.1   Activity Lifecycle

Intra-activity constraints aim to capture the so-called *activity life-cycle*, which consists of the acceptable orderings among the constitutive events marking the progression of an instance of the activity, and of the corresponding states. Hence, the activity life-cycle is typically represented by a finite state machine, where nodes represent states of the activity, and edges are labelled with events.

A simple life-cycle is shown in Fig. 6.3 (left), using the GLARE language as a basis (but notice that the concept of life-cycle is orthogonal to the specific language at hand). In this example, the life-cycle just specifies that activities are non-atomic, i.e., each activity execution spans over a time window. More specifically, whenever an activity is *candidate* for execution, a *start* event might be observed, marking the initiation of an *activity instance*. The instance is then put in the *active* state, to explicitly testify that it is currently in execution. To mark the completion of the instance, a corresponding *end* event is used. We observe that *start* and *end* are two atomic events, whereas *candidate*, *active* and *completed* are properties representing the activity instance states. The current state of each activity instance constitutes part of the global state of affairs.

The activity life-cycle requires the description of each event to contain at least two pieces of information: the event type, and the activity it is associated to. Notice also that, in principle, multiple instances of the same activity can be generated, each being associated to a specific instantiation of the corresponding life-cycle. In this work, we make the following assumption:

> For each activity, at a given moment in time at most one instance of that activity can be active.

This assumption is motivated by the fact that most activities in the CG refer to the patient, and it is unlikely that the patient is subject to two distinct instances of the same activity at the same time. Obviously, due to the presence of loops and repetitions in typical guidelines, multiple instances of the same activity could occur within a single instance. However, they will be associated to non-overlapping time windows. A further discussion on this assumption is provided below.

Checking conformance with the activity life-cycle when an event is processed breaks down to the following steps:

1. Correlate the happened event and the corresponding life-cycle instance (this comprises the creation of a new instance if a certain event occurs).
2. Check fulfilment of the "next transition" expectation: an event is accepted by the correlated life-cycle instance if it is associated to one of the outgoing transitions from the current instance state.

Table 6.1 Basic workflow patterns in GLARE, and their corresponding enabling conditions

PATTERN	REPRESENTATION	ENABLING CONDITIONS
Sequence		When A is completed, B becomes candidate
Exclusive choice		When A is completed and *cond* holds, B becomes candidate When A is completed and *cond* does not hold, C becomes candidate
Simple merge		When B is completed, D becomes candidate When C is completed, D becomes candidate
Parallel split		When A is completed, B and C become candidate
Synchronization		When B and C are completed, D becomes candidate

3. "Advance" the life-cycle instance, moving it from the current state to the next state, following the transition that corresponds to the processed event; this is executed only if the event fulfils the "next transition" expectation.

6.4.1.2 Workflow Constraints and Candidate Activities

The activities of the CG model are usually related to each other by means of inter-activity dynamic constraints, separating the allowed orderings of execution from the forbidden ones. With a procedural flavour, these constraints take the form of a workflow-like structure, which interconnects the activities by means of control-flow patterns [2] such as sequence, choice points, and parallel sections. The richness of such primitives depend on the chosen CG modelling language. A comparative evaluation of some CG modelling languages w.r.t. workflow-patterns support can be found here [22].

In general, as an execution of the CG evolves over time, the workflow determines which are the currently enabled activities, i.e., the *candidate* activities that can/must be executed next. Table 6.1 depicts the five basic control-flow patterns, their representation in GLARE, and their semantics in terms of enabling conditions, i.e., conditions that determine how the corresponding pattern enables some activity when some other activity is completed. As shown in Fig. 6.3 (left), a sequence flow departing from an activity is implicitly connected to its *completed* state, while a sequence edge pointing to an activity is implicitly connected to its *candidate* state. The intuitive semantics sketched in Table 6.1 works thanks to the assumption, stated above, that two instances of the same activity do not overlap. The presence of multiple parallel instances of the same activity would require complex correlation mechanisms to properly apply the control-flow patterns. These mechanisms are typically enforced by the process enactment engine. They rely on internal information that is not relevant for the domain per sé, and that is consequently not guaranteed to be traced and exploitable for conformance checking.

In this setting, conformance checking of control-flow constraints amounts to:

1. Properly handle the computation of candidate activities, applying the control-flow patterns semantics to the current state of affairs (which includes information about the currently completed activities).
2. Impose and verify the negative expectation about non-candidate activities: only candidate activities can be activated by means of a *start* event.
3. Ensure the proper termination of the CG execution when the trace of events is finished; the proper termination is in turn formalized by the following expectations:

   a. every active activity instance is expected to be completed before the termination;
   b. when the execution terminates, no activity can be candidate for execution.

We observe that, considering the conformance characterization provided so far, the CG procedural knowledge gives raise to a "closed" notion of conformance, where every event that is not explicitly expected is considered as forbidden, and no unforeseen activity can be executed. To partially open the workflow specification, more sophisticated forms of activity life-cycle can be introduced. For example, Fig. 6.3 (right) presents an improved version of the basic life-cycle. The new version contains an additional state and transition, to explicitly account for exceptional situations that require the prompt interruption of the running activity instance. This exceptional transition is associated to a *failure* event that leads the instance to an *aborted* terminal state. In this way, it is possible to "cancel" the execution of an activity instance under critical and exceptional circumstances, still conforming to the CG model. Notice that, in principle, the *aborted* terminal state can be associated to a different sequence flow than the one used for the *completed* state. This feature can be exploited to attach a compensation (sub)process meant to manage the exception. When no compensation process is specified, we make the assumption that the sequence flow departing from the *aborted* state is implicitly the same as the one departing from the *completed* state. The rationale behind this "robustness" principle is grounded on a practical observation about how the health operators apply the workflow part of a CG. It can happen that some actions are interrupted (aborted) for many possible reasons, and yet the execution of the CG is brought forward.

6.4.2 Integration with Declarative Knowledge

We further complicate the life-cycle model so as to enable the possibility of modelling declarative rules and constraints related to the CG, and to combine them with the procedural part. The resulting life-cycle has been first proposed in [5, 6], as a result of a close interaction with doctors and healthcare professionals.

Declarative constraints can be exploited to model underspecified portions of the CG, or to complement the CG with general, background medical knowledge (BMK), typically implicitly used by healthcare professionals to adapt the CG on a per-patient basis. For example, the BMK is employed by a physician when an alternative medicine must be found because the patient is allergic to the one mentioned in the guideline specification, or when a critical situation, threatening the life of the patient, suddenly arises. The combination of these two kinds of knowledge is a challenging task, which cannot be solved by simply isolating portions of the CG model that can be captured with a procedural flavour, and those that are better modelled with a declarative approach[5]. On the other hand, such a combination is required in order to better characterize conformance, and in particular to accept justified deviations instead of reporting them to the medical staff.

In order to show how procedural and declarative knowledge can interact in the case of BMK, we summarize in Table 6.2 some of the real-world examples put forward

---

[5] This is the typical approach followed in BPM, where the process is split into procedural and declarative fragments, or (macro)activities can be expanded by following a declarative or procedural approach (see for example the ad-hoc subprocess construct in BPMN).

in [5, 6]. These examples attest that the activities enabled by the CG procedural model could be prohibited by declarative rules, or conversely that the procedural part could enforce certain behaviours event if they are discouraged by the BMK. More specifically, three interaction modalities arise from the examples:

1. The CG supports the possibility of choosing among two different treatments, and the BMK acts as a business selection rule that helps in determining the route to be taken.
2. The BMK emends the CG, suggesting a suitable way for (temporarily) replacing the workflow prescriptions when they are deemed to be not applicable.
3. The CG defeats the BMK, imposing the prompt execution of an action even if, according to the BMK, it is in general be dangerous for the patient.

This integration gives therefore raise to a hybrid *semi-open* knowledge, where the procedural CG model must partially support the execution of unpredicted activities, as well as some deviations from its prescriptions, while the BMK must acknowledge the possibility of being defeated, honoring the motto: "domain experts always get the last word".

A deep understanding concerning the nature of this hybrid knowledge, and how its building components actually interact, is still far to be reached. Nevertheless, a first necessary step towards a proper characterization of conformance in this setting requires to revise the activity lifecycle, so as to reflect this interplay.

The revised lifecycle is shown in Fig. 6.4 (left). It is enriched with additional states and transitions, which are not only associated to events, but also to conditions that

Table 6.2 Examples of clinical behaviors induced by the interplay between procedural recommendations coming from a CG and declarative rules expressing part of the BMK, taken from [5, 6]

	CG	BMK	CG+BMK
A	Patients suffering from bacterial pneumonia must be treated with penicillin or macrolid	Do not administer drugs to which a patient is allergic	Administer macrolid to a patient with bacterial pneumonia if she is allergic to penicillin
B	Patients with post-hemorrhagic shock require blood transfusion	Do not apply therapies that are not accepted by patients. Plasma expander is a valid alternative to blood transfusion, provided that …*(omitted)*	If the patient refuses blood transfusion, in case of post-hemorrhagic shock treat her with plasma expander
C	In patients affected by unstable angina, coronary angiography is mandatory	A patient affected by advanced predialytic renal failure should not be subject to coronary angiography, because the contrast media may cause a further deterioration of the renal functions	Even in case of a predialytic renal failure, perform coronary angiography if the patient is affected by unstable angina

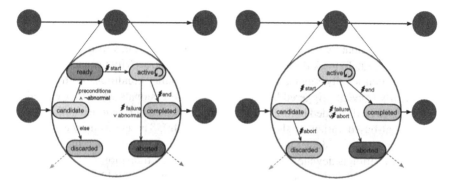

Fig. 6.4 A sophisticated activity lifecycle supporting abnormal situations and exceptions; the left diagram shows the intended lifecycle, and the right one its pure event-based version, which can be reconstructed from the analyzed trace

are checked against the current state of affairs (e.g., to verify whether the patients' data are within certain ranges). When an activity instance is *candidate*, it is not still ready to be executed. To make it *ready* for the execution, some additional conditions must be satisfied. More specifically, to be executed a candidate action must satisfy its *preconditions*, which are a part of the description of the activity. Preconditions specify whether the activity is applicable in the current state of affairs, and are evaluated on the basis of the currently available patients data and execution context. Even though preconditions are satisfied, the action cannot be executed if the current situation is "abnormal". This is captured by means of *abnormality* conditions, which are satisfied whenever the assumptions made in the CG model (e.g., *ideal* patient and context), do not hold. If the situation is not abnormal and preconditions hold, the action is *ready* to be executed. Otherwise, it is *discarded*. A *ready* activity instance can be made *active* by triggering the *start* event. Two cases are possible then: either an *end* event occurs marking that the activity instance is *completed* or an *abnormality/failure* shows up during execution, so that the action is *aborted*. As described before *failure* events mark exceptional situations that require the immediate interruption of the activity instance. The additional abnormality test is instead used to capture those situations in which the activity is started in a "normal" situation, which however becomes abnormal during the execution of the activity.

We observe that the *preconditions* are specified in the (augmented) procedural CG model, the *failure* situations depend on a specific execution, while *abnormality* circumstances are typically identified and handled by means of BMK rules. In addition, further constraints can be imposed by the BMK depending on the current context and patient's status; from the conformance point of view, this means that activity executions unforeseen by the procedural knowledge should be accepted if they are made *candidate* by the BMK.

As for conformance with this revised lifecycle, it is worth noting that its aim is not to enforce a discard/abortion of the activity instance when the corresponding state-related conditions prescribe to do so, but to check whether the actual behaviour is aligned with the ideal one. During the effective execution, healthcare professionals will decide whether the activity instance must be aborted or not, and the conformance checker will evaluate whether this course of execution deviates from the intended transitions or not. To track the actual transitions inside the activity instance lifecycle, we should then ideally replace the pre- and abnormality conditions with a corresponding *abort* event, triggered by the healthcare professionals when they consider the activity to be discarded before its execution, or aborted during its execution. This purely event-based variant is shown in Fig. 6.4 (right). The conformance problem ultimately amounts to detect and report all those instances for which the expected lifecycle transition is deviates from the actual performed transition.

Finally, notice that the *discarded* terminal state induces a third "exit point" from the activity. As for the *aborted* state, this exit point can be explicitly handled by means of additional CG/BMK rules, or be connected by default to the same outgoing sequence flow used for the *completed* state (thus ensuring robustness).

6.5   Representation of Clinical Guidelines

In Sect. 6.3 we introduced the concept of expectation: a CG could be thought of a set of rules and constraints that points out what is expected to happen next. However from the discussion in Sect. 6.4 it appears that expectations alone are not sufficient. Indeed, there is the need to reason upon the "state of affairs" when executing a CG. Such state of affairs is independent of what is expected next, and on the contrary the generation of expectations starts always from the current state. Hence, any CG in our model can be thought of as two distinct yet related descriptions: rules that specify how the happening of events affects the current state of affairs, and rules that forecast what is expected then on the basis of the current state and happened events.

Our current approach exploits two existing solutions: representation and reasoning upon the "state of affairs" is done by means of the Event Calculus [19], while expectations are represented, generated and verified by means of the Event-Condition-Expectation (ECE-) rules [7]. These two approaches can be easily integrated together, since the ECE-rules natively exploit the notion of *fluent*, core concept of the Event Calculus. From the technical viewpoint, the integration can be achieved since there exists implementations of ECE-rules and EC based on the Drools Framework.

6.5.1   Representing the Guideline Evolution with Event
        Calculus

In 1986, Kowalski and Sergot proposed the Event Calculus (EC, [19]) as a general framework to reason about time, events and change, overcoming the inadequacy of time representation in classical logic. It adopts an explicit representation of time, accommodating both qualitative and quantitative time constraints. Furthermore, it is based on (a fragment of) first-order logic, thus providing great expressiveness (such as variables and unification). Shanahan [25] intuitively characterizes the EC as "a logical mechanism that infers *what is true when*, given *what happens when* and *what actions do*".

The three fundamental concepts are that of *event*, happening at a point in *time* and representing the execution of some action, and of properties whose validity varies as time flows and events occur; such properties are called *fluents*. An EC specification is composed of two theories, each containing a set of axioms:

- a general (domain-independent) theory axiomatizing the *meaning* of the predicates supported by the calculus, i.e., the so called *EC ontology* shown in Table 6.3;
- a domain theory that *exploits* the predicates of the EC ontology to formalize the specific system under study in terms of events and their effects upon *fluents*. Our domain theory is focused on the formalization of intra- and inter-activity constraints, together with the corresponding expectations and deviations.

The domain knowledge about actions and their effects corresponds to "What actions do". The capability of an event to make a fluent true (false respectively) at some time is formalized by stating that the event *initiates* (*terminates*) the fluent. More specifically, when an event e occurs at time t, so that $initiates(e, f, t)$ and f does not already hold at time t, then e causes f to hold. In this case, we say that f is *declipped* at time t. There is also the possibility to express that some fluent holds in the initial state, using the *initially* predicate. Conversely, if $terminates(e, f, t)$ and f holds at time t, then e causes f to not hold any more, i.e., f is *clipped* at time t.

"What happens when" is the execution trace characterizing a (possibly partial) instance of the system under study. An execution trace is composed of a set of occurred events. The basic forms of EC assume that events are atomic, i.e., bound to a single time point. In particular, an execution trace is composed of a set of *happens* binary predicates, listing the occurrences of events and their corresponding timestamps.

The combination of the domain knowledge and a concrete execution trace leads to infer "what is true when", i.e., the intervals during which fluents *hold*. The $holds\_at(f, t)$ predicate of the EC ontology is specifically used to test whether f holds at time t.

Table 6.3 The basic Event Calculus ontology

Predicate	Meaning
$initially(F)$	Fluent F holds in the initial state of affairs
$initiates(Ev, F, T)$	Event Ev initiates fluent F at time T
$terminates(Ev, F, T)$	Event Ev terminates fluent F at time T
$happens(Ev, T)$	Event Ev occurs at time T
$holds\_at(F, T)$	Fluent F holds at time T
$holds\_from(F, T, T_s)$	Fluent F holds at time T since time T_s

In [6] we introduced for the first time a model of the execution of a single action, hence opening up the possibility to integrate it with the declarative knowledge. We will not report here the technicalities presented in [6]; however, we might point out that few basic fluents such as *status* (indicating possible status of an activity, such as "candidate", "active", "completed", etc.), together with events of "start", "end", "discard" and "abort" have been sufficient to fully represent the activity lifecycle discussed in Sect. 6.4.1.

6.5.2 Generating and Matching Expectations with ECE Rules

In several previous works we have explored the notion of expectations, and we have defined several different languages for defining rules that support the definition of expectation. In particular, in [7] we have introduced the Event-Condition-Expectations (ECE-) rules. Based on the rule framework Drools[6], ECE-Rules allow to link current system status (properties, and also Event Calculus fluents) and the dynamic happening of events to the generation of expectations.

An example of a rule is shown in Fig. 6.5. When a patient $pat is evaluated to be at risk of a disease $disease, with a factor judged as to be "high" and with a confidence equal or greater to the "medium" grade, then it is expected that a proper treatment is initiated within one hour from the evaluation.

This simple rule already shows the power of the ECE-Rules: the rule triggers when the evaluation of the disease risk is inserted as a event and conditions are met. As a consequence, dynamically an expectation is generated. The expectation then can be satisfied by an event representing the start of proper treatment. Note that the formalism allows to define also proper actions in case of satisfaction of the expectations (rewards) and in case of violations (possibly expected countermeasures).

```
rule "Risk factor evaluation"
when
    $pat : Patient( ... )    // patient identifier
    // evaluation of risk factor and confidence degree
    $risk : EvaluatedRisk( $phys, $pat, $disease, $factor, $conf )
    $factor == "high"
    $conf >= "medium"
then
    expect InitiateTreatment( $pat, $disease, this after[0,1hour] $risk )
        on fulfillment {         // if the treatment is initiated
            /* some increase in patient health */
        }
        on violation {           // if the treatment is not initiated
            alert( ... );
        }
end
```

Fig. 6.5 An example of ECE-Rule [7].

---

[6]http://www.jboss.org/drools/.

The choice of Drools as supporting framework for the ECE-rules is based on the Drools Chance extension, and in particular on the possibility of support various type of imperfect reasoning [26]. Indeed, the possibility of support at least fuzzy logic-based reasoning is fundamental to support the human-related nature of CGs: for example, a number of linguistic qualifiers like "high", "low" or "medium" are usually involved in guidelines specification. Moreover, imperfect reasoning is needed to cope with deadlines, specifically if humans are involved.

6.6 Related Work

There is a flourishing literature focused on conformance issues in the healthcare setting, mainly due to the impact that the execution of CGs has in terms of quality, cost savings, and effectiveness. We review some of the relevant approaches, starting with two observations. First, often the term conformance is replaced by *compliance*, so as to emphasize normative and legal aspects, or by *critiquing*, stressing the fact that the actual courses of execution are critically analysed. Second, an impressive series of works aims at providing specific, vertical solutions tailored to a single guideline or disease, and by no means we can cover this extensive literature here.

In [18], an empirical, interview-based assessment is carried out so as to understand how healthcare professionals perceive the adoption of CGs, and their usage to monitor conformance. Interestingly, the assessment of conformance with the recommendations included in the CGs is perceived by clinicians as an importat problem, with which however they do not have enough familiarity. As a recommendation for future research, they also mention the problem of putting the patient into the loop, understanding to what extent patient concordance with the CG recommendations has to be considered when assessing conformance.

The vast majority of approaches focused on conformance in the clinical setting only considers the contribution of the CGs, without dealing with how they interact with the BMK. In this respect, checking conformance is tightly related to operational decision support and conformance verification in the field of process mining [1], which is being increasingly applied to the healthcare setting [21]. Notable examples of such a cross-fertilization are [15, 16]. In [16], a graphical language for specifying declarative processes is used to capture clinical recommendations, expressing constraints about the relative occurrence of activities, as well as the data they carry. At the same time, a procedural model of a CG is simulated so as to extract possible execution scenarios. The simulated traces are then checked against the formalized recommendations so as to ascertain whether they agree or not. The approach is then extended in [15], where ontologies are exploited so as to reuse the same formalization of clinical recommendations for checking conformance of different CG models belonging to the same Open Clinical repository.

Notice that the notion of conformance used in [15, 16] is radically different from ours, because it uses as input data those extracted through simulation from the ideal

CG model, not real executions. In fact, [15, 16] can be considered as examples of techniques that show how conformance checking as intended in this paper can be complemented with techniques and tools that ascertain conformance/compliance via model checking[7]. On the one hand, formal verification applied a-priori on the CG models, before their actual executions, can help in preventing the presence of errors at runtime, and in improving the quality of models. On the other hand, they are not exhaustive, due to the fact that they do not consider specific unforeseen situations that may arise at runtime, they do not work on real patient data and contexts, and they do not consider how the BMK could be employed to dynamicall adapt the CG models on a per-patient basis. We therefore believe that both approaches are needed, so as to provide support to the healthcare professionals during the entire CG lifecycle. For more details about formal verification and model checking of CGs, the interested reader can refer to the chapter on verification in this book.

Notably, model checking techniques can be suitably employed not only for the a-priori verification of CGs, but also to tackle conformance in the way intended in this chapter. This is the case of [17], where model checking techniques are used to compare ideal actions prescribed by a CG with actual actions extracted from healthcare records that log real executions of the CG. The focus is mainly on the control-flow/temporal dimension, without taking into account resources and event data. Of particular interest is the elicitation of two lists of reasons for non-compliance, singled out by respectively considering the adherence of the actual with the expected behavior, and whether the actual behavior is supported by the patient findings. Since this second class of reasons implicitly depends on the BMK (which is used to indicate and explain why a certain action is (un)likely to be executed given certain patient findings), it would be interesting to encode the different reasons for non-compliance in our approach. This would allow us to not only report deviations back to the healthcare professionals, but also in automatically provide hints about the reasons for such deviations.

Another approach that aims at going beyond the detection of deviations is that of [3]. The authors employ Asbru to model che CG, and describe a technique to check the adherence of an observed execution to the intended model. However, they also consider preferences and policies of the institution in which the guideline is executed, and whenever a deviation is detected, they check whether the deviation can be explained by applying such additional knowledge. In this respect, policies and preferences of the institution can be considered as part of the BMK, paving the way towards the extension of our framework with preference-based reasoning.

The notion of clinical guideline conformance based on a formally defined matching between the actual and the expected behavior started in [8, 11], where the SCIFF framework, based on abductive logic programming with hypothesis confirmation, is applied to clinical guideline conformance, with application to cancer screening protocols. The possibility of exploiting the framework starting from typical procedural CG

---

[7]Notice that, even though the techniques in [15, 16] are presented as "a-posteriori" techniques, they could be considered as "a-priori" technique, because they work on the CG model, not on its real enactments.

models is tackled in [9], which presents a translation mechanism that analyzes the CG model and produces corresponding SCIFF rules. Differently from the approach here presented, the SCIFF framework tailors non-conformance to logical inconsistency, and it is therefore only able to determine whether a (partial or complete) execution trace complies with the intended model or not, without continuing with the analysis when a deviation is detected.

The general conformance framework here presented generalizes that of [5, 6] along two directions: on the one hand, we provide here a thorough analysis of the main features a generic conformance framework must provide, and on the other hand we describe a more comprehensive activity lifecycle. Interestingly, an alternative approach to our Event Calculus-based one is presented in [27], where Answer Set Programming is used to encode a preliminary version of the activity lifecycle is presented, enumerating with specific rules all the possible types of deviations that may be encountered.

Finally, we would like to point the interested reader to [24], which provides a broad analysis of the role of compliance in the healthcare setting, and its impact on the development of computerized decision-support systems for CGs.

6.7 Discussion

The adoption of Clinical Guidelines is continuously increasing, towards high quality standards in health processes. At the same time, though, healthcare professionals might run into several issues when operating in agreement with CGs, due to unforeseen situations, contextual factors, specific peculiarities of patients, administrative problems, and human decisions. When executing CGs, deviations from the expected behavior are often observed. This by no means imply a negative impact on the patient, but simply attests a discrepancy between the expected and actual execution. Detecting the presence of such deviations is nevertheless of key importance towards CG improvement on the one hand, and awareness of the patient state on the other hand.

Understanding if a CG execution deviates means to evaluate its *conformance* w.r.t to the CG model. However, the nature of CGs makes it a difficult task. One reason resides on the type of knowledge encoded in CGs: definitions, structured workflows, rules, linguistic qualifiers and temporal constraints are usually part of any CG specification. Moreover, such knowledge is expressed using both a procedural approach (e.g., the workflows), and in a declarative way (as it happens with the many rules). A second reason lies on the fact that CG are not prescriptive models: during their execution physicians and personnel continuously integrate CG with Basic Medical Knowledge, hence adding/changing/avoiding actions. A third reason is related to the socio-technical nature of CGs: e.g., deadlines for human beings might have a different semantics from deadlines in fully automated processes.

In this chapter we outlined an abstract framework for dealing with conformance, based on the notion of expectations and of matching function. The more sophisticated the matching function, more complex the type of conformance that can be verified.

However, the double-nature of CGs as being partly procedural and partly based on rules requires a deeper analysis of how these two components can inter-relate. Our proposed approach is based on an extended version of the activity life-cycle, where exceptions can occur and interrupt the execution of a single activity. We have not discussed technical solutions, but we pointed out that existing solutions might cope with the highlighted complexity.

In this chapter we have completely ignored few important dimensions, that indeed in the Business Process field are subject of an intense research activity. First of all, knowing that a deviation happened might not be sufficient: a further question is "why the deviation happened". Strictly related to this point there is the identification of the culprit for the deviation. Answer such question would require to specify in the CG specification also concepts like *responsibility, duties, permissions*, and other deontic concepts. Another question is about evaluating numerically *how much* the overall process executions deviated from the CG model. A measure of deviation would help to identify the most problematic processes, and to establish if and when corrective measures are needed. Given the specific health domain, it is reasonable to expect that any measurement function must take into account the domain semantics of the actions and of the deviations. Notice that since deviations might have also a positive impact, any measure of deviation should take into account also the produced effects.

Our current work is focused on building a unified framework where the conformance task can be accomplished. However, the nature of the hybrid reasoning techniques required by conformance is proving to be a challenging task: in particular the need of models and algorithms for perfect and imperfect reasoning at the same time is an open problem.

Acknowledgments The approaches presented in this paper are the result of discussions and collaborations with many colleagues. In particular, we would like to thank Davide Sottara, Emory Fry, Paolo Terenziani, Alessio Bottrighi, and Stefania Montani.

This work has been partially supported by the Health Sciences and Technologies - Interdepartmental Center for Industrial Research (HST-ICIR) - University of Bologna, by the DEIS Depict Project, and by the EU FP7 IP project Optique (*Scalable End-user Access to Big Data*), grant agreement n. FP7-318338.

References

1. van der Aalst, W.M.P.: Process Mining - Discovery, Conformance and Enhancement of Business Processes. Springer, Berlin (2011)
2. van der Aalst, W.M.P., et al.: Workflow patterns. Distrib. Parallel Databases **14**(1), 5–51 (2003)
3. Advani, A.A., Lo, K.-K., Shahar, Y.: Intention-based critiquing of guideline-oriented medical care. In: American Medical Informatics Association Annual Symposium (AMIA). AMIA (1998)
4. Balser, M., Duelli, C., Reif, W.: Formal semantics of Asbru-an overview.In: Proceedings of IDPT 2002 (2002)

5. Bottrighi, A., Chesani, F., Mello, P., Molino, G., Montali, M., Montani, S., Storari, S., Terenziani, P., Torchio, M.: A hybrid approach to clinical guideline and to basic medical knowledge conformance. In: Combi, C., Shahar, Y., Abu-Hanna, A. (eds.) AIME 2009. LNCS, vol. 5651, pp. 91–95. Springer, Heidelberg (2009)

6. Bottrighi, A., Chesani, F., Mello, P., Montali, M., Montani, S., Terenziani, P.: Conformance checking of executed clinical guidelines in presence of basic medical knowledge. In: Daniel, F., Barkaoui, K., Dustdar, S. (eds.) BPM Workshops 2011, Part II. LNBIP, vol. 100, pp. 200–211. Springer, Heidelberg (2012)

7. Bragaglia, S., Chesani, F., Fry, E., Mello, P., Montali, M., Sottara, D.: Event condition expectation (ECE-) rules for monitoring observable systems. In: Olken, F., Palmirani, M., Sottara, D. (eds.) RuleML - America 2011. LNCS, vol. 7018, pp. 267–281. Springer, Heidelberg (2011)

8. Chesani, F., et al.: Compliance checking of cancer-screening careflows: an approach based on computational logic. In: Computer-based Medical Guidelines and Protocols: A Primer and Current Trends. Studies in Health Technology and Informatics, vol. 139, pp. 183–192. IOS Press, Amsterdam (2008)

9. Chesani, F., Mello, P., Montali, M., Storari, S.: Testing careflow process execution conformance by translating a graphical language to computational logic. In: Bellazzi, R., Abu-Hanna, A., Hunter, J. (eds.) AIME 2007. LNCS (LNAI), vol. 4594, pp. 479–488. Springer, Heidelberg (2007)

10. Christov, S., et al.: Formally defining medical processes. Methods Inf. Med. **47**(5), 392 (2008)

11. Ciampolini, A., et al.: Using social integrity constraints for on-the-fly compliance verification of medical protocols. In: Proceedings of the 18th IEEE Symposium on Computer Based Medical Systems (CBMS 2005), pp. 503–505. IEEE Computer Society Press (2005)

12. Fridsma, D.B. (Guest ed.): Special issue on workflow management and clinical guidelines. JAMIA **22**(1), 1–80 (2001)

13. Depaire, B., Swinnen, J., Jans, M., Vanhoof, K.: A process deviation analysis framework. In: La Rosa, M., Soffer, P. (eds.) BPM Workshops 2012. LNBIP, vol. 132, pp. 701–706. Springer, Heidelberg (2013)

14. Field, M.J., Lohr, K.N. (eds.): Committee to advise the public health service on clinical practice guidelines. Clinical Practice Guidelines: Directions for a New Program. The National Academies Press, 1990

15. Grando, M.A., van der Aalst, W.M.P., Mans, R.S.: Reusing a declarative specification to check the conformance of different CIGs. In: Daniel, F., Barkaoui, K., Dustdar, S. (eds.) BPM Workshops 2011, Part II. LNBIP, vol. 100, pp. 188–199. Springer, Heidelberg (2012)

16. Grando, M.A., Schonenberg, M.H., van der Aalst, W.M.P.: Semantic process mining for the verification of medical recommendations. In: 4th International Conference on Health Informatics (HEALTHINF), pp. 5–16 (2011)

17. Groot, P., et al.: Using model checking for critiquing based on clinical guidelines. Artif. Intell. Med. **46**(1), 19–36 (2009)

18. Hutchinson, A., et al.: Towards efficient guidelines: how to monitor guideline use in primary care. Health Technol. Assess. **7**(18) (2003)

19. Kowalski, R.A., Sergot, M.J.: A logic-based calculus of events. New Gener. Comput. **4**(1), 67–98 (1986)

20. Kroes, P., et al.: Treating socio-technical systems as engineering systems: some conceptual problems. Syst. Res. Behav. Sci. **23**(6), 803–814 (2006)

21. Mans, R.S., van der Aalst, W.M.P., Vanwersch, R.J.B., Moleman, A.J.: Process mining in healthcare: data challenges when answering frequently posed questions. In: Lenz, R., Miksch, S., Peleg, M., Reichert, M., Riaño, D., ten Teije, A. (eds.) ProHealth 2012 and KR4HC 2012. LNCS, vol. 7738, pp. 140–153. Springer, Heidelberg (2013)

22. Mulyar, N., van der Aalst, W.M.P., Peleg, M.: A pattern-based analysis of clinical computer-interpretable guideline modelling languages. J. Am. Med. Inform. Assoc. **14**, 781–787 (2007)

23. Quaglini, S.: Compliance with clinical practice guidelines. Stud. Health Technol. Inform. **139**, 160–179 (2008)

24. Quaglini, S.: Compliance with clinical practice guidelines. In: Computer-based Medical Guidelines and Protocols: A Primer and Current Trends. Studies in Health Technology and Informatics, vol. 139, pp. 160–179. IOS Press, Amsterdam (2008)

25. Shanahan, M.: The event calculus explained. In: Veloso, M.M., Wooldridge, M.J. (eds.) Artificial Intelligence Today. LNCS (LNAI), vol. 1600, pp. 409–430. Springer, Heidelberg (1999)

26. Sottara, D., Mello, P., Proctor, M.: A configurable rete-oo engine for reasoning with different types of imperfect information. IEEE Trans. Knowl. Data Eng. **22**(11), 1535–1548 (2010)

27. Spiotta, M., Bottrighi, A., Giordano, L., Dupré, D.T.: Conformance analysis of the execution of clinical guidelines with basic medical knowledge and clinical terminology. In: Miksch, S., Riano, D., Teije, A. (eds.) KR4HC 2014. LNCS, vol. 8903, pp. 62–77. Springer, Heidelberg (2014)

28. Sutton, D.R., Fox, J.: The syntax and semantics of the proforma guideline modelling language. J. Am. Med. Inform. Assoc. **10**(5), 433–443 (2003)

29. Ten Teije, A., Miksch, S., Lucas, P. (eds.): Computer-based Medical Guidelines and Protocols: A Primer and Current Trends. Studies in Health Technology and Informatics, vol. 139. IOS Press, Amsterdam (2008)

30. Terenziani, P., et al.: Applying artificial intelligence to clinical guidelines: the GLARE approach. In: Ten Teije, A., Miksch, S., Lucas, P. (eds.) Studies in Health Technology and Informatics, vol. 139, pp. 273–282. IOS Press, Amsterdam (2008)

Chapter 7
Modelling and Monitoring the Individual Patient in Real Time

Catherine G. Enright and Michael G. Madden

Abstract This paper presents a framework for representing background knowledge and new data, and reasoning efficiently with this powerful combination of both knowledge and data. Domain knowledge is needed to positively bias the operation of data mining algorithms. Knowledge in the form of mathematical models can be considered sufficient statistics of all prior experimentation in the domain, embodying generic or abstract knowledge of it. We present a framework for using this knowledge in a probabilistic framework for data mining, inference, and decision making under uncertainty. Real-time data-streams, which typically contain uncertainty, are then exploited in a principled manner to individualise patient care. By combining the knowledge available in existing data streams with the expert knowledge available and an efficient inference method, we provide a powerful foundation for reasoning with uncertain and sparse data in the medical domain.

7.1 Introduction

This chapter discusses medical knowledge representation in the context of representing background knowledge, representing new data, and reasoning with both background knowledge and new data. In particular, we focus on the task of modelling patients' dynamic responses to therapies in the intensive care unit and updating those models continuously so as to enable real-time inference and decision making.

Clinicians are often inundated with data, including continuous physiological time series data, laboratory results, and patient historical records. Different clinicians put differing emphases on different parts of the information set, but it is not known how patient factors, such as their major illness and co-morbidities, affect the weight that should be put on different aspects of this data.

Early approaches to computer-based medical decision support, such as MYCIN in the 1970s [14], were based on hand-crafted expert systems, which suffered greatly from their inability to scale to large systems and the practical impossibility of being able to fully codify all aspects of human physiology. More recently, data-driven

© Springer International Publishing Switzerland 2015
A. Hommersom and P.J.F. Lucas (eds.), *Biomedical Knowledge Representation*, LNAI 9521, DOI 10.1007/978-3-319-28007-3_7

methods (initially techniques such as neural networks and more recently Support Vector Machines, e.g., [5, 17, 23, 39, 71, 73]) have had some success. However, they have two key limitations in how they are currently used: firstly, they do not generally facilitate the inclusion of domain expertise, but depend on the data for all of their information; and secondly, their reasoning is not always transparent to the medical practitioners, which is recognised to be a large barrier to their adoption [40]. Recent advances, such as the methodology described in this chapter, seek to overcome those limitations.

It is well understood that at least some domain knowledge is needed to positively bias the operation of data mining algorithms; domain knowledge also informs the essential work of data preparation and pre-processing. However, most data mining algorithms are data-driven. In 2007, Domingos [27] argued that data mining as practiced today is mostly knowledge-poor; current tools do not facilitate the incorporation and reuse of knowledge, and this is perhaps the single greatest barrier to progress.

Much of what is known about human physiology is formalised in mathematical models. Systems of ordinary differential equations (ODEs) play a prominent role in medical settings, for example in modelling physiological systems and drug dynamics. The vast majority of models found in standard textbooks, e.g. [9, 13, 59], are based on ODEs. We contend that knowledge in such a form can be considered sufficient statistics of all prior experimentation in the domain, embodying generic or abstract knowledge of it. We believe that when used in a probabilistic framework, such models provide a sound foundation for data mining, inference, and decision making under uncertainty.

ODE models typically describe general population-level behaviours. However, an individual patient's behaviour can vary considerably from the general behaviour. Patients are admitted to hospital for a large variety of reasons, they all have different pre-existing conditions and age profiles; we can therefore expect a large variability in their individual responses to treatments. To be of use for monitoring a specific patient, the mathematical model's parameters must be individualised. In the hospital setting, real-time observations of the patient can be used to do just that. In the modern Intensive Care Unit (ICU), patients are continuously monitored with array of equipment at bedsides, allowing hospitals to monitor many variables continuously and collect substantial amounts of data in Clinical Information Systems (CISs). At present, however, CISs are primarily used for record-keeping rather than decision support.

We seek to exploit this data, using systems designed for individual patient monitoring and re-purposing them to yield future improvements in clinical outcomes by individualising patient care. A key issue to deal with is that ICU data generally contains uncertainty: it may be noisy as it can be subject to measurement error and/or simple transcription errors, and data may be missing. In addition, the frequency of the data may be sparse relative to the dynamics of the underlying system thus making it difficult to individualise the parameters.

In order to reason with uncertain data streams on a highly variable patient cohort, we have developed a probabilistic framework [30–32] that will be summarised in this chapter. Our methodology, PRIM (Probabilistic Real-time Intelligent Monitor), makes use of existing knowledge in the form of mathematical equations and

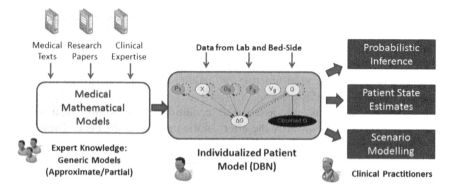

Fig. 7.1 PRIM (Probabilistic Real-Time Intelligent Monitor) is a framework that encodes domain knowledge in the form of ODEs as probabilistic graphical models that are adapted based on observed data.

encapsulates it in a dynamic Bayesian network (DBN) setting which can exploit the real-time data streams to individualise model parameters to the patient. Figure 7.1 provides a graphical representation of our framework. PRIM can handle both data and model uncertainty in a principled manner, can be used for temporal data mining with noisy and missing data, and can be used to re-estimate model parameters automatically using data streams.

In this chapter, we first present a brief background on DBNs and particle filtering, as they form the basis of our PRIM framework. Then in Sect. 7.3, we look at recent approaches to probabilistic medical knowledge representation. In Sect. 7.4, we explain our methodology for building a PRIM framework from a set of ODEs and in Sect. 7.5, we present our Adaptive-Time Particle Filtering algorithm. This algorithm is more efficient than standard fixed-time step particle filtering. In Sect. 7.6, we discuss the challenges of monitoring and controlling blood glucose in ICU patients and in Sect. 7.7 we apply our PRIM framework to this task. We show that PRIM out-performs a previous approach and demonstrate that the method is effective at re-estimating model parameters and reasoning with the sparse and potentially unreliable data available at the bed-side.

7.2 Background and Notation

7.2.1 Bayesian Networks

Bayesian Networks are directed acyclic graphs where each variable to be considered is represented by a node. Bayesian Networks can be considered to be a representation of independence relationships between the nodes. If an arc exists from node X to node Y, X is said to be a parent of Y. The absence of an arc between two nodes indicates they do not influence each other directly and are conditionally independent. In a

Bayesian Network, each node is conditionally independent of its non-descendants in the graph given the values of all its parents.

Many BN structures can represent the same independence relationships. However, it is recommended [50, 65] that the structure reflects causal order so that causes are parents of effects. Non-causal ordering can require more arcs and result in a less compact topology [50, 65].

Each node X_j has an associated conditional probability distribution $P(X_j | Parents(X_j))$ to quantify the effect of the parents on the node. These distributions are referred to as the conditional probability tables (CPTs). The network structure and the conditional probability tables can be viewed as a representation of the full joint probability distribution for each variable. Each entry in the joint distribution is represented by the product of the appropriate elements of the conditional probability tables. The joint probability of a set of variables can be determined by

$$P(x_1, \ldots, x_n) = \prod_{j=1}^{n} P(x_j | parents(X_j)) \tag{7.1}$$

where x_1 denotes a particular assignment to the variable X_j and $parents(X_j)$ denotes the specific values of the variables in $Parents(X_j)$.

Nodes in a Bayesian Network may be continuous or discrete. Nodes can be either observed or hidden. One purpose of a BN can be to infer probable values for the hidden nodes. Observed nodes are nodes for which we have an observation of its true state, e.g. a measurement for a patients glucose level at a particular time. Hidden nodes cannot be directly observed, e.g. the patients sensitivity to insulin. We can, however, infer a probable value for the patients insulin sensitivity using the measured glucose levels.

The graphical representation used in this chapter is shown in Fig. 7.2. In this representation observed nodes are shaded black and hidden nodes are shaded grey.

7.2.2 Dynamic Bayesian Networks

DBNs, which are used in our probabilistic framework, are Bayesian Networks that represent temporal systems, i.e. where the past state influences the current state.

DBNs were originally introduced by Dean and Kanazawa [24]. The purpose of a DBN is to infer probable values for the hidden variables as they evolve over time. DBNs discretise time and we denote each time step with the index i. If we un-roll the DBN it yields a BN structure repeated over time, the joint distribution therefore follows from Eq. (7.1) and over T time-slices can be given by:

$$P(Z_{0:T}) = \prod_{i=1}^{T} \prod_{j=1}^{N} P(Z_i^j | parents(Z_i^j)) \tag{7.2}$$

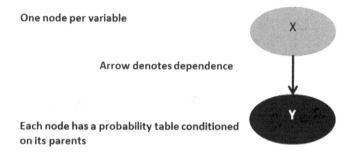

One node per variable

Arrow denotes dependence

Each node has a probability table conditioned
on its parents

Fig. 7.2 Basic concepts and representation of a Bayesian Network. Hidden nodes are shown here
in grey. Observed nodes are shown in black.

We partition the nodes into input nodes (denoted by I_i), hidden nodes (denoted by X_i),
and observation nodes (denoted by Y_i). Input nodes are observed and are typically
parents of the hidden X_i nodes. The hidden nodes are in turn parents of the observed
Y_i nodes. In specifying a DBN three sets of probability distributions are required:

1. The initial state distribution $P(X_0)$,
2. The sensor/observation models $P(X_i|I_i)$ and $P(Y_i X_i)$,
3. The transition model $P(X_{i+1}|X_i)$.

DBNs are first-order Markov in the sense that the state at time step $i + 1$ is assumed
to depend only on the state at time step i. DBNs are generally assumed to have a fixed
time step. The modeller chooses a natural fixed time step size in order to specify the
model structure and the transitional probability tables.

   Here, DBNs are assumed to be time invariant, i.e., their structure does not change
over time, as opposed to non-stationary DBNs proposed by Robinson and Hartemink
[63]. Detailed discussions on DBNs can be found in [50, 57, 65].

7.2.2.1   Graphical Representation

We represent DBNs using a compact format shown on the left in Fig. 7.3. Hidden
nodes are shown in grey here; different shading for different node types is used later.
Observed nodes are shown in black. Dependencies within a time-slice are indicated
with a solid arc. Inter-slice dependencies are indicated by a dotted line. On the right-
hand side the un-rolled DBN is presented. From this version, it is clear that a DBN
is a Bayesian Network with a repeating structure for each time slice, with arcs from
one time slice to the next.

7.2.2.2   DBN Creation

Both DBN structure and parameters can be learned from data [36, 50, 65]. However most DBNs are constructed by hand, using knowledge elicited from domain
experts [22]. This knowledge elicitation process is difficult and time consuming

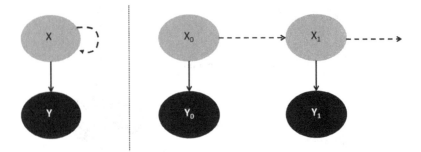

Fig. 7.3 Two different representations of a simple DBN. The compact representation on the left hand side is used in the remainder of this chapter. Hidden nodes are shown here in grey. Observed nodes are shown in black. Dependencies within a time-slice are indicated with a solid arc. Inter-slice dependencies are indicated by a dotted line. The un-rolled representation on the right is also commonly used.

[37, 55]. In the PRIM framework, this knowledge elicitation bottleneck is bypassed by using existing summarised domain knowledge in the form of ordinary differential equations.

7.2.2.3 Inference

There are four basic inference tasks that can be solved in a DBN [65]:

- Filtering: Keeping track of the current state. This is the task of computing the posterior distribution given all the evidence to date, i.e. $P(X_i|y_{1:i})$.
- Prediction: Computing the posterior distribution over future states, i.e. $P(X_{i+k}|y_{1:i})$ for some $k > 0$.
- Smoothing: Computing the posterior distribution over past states, i.e. $P(X_k|y_{1:i})$. for some $k > 0$ such that $0 <= k < i$. The smoothed estimate will be more accurate as it incorporates more evidence.
- Most Likely Explanation: Determining the most likely sequence of states to have generated a sequence of observations, i.e. $\arg\max_{x_{1:i}} P(x_{1:i}|y_{1:i})$.

For our purposes we are interested in 1 and 2 above, Filtering and Prediction. Exact inference is only possible in simple DBNs. For more complex DBNs approximate filtering and prediction can be performed using a fixed time step particle filtering algorithm, as explained next.

7.2.3 Particle Filtering

Particle Filtering is the sequential Monte Carlo method by which we infer the most probable states of the DBN nodes. In this work, a standard particle filtering algorithm developed for control theory by Gordon et al. [38] is used.

A particle contains a value for every node in the network in both the current and previous time slice. Thus, each particle has values instantiating all nodes in the network, where each node is consistent with all other nodes and with the evidence (nodes for which actual values are observed). Taken together, the particles can be used to assess most likely values of nodes and their distributions.

Where an observation exists at the current time slice, its value is used, otherwise a random value is chosen from the nodes distribution. Each particle is weighted to determine the probability of this set of node values given the observations. For each time slice the particles are summarized to return the weighted mean and weighted standard deviation for each node. Prior to processing the next time slice, the set of particles are re-sampled, i.e. individual particles are either multiplied or suppressed. The probability that a sample is selected is proportional to its weight. Higher-weight samples will spawn multiple copies, whereas lower-weight samples will die-off. The purpose of the re-sampling step is to focus the set of samples on the high-probability regions of the state space. The standard algorithm uses fixed time steps. As will be shown later, this can sometimes be inefficient. In Sect. 7.5, we present an alternative, that adapts the time step automatically as required.

7.3   Recent Approaches to Probabilistic Medical Knowledge Representation

BNs and DBNs have previously been used in the medical setting. An excellent introduction to the field is provided by Lucas et al. [55]. Aleks et al. [2] describe an application of DBNs to analysing ICU data. They demonstrated accurate detection and removal of artefacts in the arterial-line blood pressure sensor data. Charitos et al. [18] developed a DBN to successfully diagnose ventilator-associated pneumonia in ICU Patients. Research from the MIMIC II project includes applying a Kalman Filter to estimate blood pressure and heart rate derived from the ABP waveform in the presence of high levels of persistent noise and artefact [53], using a Bayesian Network to estimate fluid requirements in the ICU [16] and using a Bayesian network to model the cardiovascular system [62]. These BNs and DBNs have mostly only used discrete variables; our work contains both discrete and continuous variables.

Techniques have been developed to learn both BN and DBN structure and parameters from data. More recently techniques for combining expert knowledge and automated learning for building BN structure [35, 61] have been published. However most models, including the ones noted here, are manually constructed using knowledge elicited from domain experts [22, 55]. This is a time consuming task [35, 55]. Knowledge elicitation therefore remains a bottleneck; this is clear in the paper of van Gerven et al. [37], for example, which provides an excellent demonstration of the steps required to build a DBN model for prognosis of carcinoid patients. In order to bypass this bottleneck, our PRIM methodology automatically constructs DBNs from mathematical models, since mathematical models can be considered to embody existing expert knowledge. Chase et al. provide a strong argument for using physiological mathematical models in the critical care environment [21] and give examples where physiological models already form the basis of applications to manage sedation [64], cardiovascular diagnosis and therapy [66], mechanical ventilation [67], and the diagnosis of sepsis [12]. They argue that mathematical models offer significant physiological insight into patient status and behaviour.

Work has previously been carried out using mathematical models in both Bayesian Networks and DBNs. Bellazzi et al. [7] provide a good comparison of some of these methods. While some focus on predicting individual model parameters which are then used off-line [6] others discretise the state-space [42] and so do not explicitly incorporate the model equations in their original form. Voortman et al. [72] propose building causal graphs from time-series data and exploiting the ODEs to impose constraints on the model structure. In the separate, but related, topic of simulating human physiology, Abkai and Hesser [1] recognised the benefits of using both deterministic and probabilistic models. However unlike our approach which is explained in Sect. 7.4, they separate the ordinary differential equation solvers and the DBN models.

Evers and Lucas [33] recently proposed constructing DBNs for Linear Dynamic Systems. They too recognise that using existing models can significantly reduce the knowledge engineering effort required when building DBNs. Linear Dynamic Systems are amenable to efficient simulation, since the exact solution is available in a closed form. In contrast, the PRIM framework deals with non-linear systems which typically cannot be solved exactly, and so must be treated using numerical solvers as will be explained in Sect. 7.4.

Anderson and Højbjerre [4] have shown the use of SDEs (Stochastic Differential Equations) in combination with graphical models. They reworked the Minimal Model of Bergman et al. [11] into a DBN model. They transformed the Bergman model into SDEs and in a similar manner to this work, they then used a graphical model to estimate the model parameters and handle measurement uncertainty. In the SDE formulation, noise appears explicitly as a term in the equation. The solution is understood to be itself a stochastic process. To simulate such solutions numerically, one may use methods such as the Euler-Maruyama approach (see, e.g., [49]) to generate approximate solutions for a given set of random walks representing the Wiener processes. The approach used in PRIM is more direct; the model is given in the form of deterministic ODEs and mapped directly to the DBN which then incorporates the effects of noise, and generates solutions using a numerical technique such as the (standard) Euler approach. The PRIM approach does not require a transformation of a system of ODEs to SDEs prior to constructing the DBN. This is important because the vast majority of the mathematical models available are structured as ODEs, not SDEs.

7.4 Building a Probabilistic Framework with Mathematical Models

Typically mathematical models, in the form of ordinary differential equations, describe general population-level behaviours. In order to describe individuals, model parameters must be re-calibrated using observations of the individual. However, in most real-life situations, these observations contain uncertainty. They can be subject to measurement error or simple transcription errors. Data may be missing. Relevant quantities may not be measured or recorded. Observations may be sparse relative to the dynamics of the underlying system thus making it difficult to individualise the parameters.

Our probabilistic approach, using DBNs, offers an efficient framework for re-estimating model parameters dynamically over time, based on accumulated evidence. The knowledge elicitation bottleneck associated with manual DBN construction is bypassed by basing the DBN on readily available ODE models.

Next we show our methodology for automatically constructing a DBN framework from a given ODE model.

7.4.1 Methodology for Constructing DBNs from ODEs

When using ODEs to model any non trivial real-world situation, it is usually the case that the systems are so complex that the solution is not available in a closed form. Instead, numerical methods that estimate the solution at discrete points in time are employed. The simplest technique for initial value problems (IVPs) is Euler's method, see for example, [45].

Consider the following IVP: find $N(t)$ such that $N(t_0)$ is given, and

$$\frac{dN}{dt} = f(N, t) = f(N, t; A, P_1, P_2, \ldots, P_m), \quad \text{for all} \quad t > t_0,$$

where N may be scalar-valued (for a single equation) or vector-valued (for a coupled system). Other terms in f are a time-varying coefficient A and model parameters $P_1, \ldots, P_m$.

We will find approximations to N at times $t_1, t_2, t_3, \ldots$. Let us denote by N_i the approximate for $N(t_i)$. Setting $h_i = t_{i+1} - t_i$, Euler's method is

$$N_{i+1} = N_i + h_i f(N_i, t_i) \quad \text{for} \quad i = 0, 1, \ldots. \tag{7.3}$$

Thus the rate of change of N at step i is

$$f(N_i, t_i) = \frac{N_{i+1} - N_i}{h_i} =: \Delta N_i, \tag{7.4}$$

and we can rewrite (7.3) as

$$N_{i+1} = N_i + h_i \Delta N_i \quad \text{for} \quad i = 0, 1, \ldots. \tag{7.5}$$

This approximation is first-order accurate in the sense that error, $|N(t_i) - N_i|$, is proportional to $\max |h_i|$.

Fig. 7.4 Nodes N and ΔN
are deterministic nodes
implementing Eqs. (7.4) and
(7.5) respectively. Solid
arrows connect nodes within
a time slice; dashed arrows
connect nodes between time
slices.

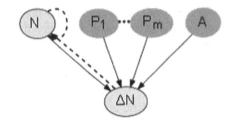

When we map the ODEs to a DBN, we set the DBN's discrete time steps to be duration h_i also. We encapsulate an Euler approximation by mapping Eqs. (7.4) and (7.5) directly to two deterministic nodes, ΔN and N in the DBN, as illustrated in Fig. 7.4.

As the figure shows, Node ΔN is a deterministic node, and its parent nodes are set to be all the terms needed to solve $f(N_i, t_i)$, in the same time slice of the DBN.

Node N is also a deterministic node. In each time slice, it evaluates the current value of N_{i+1} using Eq. (7.5), hence its parents are set to be itself and node ΔN from the previous time slice. (Note that inter-time slice arcs are shown in dashed arrows in Fig. 7.4.)

In the DBN, the model parameters, $P_1, \ldots, P_m$, are represented as continuous nodes. This procedure may be applied to a system of ODEs, by creating a sub-net for each equation and adding dependencies between them, as dictated by terms appearing in the equations.

7.4.2 Expanding the DBN to Represent Measurement Uncertainty

The DBN provides a natural framework to reason with noisy data. The observed value of the variable to be approximated is assumed to contain a certain amount of measurement error. As can be seen in Fig. 7.5, each observed measurement (for

Fig. 7.5 Extra evidence
nodes (black) are added to
model the relationship
between observed and true
values.

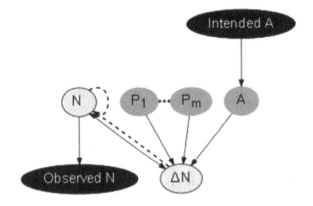

example *ObservedN*) is modelled as a continuous distribution whose mean is its parent node (N), the true variable value and whose standard deviation represents the measurement uncertainty. Similarly, each actual input (A) to a system differs from the intended input (*IntendedA*), which is observed, and so a clear distinction is created in the DBN. The true value (A) is represented as a conditional distribution whose mean is the intended value.

7.4.3 Expanding the DBN to Re-Estimate Parameters

Model parameters $P_1, \ldots, P_m$, are allowed to vary over time. In Fig. 7.6, they are represented as continuous nodes. Distributions on the initial state model can be viewed as the distribution of the population values. These population values can be learned from the data or obtained from the published literature. All model parameters are allowed to vary in each time step by including a conditional dependency on its value in the previous time, as shown in Fig. 7.6; they can therefore converge to values appropriate to the individual case over time, based on evidence from the temporal data stream.

7.4.4 Selection of DBN Parameters

As noted in Sect. 7.4.3 above, model parameters are represented as continuous nodes and the initial state model distribution can be viewed as the distribution of the population values. These population values are often published along with the ODE models and can therefore be taken from the literature. In the case where there are no published values, the parameters can be learned from the data. Using data from a large number of subjects, both the sensor model and the transition model parameters can be learned using an Expectation Maximization (EM) algorithm [25].

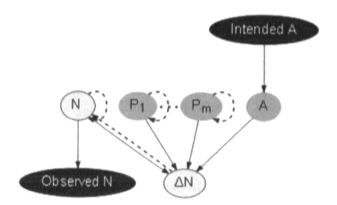

Fig. 7.6 Extra inter-slice arcs on nodes $P_1, \ldots, P_m$ to allow parameters to be tuned to the evidence over time.

7.4.5 Handling Numerical Errors

In previous work we evaluated the approach on abstract models where the true solution is known [29, 30]. We found that in the cases where data error dominates over numerical error, the most accurate results are obtained using a minimal number of time steps. The time step length should be chosen small enough to ensure stability of the underlying ODE model, but as large as possible to ensure a minimal number of steps in between observations.

The Euler method presented above is first-order accurate in the sense that the numerical error is proportional to $h_i = t_{i+1} - t_i$. Therefore, decreasing h_i reduces the numerical error, but of course leads to increased run times. A standard technique for obtaining a more accurate solution while using the same step size is to use a higher order method. We have looked at how a higher order solver, a Runge-Kutta solver, can be incorporated in our DBN framework in previous work; for details, please refer to [29, 30]. We found that incorporating an RK2 or higher order solver can increase the numerical accuracy, that is, it can reduce the error that is introduced into the simulation because we are using an approximate solution to the differential equation rather than the true solution.

In stiff examples, significant efficiency benefits are gained using the higher-order RK2 solver because larger step sizes can be used. For systems that are not stiff, there are no benefits to be gained by using higher-order schemes. In the next section, we present an approach that leads to efficiency improvements in both stiff and non-stiff problems.

7.5 Adaptive-Time Particle Filtering

Inference in DBNs is often carried out using a standard fixed-time step particle filtering algorithm [38]. Careful consideration must be given to step-size selection. The step size must be chosen to be sufficiently small so that numerical error is not significant. However, reducing step sizes results in increased computation, so a balance must be struck between a practical run-time and numerical accuracy. As has been noted earlier, for non-stiff systems this is not necessarily a concern; however, for stiff problems very small step sizes may be required and inference quickly becomes inefficient. An alternative approach, that involves adapting the step size according to the dynamics at each step, is therefore proposed.

We have proposed an algorithm for particle filtering that allows for non-fixed step sizes [30]. We call this algorithm Adaptive-Time Particle Filtering. It is comprised of two parts, as described in the sub-sections to follow. First, an approach where each particle is allowed adapt the step size independently according to its own dynamics is presented. Once we have a scheme that allows for variable time steps, we implement a mechanism for automatically choosing those time steps.

7.5.1   Adapting the Time Step

In the standard fixed-time step DBN, when filtering and prediction are carried out, the results are reported at each step. With our Adaptive-Time Particle Filtering, the user can specify the intervals at which the results should be reported. In certain situations, the adaptive algorithm may choose very small step sizes to capture rapidly changing dynamics, for example 0.01 min, but the user may only be interested in the predicted values at a larger time interval, for example, every 10 min. The user can specify this summary interval or a set of summary times. Each particle is propagated independently to the next summary time, allowing each particle adapt the step size for the dynamics that result from its particular set of values. In fixed-time step particle filtering, if the granularity of the evidence time stamp does not match the fixed-time step, it must be approximated to the nearest step. One advantage of our adaptive approach is that exact time stamps can be used.

For our algorithm, evidence is divided into two types; continuous and instantaneous. Continuous evidence is defined as evidence that remains constant until a new value is reported. On the other hand, instantaneous evidence is defined as evidence with a value at a particular moment in time. Where new instantaneous evidence or changes in continuous evidence occur, a summary step is invoked. At each summary step, the particles are weighted based on the evidence, and re-sampling ensures that the samples with the higher weights are more likely to be propagated to the next step.

A formal description of the inference algorithm is shown in Algorithm 1. In the algorithm, S denotes the set of particles. The times at which summaries are reported are denoted $\{R_0, \ldots, R_K\}$. Between summaries, the time steps are $\{t_0, t_1, \ldots\}$;; note that these may be different for different particles.

7.5.2   Choosing the Step Size

The step size control mechanism used is shown in Algorithm 2. It is based on a procedure outlined by Butcher [15, §202] and demonstrated by Nhan [58], that aims

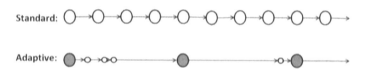

Fig. 7.7 Illustration of time-stepping in fixed step particle filtering and Adaptive-Time Particle Filtering. Traditionally, inference is performed at fixed intervals. With Adaptive-Time Particle Filtering, summary steps (gray) can be specified at any fixed interval and are used to report the values of hidden variables at regular intervals. In between summary steps, the particle filtering algorithm adjusts to use step sizes appropriate to the dynamics at each step.

Algorithm 1. Adaptive-Time Particle Filtering **returns** Q, a vector of summarised particles for each summary step

---

Inputs:
F : finish time
N : number of particles
$\{R_0, \ldots, R_K\}$ summary times
Local Variables:
S : a vector of particles of size N
W : a vector of weights of size N
Q : a vector of summarised particles
$\bar{h}$: proposed step size; $\bar{h} \leftarrow R_1 - R_0$
$t_0 = 0; i \leftarrow 0; k \leftarrow 0$

while $R_{k+1} < F$ **do**
  for $p = 1 \to |S|$ **do**
    $i \leftarrow 0$
    $t_i = R_k$
    while $t_i \leq R_{k+1}$ **do**
      repeat
        $S_p \leftarrow$ sample from $P(x_t|x_{t-1})$ {Scaled according to the step size}
        $(tol OK, \bar{h}) \leftarrow$ Check Tolerance($\bar{h}$)   {See Algorithm 2}
        if $tol OK$ **then**
          $t_{i+1} \leftarrow t_i + \bar{h}$ {Set proposed step size for the next step}
        else
          $t_i \leftarrow t_{i-1} + \bar{h}$ {Try again with a smaller step}
        end if
      until $tol OK$
      $i \leftarrow i + 1$
    end while
  end for
  $W \leftarrow P(y_{i+1}|x_{i+1})$ {Weight particles based on evidence}
  $Q \leftarrow$ summarise S based on W {Store weighted mean and standard deviation of all particles}
  $S \leftarrow$ re-sample S based on W {Select most likely particles for next iteration}
  $k \leftarrow k + 1$
end while
return Q

---

to control the truncation error introduced at each time step. To do this, we must estimate the local error. The error is estimated using the delta nodes described in Sect. 7.4. This estimated error is compared to a prescribed tolerance. If the tolerance is met, the current step is accepted and a new step size is proposed for the next step, which may be bigger. If the tolerance is exceeded, the current step is rejected and a reduced step size proposed.

In order to control the numeric error introduced at each time step, we must estimate the local error. Butcher [15] shows that a good estimate of the local error is

$$\frac{h_i^2}{2}\mathcal{E}, \quad \text{where} \quad \mathcal{E} = \frac{|(f(N_{i+1}, t_{i+1}) - f(N_i, t_i))|}{h_i}.$$

In the notation of Sect. 7.4:

$$\mathscr{E} = \frac{|\Delta N_{i+1} - \Delta N_i|}{h_i}.$$

Note, however, that for a coupled system, N is a vector valued quantity. Since we wish to control the largest error in any component in the system, we set

$$\mathscr{E} = \frac{\max |\Delta N_{i+1} - \Delta N_i|}{h_i}.$$

We aim to keep the estimated error below a prescribed tolerance, τ. If the tolerance is met, the current step is accepted and a new step size is proposed for the next step, which may be bigger or smaller.

The term $\sqrt{2\tau/\mathscr{E}}$ is an estimate of the maximum step size that would ensure the tolerance is met: any step size less than or equal to this is likely to yield a numerical approximation with the desired accuracy. So that the choice is unlikely to overestimate the step size and hence trigger an unnecessary extra step, we set the new step size to be $q\sqrt{2\tau/\mathscr{E}}$ where $q \in (0, 1)$ is a user-chosen parameter. Values in the range 0.6–0.9 work well. In our examples in this paper we set $q = 0.9$.

When the solution switches from a region in which its derivative changes rapidly to a region in which its derivative changes slowly, the algorithm will increase the step size in order to maintain efficiency. However, as noted by Butcher [15], if the step size changes rapidly then the error will be adversely affected. Therefore, we control the rate at which the step size increases with the parameter $M_1 > 1$, the maximum factor by which the current step size will be increased. The proposed step size is the smaller of the estimated step size based on achieving the desired error i.e., $q\sqrt{2\tau/\mathscr{E}}$, and $h_i M_1$. In this paper we set $M_1 = 1.5$.

If the tolerance is exceeded, the current step is rejected and a reduced step size proposed. Once again the proposed step size is estimated as $q\sqrt{2\tau/\mathscr{E}}$. To ensure a reduced step size is always recommended we introduce M_2 and set $M_2 < 1$. The algorithm recommends the smaller of the estimated step size $q\sqrt{2\tau/\mathscr{E}}$, and a factor of the current step size $h_i M_2$. In our examples in this paper we set $M_2 = 0.9$.

In [30], we present the results of sensitivity tests on q, M_1 and M_2, in summary, they show that the algorithm is reliable for any set of values satisfying $0.6 \le q \le 0.9$, $M_1 > 1$, and $M_2 < 1$.

Previously, we evaluated this approach on a test model where the true solution was known and showed that it is both efficient and easier to use than the fixed time step approaches [29, 30]. In the next section we apply this framework to monitor blood glucose levels in ICU patients.

Algorithm 2. Check Tolerance(h_i) **returns** Boolean to indicate if tolerance check passes and a proposed step size $\bar{h}$

Inputs:
h_i : previous step size
τ : Prescribed tolerance
$\Delta N_{i+1}, \Delta N_i$: Vectors of delta nodes
Local Variables:
M_1 : Maximum factor by which step size is increased
M_2 : Factor by which step size will decrease if tolerance is not met.
q : Safety factor so the step size is just less than the maximum recommended

$\mathscr{E} \leftarrow \max |\Delta N_{i+1} - \Delta N_i| / h_i$
if $\left(h_i^2 \mathscr{E}/2\right) < \tau$ **then**
   $\bar{h} \leftarrow \min\left(q\sqrt{2\tau/\mathscr{E}}, h_i M_1\right)$ {Tolerance met; suggest step size for next step}
   $tolOK = true$
else
   $\bar{h} \leftarrow \min\left(q\sqrt{2\tau/\mathscr{E}}, h_i M_2\right)$ {Tolerance not met; suggest smaller step size}
   $tolOK = false$
end if
return $(tolOK, \bar{h})$

7.6 Application to Monitoring Blood Glucose

7.6.1 Hyperglycaemia in the ICU

In an ICU, patients often experience stress-induced hyperglycaemia [56]. Kavanagh and McCowen [48] provide an excellent summary of the clinical problem. Stress-induced hyperglycaemia in ICU patients is caused by increased concentrations of stress hormones (adrenaline, growth hormone, glucocorticoid and glucagon), the use of medications such as exogenous glucocorticoids and catecholamines and the administration of intravenous dextrose, in parenteral nutrition and antibiotic solutions [56]. The consequences of elevated glucose levels may be manifested at the molecular or cellular level, combining to cause tissue abnormalities that include sepsis, impaired wound healing, and neuromyopathy (disease of both muscles and nerves) [48]. It has been shown that hyperglycaemia is associated with increased mortality and increased morbidity in critically ill patients [10].

To prevent hyperglycaemia in the ICU, exogenous insulin is administered. Due to its quick action and short half-life, intravenous (IV) insulin is the preferred choice for rapid correction of hyperglycaemia [3]. Determining the optimal target range for blood glucose and the optimal approach to controlling blood glucose levels in critically ill patients is however still a matter for debate.

Tight control of plasma glucose levels (80–110 mg/dl) has previously been demonstrated to improve outcome in a predominantly surgical population of critically ill patients [10]. In contrast, the more recent NICE-SUGAR study found a blood glucose target of less than 180 mg/dl resulted in lower mortality than did a tight target of 81–108 mg/dl [44]. Kansagara et al. [47] recently conducted a review of 21 trials, including the two mentioned above, to evaluate the benefits and harms of intensive insulin therapy (IIT) in hospitalized patients. They conclude "No consistent evidence demonstrates that IIT targeted to strict glycaemic control compared with less strict glycaemic control improves health outcomes in hospitalized patients. Furthermore, IIT is associated with an increased risk for severe hypoglycaemia". Even one episode of hypoglycaemia has been shown to increase mortality in critically ill patients [51]. Therefore, despite several trials, considerable uncertainty still exists regarding the optimal glucose range and how best to achieve it. Even when a target range is selected, achieving this target range, while preventing both hypoglycaemia and hyperglycaemia, is difficult.

7.6.1.1 Targeting a Glucose Range

As mentioned, exogenous insulin is administered intravenously to critically ill patients to regulate blood glucose levels. This insulin dosage must be balanced with the glucose that is administered both enterally (i.e. via the gastrointestinal tract) and parenterally (i.e. intravenously) as part of nutritional feeds. Blood glucose levels are measured regularly and depending on the measured glucose levels the insulin dosages are adjusted.

Typically, in a busy ICU, there are a number of ways in which glucose is measured. Most require a sample of blood to be drawn from the patient which can be uncomfortable for the patient and is labour intensive for the nursing staff. The most accurate glucose measurements are obtained by sending arterial blood samples to the laboratory for testing [19]. However there can be a time delay of many hours in getting the results. A patients condition can change dramatically in this time period. Point of Care (POC) methods are more common. Very accurate results are obtained using Arterial Blood Gas Analysers (ABG) located in the ICU [8] when the sample is analysed within 10 min of the blood draw. In some ICUs finger-stick glucose measurements are used, despite the fact that they have been shown to be inaccurate for critically ill patients [46]. Not only is the technique prone to large measurement error but poor peripheral perfusion (e.g., circulatory shock) can result in a lower glucose value in capillary than venous blood [60]. We use both lab glucose measurements and ABG glucose measurements for our analysis. The glucose level reported by the lab techniques and the ABG machines is plasma glucose. Plasma glucose is measured in mg/dl or mmol/l.

The frequency at which plasma glucose is measured is a key factor in regulating glucose [19]. Frequent, accurate, and timely glucose measurements are required for appropriate infusion dosing [19, 34]. An unstable patient may be monitored hourly, but a stable patient's glucose may only be measured every 4 h. Insulin is a very fast-acting hormone; its half-life in the blood stream is only a few minutes. Even hourly measurements could be considered infrequent when compared with the dynamics of insulin and glucose. However, the need for regular measurements must be balanced with the patients comfort and the work-load of the staff. Although continuous blood monitors are available they are expensive and not as accurate as ABG or Lab results. They are not widely used in the ICU setting [19].

7.6.1.2   Considerations When Modelling Glycaemia

Because of the importance of avoiding hyperglycaemia and hypoglycaemia and the difficulty in getting frequent accurate glucose measurements, a model that tracks and predicts a patients glucose levels in real-time is needed. There are a number of factors that must be considered in designing such a model, as described next.

Inter-Patient Variability: Substantial variability has been noted in the responses of different patients to insulin and glucose infusions [20, 43]. This is due to a variety of reasons. These include the reason for which the patient was admitted to the ICU; for example, a patient with sepsis is more likely to have hyperglycaemia than a patient who was admitted following cardiac surgery [19]. Severity of illness is known to affect glucose metabolism [54]. There may also be interactions with other medications being taken by the individual; for example, steroids can sometimes reduce insulin sensitivity [19]. Pre-existing conditions such as diabetes also affect the patients response to insulin and glucose. For such reasons, substantial variability is seen in the responses of different patients to insulin infusions. It is therefore necessary to develop a model that can be calibrated to a wide variety of patients.

Intra-Patient Instability: Patients in an ICU tend to be unstable: their individual insulin sensitivity can fluctuate as their condition changes. In fact, glucose variability has been shown to be a significant independent predictor of ICU and hospital mortality [28]. Patient parameters must therefore be continually re-estimated in real-time to account for both sudden and slow changes.

Inaccurate and Incomplete Data: As mentioned, plasma glucose measurements are subject to instrumentation error [46, 60]. There may also be inaccuracies in the recording of data. Typically results are manually entered into clinical databases. Times and quantities may be approximated or misreported. Data may be missing, e.g., glucose from medications administered in a glucose solution may not be recorded.

7.7   Probabilistic Framework to Monitor Blood Glucose

To apply the PRIM framework to the task of monitoring blood glucose, we first take an existing ODE model from the literature, incorporate it in a DBN and then reason with the data available at the bed-side. In this case, we use blood glucose measurements, administered insulin and administered glucose. The resulting methodology in shown in Fig. 7.8.

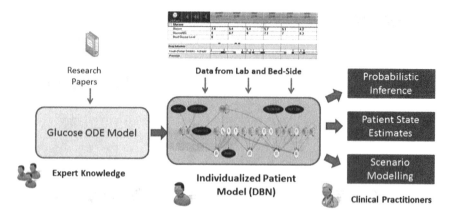

Fig. 7.8 The PRIM framework as applied to monitoring blood glucose levels

7.7.1 The System of ODEs

The starting point for constructing the DBN is the ICU-Minimal Model (ICU-MM) of Van Herpe et al. [69]. It is a model for predicting plasma glucose levels in critically ill patients who are in receipt of a glucose and insulin infusion. It is described by a system of four differential equations:

$$\frac{dG}{dt}(t) = \left(P_1 - X(t)\right)G(t) - P_1 G_b + \frac{F_G}{V_G}, \tag{7.6a}$$

$$\frac{dX}{dt}(t) = P_2 X(t) + P_3\left(I_1(t) - I_b\right), \tag{7.6b}$$

$$\frac{dI_1}{dt}(t) = \alpha \max\left(0, I_2(t)\right) - n(I_1(t) - I_b) + \frac{F_I}{V_I}, \tag{7.6c}$$

$$\frac{dI_2}{dt}(t) = \beta\gamma\left(G(t) - h\right) - n I_2(t). \tag{7.6d}$$

Here, G is the plasma glucose level, X is the effect insulin has on the plasma glucose, I_1 is the plasma insulin level and I_2 the endogenous insulin produced by the pancreas. A detailed description of the model terms can be found in Van Herpe et al. [69].

7.7.2 The DBN Derived from the ODEs

Using our procedure, that was described in Sect. 7.4, the DBN structure is derived from the ICU-MM. Each equation is mapped to a subnet in the DBN. The DBN contains both hidden and observed nodes. Hidden (continuous or discrete) random nodes are dark grey, observed nodes are black and deterministic nodes are light grey.

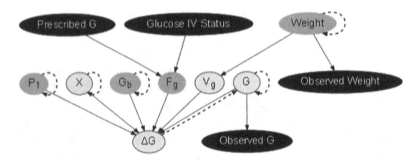

Fig. 7.9 Subnet of DBN for Eq. (7.6a) of ICU-MM

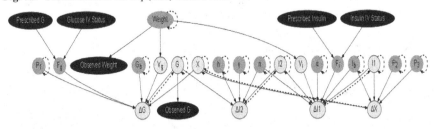

Fig. 7.10 The ICU-MM system of differential equations mapped to a DBN.

Delta nodes capture changes in quantities over time. These changes are calculated using the differential equations of the ICU-MM (7.6). Each delta node has, as parent nodes, the various terms needed to solve the appropriate differential equation.

To illustrate this, Fig. 7.9 shows the section of the DBN that is related to Eq. (7.6a) of the ICU-MM. Here, the ΔG node determines the per time step change in plasma glucose levels. The current plasma glucose level is determined based on the glucose level and ΔG calculated in the previous time slice. Each of the terms in the differential equation for G is represented as a parent node of ΔG.

The DBN is expanded as described in Sect. 7.4. Model parameters are allowed to vary over time. Their initial mean values are based on the literature [41, 68–70]. Each model parameter is allowed to vary in each time step by including a conditional dependency on its value in the previous time. In this way, they can converge to values appropriate to the individual case over time, based on the evidence. The model parameter means are shown, along with the standard deviations for the initial state and transition models, in Table 7.1.

Model parameters are represented as truncated Gaussian nodes, in order to constrain the DBN to postulate values that are not unrealistic for nodes. For example, the true value for P_1 cannot be a negative value, only positive values are possible.

Limits were also placed on some deterministic nodes using min/max functions. For example, it is not possible to have a negative quantity of glucose in plasma, so a limit is placed on node G to reflect this.

The observed value for plasma glucose (*Observed G* in the DBN) is assumed to contain a certain amount of measurement error. It is therefore modelled with a

Table 7.1 Conditional probability tables for the model parameters of the ICU-MM.

Node	Mean	Standard deviation		Range
		Initial state model	Transition model	
G_b	G_0	40	0.05	0+
I_b	$-13 + 0.22 \times IBW_R$ (see[a])	5	0.005	0+
P_1	-0.0131 per min	0.013	0.005	-1:0
P_2	-0.0135 per min	0.013	0.002	-1:0
P_3	2.9E-6 ml/(min2U)	2.0E-6	1.0E-6	0:1
h	136 mg/dl	30	0.1	0:360
n	0.013 per min	0.1	0.001	0:1
α	3.11	0.5	0.01	0+
γ	0.00536 per min	1.0E-5	1.0E-5	0:1
$Weight$	$Observed\ Weight_0$	1	0.1	0+

[a] IBW_R as defined in [68] refers to the body weight relative to the ideal body weight (defined in the Metropolitan Life Insurance Tables) expressed as a percentage

Gaussian distribution whose mean is its parent node, the actual plasma glucose level, G. Likewise, the data from the ICU reflects the prescribed intravenous infusion rates for insulin and glucose; the actual administered rates may be different. Therefore, the actual rates are modelled with Gaussian distributions whose means are the prescribed rates. I.V. status nodes are introduced to indicate if the patient is in receipt of an infusion. When the I.V status is on, the actual rates are modelled with Gaussian distributions whose means are the prescribed rates. In this way, data uncertainty is handled. When the I.V status is off, the actual rates are zero; they do not differ from the prescribed rates. Note that while we use Gaussian distributions in this model, other distributions could be used where suitable.

In a similar manner, a subnet for each of the other Eqs. (7.6b–7.6d) is added to the DBN. The full DBN is shown in Fig. 7.10.

The nodes V_g and V_i are modelled as deterministic nodes. Their values are calculated as $1.6 \times weight$ and $120 \times weight$ respectively.

7.7.3 Evaluation

7.7.3.1 Description of the Data

For comparative evaluation of the methods, data was used from patients in the ICU of University Hospital Galway (UHG). Two distinct datasets were used. Firstly data from historical patient records were used. The dataset was previously described in [32]. The patients were not on specific insulin therapy trials, so the dataset only contains routine measurements. Accordingly, plasma glucose measurements are infrequent and sporadic. At times, changes in the plasma glucose cannot be explained with the data available; this may be because either information is incomplete (e.g., if the patient was administered glucose that was not recorded) or measurements are inaccurate (e.g., due to data-entry errors or measurement assay). However, this dataset provides a realistic sample of the routine data available in a busy ICU where a system, such as the one described here, could eventually be deployed for patient monitoring and simulations of the effects of therapies. Data from patients with the following characteristics was selected:

- Sepsis as a primary diagnosis
- Non-diabetic
- Not in receipt of steroids
- No major organ failure
- Only in receipt of parenteral nutrition.

The second dataset, a subset of which was first used in [31], was actively gathered rather than being drawn from historical patient records. Once again the patients were not on specific insulin therapy trials. Glucose measurements were taken hourly for a 12 h period for 9 patients. Care was taken to ensure the correct time stamp was entered on all relevant data records. As the medical student taking the extra measurements was only available for a short period of time, the patient selection criteria were relaxed. The patient characteristics for this group were:

- Sepsis as a primary diagnosis
- Non-diabetic
- No major organ failure

Permission for extracting and gathering this data was given by the Galway Research Ethics Committee, UHG. All records were anonymised and stored on encrypted drives.

7.7.3.2   Results from Monitoring for an Individual Patient

For the purposes of this discussion, a reasonably stable patient (Patient 30) from the first dataset is selected. Inference is performed using adaptive-time particle filtering.

As can be seen in Fig. 7.11, the observations for plasma glucose are intermittent; the DBN therefore makes internal predictions of plasma glucose levels in between observations. The accuracy of the predictions can be evaluated by comparing the predicted value at the time of a measurement to the actual value, prior to the DBN incorporating the actual value as evidence. It should be noted that the measurement may not be perfectly accurate. For example, at approximately 34 h the glucose measurement jumps to over 200 mg/dl despite the fact that there is no change in the infusions. It is likely that this, and the drop to 130 mg/dl at approximately 43 h, are both incorrect measurements.

In Fig. 7.11, the dark lines are the mean values inferred by the DBN at each minute, and the lighter shaded areas show one standard deviation, to give a sense of the uncertainty associated with each prediction. One can observe that the mean value often jumps when a new observation becomes available. There are factors that are not captured in the model that influence plasma glucose levels. Because of these, mean values predicted by the model can drift from reality in between observations. When a new observation is available, the model tends to realign with it. It is informative to consider how the standard deviations vary over time. Because the DBN always assumes variability of values over time, and because observations of plasma glucose levels are available only intermittently, as the time since the last observation increases, the range of possible values increases, so the uncertainty of the predictions also increases. Whenever an observation is provided, the DBN's plasma glucose prediction realigns to a value close to this, and its uncertainty collapses.

7.7.3.3   Comparison to ODEs with Parameter Re-Estimation

Van Herpe et al. re-estimate the model parameters by using an unconstrained non-linear optimisation algorithm [52]. Attempts to apply that specific approach on our dataset, which has less frequent evidence, were unsuccessful; the optimisation algorithm frequently failed to converge. Therefore, a variant on the method is used [26]

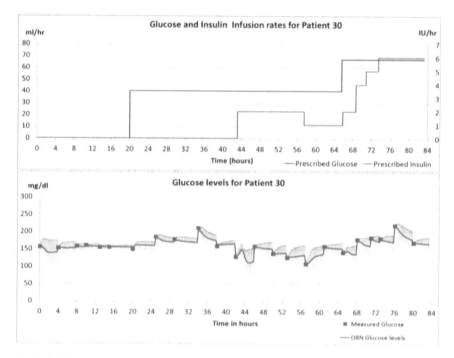

Fig. 7.11 The top graph shows the prescribed insulin and glucose infusion rates. The lower graph shows the measured glucose levels as boxes and the predicted mean plasma glucose level in blue along with a shaded area showing the predicted standard deviation.

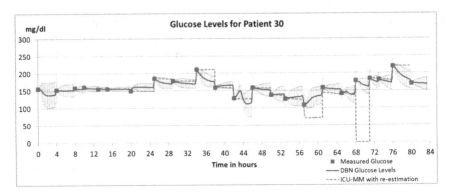

Fig. 7.12 The glucose predictions from the DBN compared to an Euler approximation with an optimisation algorithm for parameter re-estimation shown as dashed green line.

which allows bounds to be placed on the parameters to be re-estimated. As our glucose measurements are less frequent, all measurements within the previous 24 h are used each time parameters are re-estimated. The dashed line in Fig. 7.12 shows the trajectory for the ODEs with re-estimation.

It can be observed in Fig. 7.12 that the Euler approximation with the optimisation algorithm performs rather poorly for patient 30. The set of parameters selected by the algorithm do not allow the model to respond to the changes in the infusions. At 68 h, it predicts a glucose level of zero which is not realistic.

7.7.3.4   DBN Results for Twelve Patients

Figure 7.13 and Table 7.2 show a comparison of the average root mean squared error, calculated using the difference between the actual glucose measurements and glucose predictions, for twelve ICU patients, chosen at random. In 10 out of 12 cases our DBN method out-performs the other method, very substantially so in some cases, such as Patient 101, where the ODE solution gives an error of 48.57 % but our DBN method produces a much lower error of 12.28 %. In the case of Patient 60, the optimisation algorithm could not find appropriate parameters, whereas the DBN framework was able to make predictions, albeit with a high RMSE of 37.05 %. Hence the ODE result for P60 is not plotted in Fig. 7.13.

It should be noted that while we are comparing the RMSE of predictions relative to measured values, the measured values are not always perfectly accurate.

These results highlight the advantages of incorporating the ODE system in a DBN framework. The DBN framework adjusts parameters as soon as it receives the first piece of evidence, in contrast to methodologies that require a calibration window containing a number of observations. The DBN reacts to both gradual and sudden changes in model parameters as it tracks a range of possible trajectories.

Table 7.2 Average RMSE for 12 patients, comparing results using a DBN with adaptive-time steps and the results from the Euler approximation with parameter re-estimation.

Patient	RMSE	
	ICU-MM DBN	ODE with Re-estimation
P23	11.42 %	16.17 %
P91	20.28 %	41.18 %
P30	17.00 %	33.33 %
P40	32.83 %	45.49 %
P61	15.03 %	19.90 %
P24	16.45 %	29.60 %
P64	7.43 %	17.81 %
P09	17.39 %	20.40 %
P01	24.54 %	21.41 %
P102	12.58 %	19.19 %
P101	12.28 %	48.57 %
P60	37.05 %	NaN
Average	18.69 %	

The framework accounts for data uncertainty and model uncertainty in a principled manner.

By performing inference with the Adaptive-Time Particle Filter introduced in Sect. 7.5, these benefits are gained much more efficiently.

While 60 1-minute time steps are required per patient per hour using the standard fixed time steps approach, an average of 12 adaptive time steps per patient per hour are executed by the adaptive algorithm. The average number of steps executed per

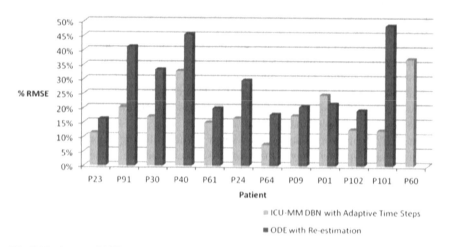

Fig. 7.13 Average RMSE for 12 patients, comparing results using a DBN with adaptive-time steps and the results from the Euler approximation with parameter re-estimation.

Table 7.3 Average number of adaptive steps per hour for each patient compared to 60 fixed 1-minute step: this shows that the new adaptive time step algorithm yields significant time savings.

Fixed steps	P23	P91	P30	P40	P61	P09	P01	P64	P24	P101	P102	P60
60	12	14	11	12	13	13	11	17	10	9	12	14

patient per hour is shown in Table 7.3. The fixed time step approach requires 5 times the number of adaptive time steps. Using the adaptive time approach inference is performed much more efficiently without compromising the accuracy of the predictions. In general, analysing data from sensor streams in real time imposes computational constraints because data must be processed as they arrive, so time savings like this can be important.

7.8 Conclusions

This chapter has discussed recent advances in representing background knowledge, representing new data, and reasoning with both background knowledge and new data, in order to enable real-time inference and decision making.

Much knowledge of human physiology is formalised as systems of differential equations. In this chapter we have described recent work for making use of this knowledge in a probabilistic framework (PRIM) that can be used to monitor patients in real-time.

The PRIM methodology is applied to monitor critically ill patients plasma glucose levels in response to insulin and glucose infusions. With the data available, which is sporadic and may be inaccurate and incomplete, the framework out-performs a previous approach demonstrating that the method is effective at re-estimating model parameters and reasoning with sparse and potentially unreliable data.

PRIM adjusts parameters as soon as it receives the first piece of evidence, in contrast to methodologies that require a calibration window containing a number of observations. It reacts to both gradual and sudden changes in model parameters as it tracks a range of possible trajectories. It accounts for data uncertainty and model uncertainty in a principled manner.

The PRIM framework also includes a new particle filtering algorithm that uses time steps that adapt according to the dynamics at each time step. In fact, each particle follows its own adaptive-time scheme, leading to advantages in both efficiency and accuracy. In fast-slow systems, there are periods where very small steps must be used to capture rapidly changing dynamics, but large steps are more suitable during periods of slow change. No one step size is optimal. In examples where the underlying ODE system is stiff and fixed step sizes are being used, they must be very small. This quickly becomes very inefficient even when using solvers of orders higher than one. Our adaptive-time particle filtering algorithm addresses these inefficiencies by allowing the time step size to adapt automatically. Another advantage in the adaptive approach is that time steps are automatically aligned with the exact time stamp of the evidence. In traditional fixed time step approaches, evidence must be approximated to the nearest fixed step, introducing further uncertainty.

By combining the knowledge available in existing data streams with the expert knowledge available in the form of differential equations and an efficient inference method, we believe that this can provide a powerful foundation for reasoning with uncertain and sparse data in the medical domain.

Acknowledgments This material is based upon works supported by the Science Foundation Ireland under Grant No. 08/RFP/CMS1254.

References

1. Abkai, C., Hesser, J.: Virtual intensive care unit (ICU): real-time simulation environment applying hybrid approach using dynamic bayesian networks and ODEs. Stud. Health Technol. Inform. **142**, 1–6 (2009)
2. Aleks, N., et al.: Probabilistic detection of short events, with application to critical care monitoring. In: Proceedings of NIPS 2008: 22nd Annual Conference on Neural Information Processing Systems, pp. 49–56, Vancouver, Canada (2008)
3. Alexanian, S.M., McDonnell, M.E., Akhtar, S.: Creating a perioperative glycemic control program. In: Anesthesiology Research and Practice (2011)
4. Andersen, K.E., Højbjerre, M.: A bayesian approach to bergmans minimal model. In: Proceedings of the Ninth International Workshop on Artificial Intelligence and Statistics, pp. 236–243 (2003)
5. Barbini, E., et al.: A comparative analysis of predictive models of morbidity in intensive care unit after cardiac surgery part I: model planning. BMC Med. Inform. Decis. Mak. **7**, 35 (2007)
6. Bellazzi, R.: Drug delivery optimization through bayesian networks. In: Proceedings of the Annual Symposium on Computer Application in Medical Care, pp. 572–578. American Medical Informatics Association (1992)
7. Bellazzi, R., Magni, P., De Nicolao, G.: Dynamic probabilistic networks for modelling and identifying dynamic systems: a MCMC approach. Intell. Data Anal. **1**, 245–262 (1997)
8. Bénéteau-Burnat, B., et al.: Evaluation of the blood gas analyzer gem PREMIER 3000. Clin. Chem. Lab. Med. **42**, 96–101 (2004)
9. Berg, H.V.D.: Mathematical Models of Biological Systems. Oxford University Press, Oxford (2011)
10. Van den Berghe, G., et al.: Intensive insulin therapy in critically ill patients. N. Engl. J. Med. **345**(19), 1359 (2001)
11. Bergman, R.N., Phillips, L.S., Cobelli, C.: Physiologic evaluation of factors controlling glucose tolerance in man: measurement of insulin sensitivity and beta-cell glucose sensitivity from the response to intravenous glucose. J. Clin. Invest. **68**, 1456–1467 (1981). PMC370948
12. Blakemore, A., et al.: Model-based insulin sensitivity as a sepsis diagnostic in critical care. J. Diab. Sci. Technol. **2**, 468–477 (2008)
13. Britton, N.F.: Essential Mathematical Biology. Springer, London, New York (2003)
14. Buchanan, B.G., Shortliffe, E.H.: Rule Based Expert Systems: the Mycin Experiments of the Stanford Heuristic Programming Project (The Addison-Wesley series in Artificial Intelligence). Addison-Wesley Longman Publishing Co., Reading, MA (1984)
15. Butcher, J.C.: Numerical Methods for Ordinary Differential Equations, 2nd edn. Wiley, Hoboken (2008)

16. Celi, L.A., et al.: An artificial intelligence tool to predict fluid requirement in the intensive care unit: a proof-of-concept study. Crit. Care **12**(6), R151 (2008)
17. Cevenini, G., et al.: A comparative analysis of predictive models of morbidity in intensive care unit after cardiac surgery part II: an illustrative example. BMC Med. Inform. Decis. Mak. **7**, 36 (2007)
18. Charitos, T., et al.: A dynamic bayesian network for diagnosing ventilator-associated pneumonia in ICU patients. Expert Syst. Appl. **36**(2), 1249–1258 (2009)
19. Chase, J.G., et al.: Model-based glycaemic control in critical care a review of the state of the possible. Biomed. Signal Process. Control **1**(1), 3–21 (2006)
20. Chase, J.G., et al.: Tight glycemic control in critical care - the leading role of insulin sensitivity and patient variability: a review and model-based analysis. Comput. Methods Programs Biomed. **102**, 156–171 (2011)
21. Chase, J.G., et al.: Physiological modeling, tight glycemic control, and the ICU clinician: what are models and how can they affect practice? Ann. Intensive Care **1**, 11 (2011)
22. Chatterjee, S., Russell, S.: Why are DBNs sparse? In: International Conference on Artificial Intelligence and Statistics, pp. 81–88, Sardinia (2010)
23. Chen, H.Y., et al.: Prediction of tacrolimus blood levels by using the neural network with genetic algorithm in liver transplantation patients. Ther. Drug Monit. **21**(1), 50–56 (1999)
24. Dean, T., Kanazawa, K.: A model for reasoning about persistence and causation. Comput. Intell. **5**(2), 142–150 (1989)
25. Dempster, A.P., et al.: Maximum likelihood from incomplete data via the EM algorithm. J. R. Stat. Soc. Ser. B (Methodological) **39**(1), 1–38 (1977)
26. D'Errico, J.: Matlab function fminsearchbnd (2006)
27. Domingos, P.: Toward knowledge-rich data mining. Data Min. Knowl. Disc. **15**, 21–28 (2007)
28. Egi, M., et al.: Variability of blood glucose concentration and short-term mortality in critically ill patients. Anesthesiology **105**, 244–252 (2006)
29. Enright, C.G.. A Probabilistic Framework Based on Mathematical Models with Application to Medical Data Streams. Ph.D thesis, National University of Ireland, Galway (2012)
30. Enright, C.G., et al.: Bayesian networks for mathematical models: techniques for automatic construction and efficient inference. Int. J. Approximate Reasoning **54**, 323–342 (2013)
31. Enright, C.G., Madden, M.G., Madden, N., Laffey, J.G.: Clinical time series data analysis using mathematical models and DBNs. In: Peleg, M., Lavrač, N., Combi, C. (eds.) AIME 2011. LNCS, vol. 6747, pp. 159–168. Springer, Heidelberg (2011)
32. Enright, C.G., et al.: Modelling glycaemia in ICU patients: a dynamic Bayesian network approach. In: Proceedings of BIOSIGNALS-2010, Part of the 3rd International Joint Conference on Biomedical Engineering Systems and Technologies, pp. 452–459, Valencia (2010)
33. Evers, S., Lucas, P.J.F.: Constructing bayesian networks for linear dynamic systems. In: The 8th Bayesian Modelling Appications Workshop, UAI 2011, pp. 26–33, Barcelona (2011)
34. Fahy, B.G., Sheehy, A.M., Coursin, D.B.: Glucose control in the intensive care unit. Crit. Care Med. **37**, 1769–1776 (2009)
35. Flores, J.M., et al.: Incorporating expert knowledge when learning bayesian network structure: a medical case study. Artif. Intell. Med. **53**, 181–204 (2011)
36. Friedman, N., Murphy, K., Russell, S.: Learning the structure of dynamic probabilistic networks. In: Proceedings of the Fourteenth Conference on Uncertainty in Artificial Intelligence, pp. 139–147 (1998)
37. van Gerven, M.A.J., Taal, B.G., Lucas, P.J.F.: Dynamic bayesian networks as prognostic models for clinical patient management. J. Biomed. Inform. **41**(4), 515–529 (2008)
38. Gordon, N.J., Salmond, D.J., Smith, A.F.M.: Novel approach to nonlinear/non-gaussian bayesian state estimation. IEE Proc. F (Radar and Signal Processing) **140**(2), 107–113 (1993)
39. Hanson III, C.W., Marshall, B.E.: Artificial intelligence applications in the intensive care unit. Crit. Care Med. **29**, 427 (2001)
40. Hart, A., Wyatt, J.: Evaluating black-boxes as medical decision aids: Issues arising from a study of neural networks. Med. Inform. **15**, 229–236 (1990)

41. Haverbeke, N., et al.: Nonlinear model predictive control with moving horizon state and disturbance estimation application to the normalization of blood glucose in the critically ill. In: Proceedings of the 17th IFAC World Congress (2008)
42. Hejlesen, O.K., et al.: DIAS the diabetes advisory system: an outline of the system and the evaluation results obtained so far. Comput. Methods Programs Biomed. **54**(1), 49–58 (1997)
43. Hovorka, R., et al.: A simulation model of glucose regulation in the critically ill. Physiol. Meas. **29**(8), 959–978 (2008)
44. The NICE-SUGAR Study Investigators.: Intensive versus conventional glucose control in critically ill patients. N. Engl. J. Med. **360**(13), 1283–1297 (2009)
45. Iserles, A.: A First Course in the Numerical Analysis of Differential Equations. Cambridge University Press, Cambridge (2008)
46. Kanji, S., et al.: Reliability of point-of-care testing for glucose measurement in critically ill adults. Crit. Care Med. **33**, 2778–2785 (2005)
47. Kansagara, D., et al.: Intensive insulin therapy in hospitalized patients: a systematic review. Ann. Intern. Med. **154**, 268–282 (2011)
48. Kavanagh, B.P., McCowen, K.C.: Glycemic control in the ICU. N. Engl. J. Med. **363**(26), 2540–2546 (2010)
49. Kloeden, P.E.: Numerical Solution of Stochastic Differential Equations, 3rd edn. Springer, Berlin, New York (1999)
50. Koller, D., Friedman, N.: Probabilistic Graphical Models: Principles and Techniques. The MIT Press, Cambridge (2009)
51. Krinsley, J.S., Grover, A.: Severe hypoglycemia in critically ill patients: risk factors and outcomes. Crit. Care Med. **35**, 2262–2267 (2007)
52. Lagarias, J.C., et al.: Convergence properties of the nelder-mead simplex method in low dimensions. SIAM J. Optim. **9**(1), 112–147 (1998)
53. Li, Q., Mark, R.G., Clifford, G.D.: Artificial arterial blood pressure artifact models and an evaluation of a robust blood pressure and heart rate estimator. BioMed. Eng. Online **8**(1), 13 (2009)
54. Lind, L., Lithell, H.: Impaired glucose and lipid metabolism seen in intensive care patients is related to severity of illness and survival. Int. J. Crit. Coron. Care Med. **5**, 100–105 (1994)
55. Lucas, P.J.F., van der Gaag, L.C., Abu-Hanna, A.: Bayesian networks in biomedicine and health-care. Artif. Intell. Med. **30**(3), 201–214 (2004)
56. McCowen, K.C., Malhotra, A., Bistrian, B.R.: Stress-induced hyperglycemia. Crit. Care Clin. **17**(1), 107–124 (2001)
57. Murphy, K.P.: Dynamic Bayesian Networks: Representation, Inference and Learning. Ph.D thesis, Department of Computer Science, UC Berkeley (2002)
58. Nhan, A.T.: Numerical solutions of models for glucose and insulin levels in critically ill patients. MA thesis, National University of Ireland, Galway, June 2011
59. Ottesen, J.T., Olufsen, M.S., Larsen, J.K.: Applied mathematical models in human physiology. In: SIAM: Society for Industrial and Applied Mathematics, 1 edn, February 2004
60. Pitkin, A.D., Rice, M.J.: Challenges to glycemic measurement in the perioperative and critically ill patient: a review. J. Diab. Sci. Technol. **3**(6), 1270–1281 (2009)
61. Radstake, N., Lucas, P.J.F., Velikova, M., Samulski, M.: Critiquing knowledge representation in medical image interpretation using structure learning. In: Riaño, D., ten Teije, A., Miksch, S., Peleg, M. (eds.) KR4HC 2010. LNCS, vol. 6512, pp. 56–69. Springer, Heidelberg (2011)
62. Roberts, J.M., et al.: Bayesian networks for cardiovascular monitoring. In: Engineering in Medicine and Biology Society, EMBS 2006, 28th Annual International Conference of the IEEE, pp. 205–209 (2006)
63. Robinson, J.W., Hartemink, A.J.: Non-stationary dynamic bayesian networks. In: Advances in Neural Information Processing Systems, pp. 1369–1376 (2008)
64. Rudge, A.D., et al.: Physiological modelling of Aagitationsedation dynamics. Med. Eng. Phys. **28**, 629–638 (2006)
65. Russell, S., Norvig, P.: Artificial Intelligence: a Modern Approach, 2nd edn. Prentice Hall, Upper Saddle River (2002)

66. Starfinger, C., et al.: Model-based cardiac diagnosis of pulmonary embolism. Comput. Methods Programs Biomed. **87**(1), 46–60 (2007)
67. Sundaresan, A., et al.: A minimal model of lung mechanics and model-based markers for optimizing ventilator treatment in ARDS patients. Comput. Methods Programs Biomed. **95**(2), 166–180 (2009)
68. Van Herpe, T.: Blood Glucose Control in Critically Ill Patients: Design of Assessment Procedures and a Control System. Ph.D thesis, Katholieke Universiteit Leuven, Belgium (2008)
69. Van Herpe, T., et al.: A minimal model for glycemia control in critically ill patients. In: Engineering in Medicine and Biology Society, EMBS 2006. 28th Annual Conference of the IEEE, pp. 5432–5435. IEEE (2006)
70. Van Herpe, T., et al.: Prediction performance comparison between three intensive care unit glucose models. In: Proceedings of the 7th IFAC Symposium on Modelling and Control in Biomedical Systems, Aalborg, Denmark (2009)
71. Van Looy, S., et al.: A novel approach for prediction of tacrolimus blood concentration in liver transplantation patients in the intensive care unit through support vector regression. Crit. Care **11**, R83 (2007)
72. Voortman, M., Dash, D., Druzdzel, M.J.: Learning why things change: the difference-based causality learner. In: Proceedings of the 26th Annual Conference on Uncertainty in Artificial Intelligence (2010)
73. Zhang, Y., Szolovits, P.: Patient-specific learning in real time for adaptive monitoring in critical care. J. Biomed. Inform. **41**(3), 452–460 (2008)

Assessment of Health
and Personalisation

Chapter 8
Personalised Medicine: Taking a New Look at the Patient

Marco Scutari

Personalised medicine strives to identify the right treatment for the right patient at the right time, integrating different types of biological and environmental information. Such information come from a variety of sources: omics data (genomic, proteomic, metabolomic, etc.), live molecular diagnostics, and other established diagnostics routinely used by medical doctors [6]. Integrating these different kinds of data, which are all high-dimensional, presents significant challenges in knowledge representation and subsequent reasoning [4, 18]. The ultimate goal of such a modelling effort is to elucidate the flow of information that links genes, protein signalling and other physiological responses to external stimuli such as environmental conditions or the progress of a disease.

Omics data, which include single-nucleotide polymorphisms (SNPs), protein and gene regulatory networks, are investigated using high-throughput platforms such as the ones developed for the Human Genome project [2, 14]. Systems biology studies the relationships among the elements in omics data as they change in the presence of genetic and environmental perturbations, extending techniques that were previously used on a smaller scale [13]. Such knowledge can improve our ability to understand and predict the behaviour of complex biological systems, but requires careful handling in integrating different sources. On its own, each type of data often contains too much noise for single biological signals to be identifiable, much less their interplay. Pooling the information available across omics data (e.g. sequencing and expression information about relevant genes, possibly under different treatment regimens) provides an option to increase statistical power and produce reliable knowledge representation models [10].

The role of live molecular diagnostics, and to some extent of traditional diagnostics, is to complement omics data with longitudinal measures of the patient's condition that are easier and cheaper to collect. Several examples of the modelling and implementation techniques involved are covered in the previous sections. Integrating such diagnostics is essential because genetic information correlate only imperfectly with protein levels [8], which in turn are very noisy predictors of most pathologies.

Applications of personalised medicine fall roughly in three groups. Firstly, drug discovery and development can be made more efficient and effective [6]. On the

© Springer International Publishing Switzerland 2015
A. Hommersom and P.J.F. Lucas (eds.), *Biomedical Knowledge Representation*, LNAI 9521, DOI 10.1007/978-3-319-28007-3_8

one hand, omics data can provide feedback at early stages of drug discovery by replacing the traditional trial-and-error approach with a hypothesis-driven one based on a formal knowledge representation model. On the other hand, omics data can also be used to improve clinical trial design by guiding patients selection and stratification based on predicted drug toxicity and non-responders profiles. This is likely to prove more effective than defining populations in terms of race or ethnicity, since only 5–10 % of the total human genetic variance occurs between different ethnic groups [1] and boundaries between different populations are often not clear.

Secondly, several aspects of the diagnostic process can be improved. For example, the normal behaviour of a biological system can be better defined at the molecular level than using non-specific clinical signs. As a result, pathologies can be classified with greater precision based on a molecular taxonomy [6]; previously unknown differences have been highlighted in breast cancer [7] and leukaemia [17] in this way. Furthermore, genetic tests need to be improved in their sensitivity and specificity; they are challenging to perform reliably and interpret correctly, and they focus predominantly on rare diseases [9].

Thirdly, personalised medicine allows treatment for many diseases to be tailored to each patient to an unprecedented degree. For example, adverse reactions to specific compounds can be predicted with greater accuracy, and non-responders can be identified without actually starting a therapy that may or may not be effective.

To investigate and implement personalised medicine in practice, many challenges need to be overcome at the modelling level; some of them will be covered in the following chapter. First and foremost, a working knowledge representation model must be established to facilitate reasoning on high-dimensional, heterogeneous data. Currently, probabilistic graphical models (Bayesian networks in particular) seem to be a popular approach [3, 5, 12]. Their ability to provide at the same time an intuitive understanding of the data to biologists and medical doctors (through the graph structure) and a rigorous probabilistic framework to statisticians and computer scientists makes them an ideal tool for this task.

Moreover, specific distributional assumptions are required to accurately describe both omics and diagnostics data effectively. Gaussian and discrete Bayesian networks from classic literature [16] present important limitations in modelling omics data, as do more general models such as chain graphs. For instance, assuming normality for gene expressions will almost certainly result in a biased model, because expression levels are usually highly skewed. Likewise, ignoring the ordering of the alleles in SNP data disregards information which is known to be fundamental in quantitative genetics. Ideally, probabilistic assumptions should also support the inclusion of available prior information from different sources, as in Schadt et al. [15].

A related issue is the computational complexity of both model estimation and subsequent inference, which poses severe limits to the use of flexible distributional assumptions in Bayesian networks and to the scope of the questions these networks can answer. The use of prior information can speed up model estimation by reducing the set of the models under consideration, even though it may introduce bias as well if the phenomenon we are modelling is not well understood. Another possible solution is to perform feature selection as a pre-processing step, thus speeding up inference as well. In the context of Bayesian networks, Markov blankets provide a natural way to do so while retaining as much information as possible [11]. However, given the complexity of the data used in personalised medicine, the cost of feature selection is often as high as that of model estimation.

In conclusion, while there are many open problems to address, an effective use of knowledge representation is crucial in implementing reliable personalised medicine protocols. Omics and other established diagnostics provide a wealth of data, which calls for appropriate modelling spanning techniques from statistics, computer science and quantitative biology.

References

1. Cavalli-Sforza, L.L., Feldman, M.W.: The application of molecular genetic approaches to the study of human evolution. Nat. Genet. **33**, 266–275 (2003)
2. Collins, F.S., Morgan, M., Patrinos, A.: The human genome project: lessons from large-scale biology. Science **300**(5167), 186–290 (2003)
3. Cooper, G.F., et al.: An efficient bayesian method for predicting clinical outcomes from genome-wide data. In: AMIA Annual Symposium Proceedings, pp. 127–131 (2010)
4. Emmer-Streib, F.: Personalized medicine: has it started yet? A reconstruction of the early history. Front. Genet. **3**(313), 1–4 (2013)
5. Friedman, N., Linial, M., Nachman, I.: Using Bayesian networks to analyze expression data. J. Comput. Biol. **7**, 601–620 (2000)
6. Ginsburg, G.S., McCarthy, J.J.: Personalized medicine: revolutionizing drug discovery and patient care. Trends Biotechnol. **19**(12), 491–496 (2001)
7. Golub, T.R., et al.: Molecular classification of cancer: class discovery and class prediction by gene expression monitoring. Science **286**(5439), 531–537 (1999)
8. Gygi, S.P., et al.: Quantitative analysis of complex protein mixtures using isotope-coded affinity tags. Nat. Biotechnol. **17**, 994–999 (1999)
9. Hamburg, M.A., Collins, F.S.: The path to personalized medicine. New Engl. J. Med. **363**, 301–304 (2010)
10. Ideker, T., et al.: Integrated genomic and proteomic analyses of a systematically perturbed metabolic network. Science **292**(5518), 929–934 (2001)
11. Koller D., Sahami M.: Toward optimal feature selection. In: Proceedings of the 13th International Conference on Machine Learning (ICML), pp. 284–292 (1996)
12. Mourad, R., Sinoquet, C., Leray, P.: A hierarchical bayesian network approach for linkage disequilibrium modeling and data-dimensionality reduction prior to genome-wide association studies. BMC Bioinform. **12**(16), 1–20 (2011)
13. Sachs, K., et al.: Causal protein-signaling networks derived from multiparameter single-cell data. Science **308**(5721), 523–529 (2005)
14. Sawicki, M.P., et al.: Human genome project. Am. J. Surg. **165**(2), 258–264 (1993)
15. Schadt, E.E., et al.: An integrative genomics approach to infer causal associations between gene expression and disease. Nat. Genet. **37**(7), 710–717 (2005)
16. Scutari, M., Strimmer, K.: Introduction to graphical modelling. In: Balding, D.J., Stumpf, M., Girolami, M. (eds.) Handbook of Statistical Systems Biology. Wiley, Hoboken (2011)
17. Waring, J.F., et al.: Microarray analysis of hepatotoxins in vitro reveals a correlation between gene expression profiles and mechanisms of toxicity. Toxicol. Lett. **120**(1–3), 359–368 (2001)
18. Weston, A.D., Hood, L.: Systems biology, proteomics, and the future of health care: toward predictive, preventative, and personalized medicine. J. Proteome Res. **3**(2), 179–196 (2004)

Chapter 9
Graphical Modelling in Genetics and Systems Biology

Marco Scutari

Abstract Graphical modelling in its modern form was pioneered by Lauritzen and Wermuth [43] and Pearl [56] in the 1980s, and has since found applications in fields as diverse as bioinformatics [28], customer satisfaction surveys [37] and weather forecasts [1]. Genetics and systems biology are unique among these fields in the dimension of the data sets they study, which often contain several thousand variables and only a few tens or hundreds of observations. This raises problems in both computational complexity and the statistical significance of the resulting networks, collectively known as the "curse of dimensionality". Furthermore, the data themselves are difficult to model correctly due to the limited understanding of the underlying phenomena. In the following, we will illustrate how such challenges affect practical graphical modelling and some possible solutions.

9.1 Background and Notation

Graphical models [39, 56] are a class of statistical models composed by a set $\mathbf{X} = \{X_1, X_2, \ldots, X_p\}$ of *random variables* describing the quantities of interest and a *graph* $\mathscr{G} = (\mathbf{V}, E)$ in which each *node* or *vertex* $v \in \mathbf{V}$ is associated with one of the random variables in $\mathbf{X}$. The *edges* $e \in E$ are used to express direct dependence relationships among the variables in $\mathbf{X}$. The set of these relationships is often referred to as the *dependence structure* of the graph. Different classes of graphs express these relationships with different semantics, which have in common the principle that graphical separation of two vertices implies the conditional independence of the corresponding random variables [56]. Examples most commonly found in literature are *Markov networks* [21, 72], which use undirected graphs; *chain graphs* [17], which use partially directed graphs; and *Bayesian networks* [41, 53], which use directed acyclic graphs.

In principle, there are many possible choices for the joint distribution of $\mathbf{X}$, depending on the nature of the data and the aims of the analysis. However, literature has focused mostly on two cases: the *discrete case* [33, 72], in which both $\mathbf{X}$ and the

© Springer International Publishing Switzerland 2015
A. Hommersom and P.J.F. Lucas (eds.), *Biomedical Knowledge Representation*, LNAI 9521, DOI 10.1007/978-3-319-28007-3_9

X_i are multinomial random variables, and the *continuous case* [31, 72], in which **X** is multivariate normal and the X_i are univariate normal random variables. In the former, the parameters of interest are the *conditional probabilities* associated with each variable, usually represented as conditional probability tables; in the latter, the parameters of interest are the *partial correlation coefficients* between each variable and its neighbours in $\mathcal{G}$.

The estimation of the structure of $\mathcal{G}$ is called *structure learning* [21, 39], and consists in finding the graph that encodes the conditional independencies present in the data. Ideally it should coincide with the dependence structure of **X**, or it should at least identify a distribution as close as possible to the correct one in the probability space. Several algorithms have been presented in literature for this problem. Despite differences in theoretical backgrounds and terminology, they can all be traced to three approaches: *constraint-based* (which are based on conditional independence tests), *score-based* (which are based on goodness-of-fit scores) and *hybrid* (which combine the previous two approaches). For some examples, see Castelo and Roverato [11], Friedman et al. [29], Larrañaga et al. [42] and Tsamardinos et al. [71]. All these structure learning algorithms operate under a set of common assumptions:

- there must be a one-to-one correspondence between the nodes in the graph and the random variables in **X**; this means in particular that there must not be multiple nodes which are deterministic functions of a single variable;
- observations must be independent. If some form of temporal or spatial dependence is present, it must be specifically accounted for in the definition of the network, as in *dynamic Bayesian networks* [39];
- every combination of the possible values of the variables in **X** must represent a valid, observable (even if really unlikely) event.

On the other hand, the structure of the network can also be specified from prior knowledge of the phenomenon underlying the data; in this case the graphical model implements an *expert system* [12, 16]. This is rarely done in practice, especially in genetics and systems biology, because available information are typically scarce or unreliable. It is far more common to use such information to inform the choices made by a structure learning algorithm, thus making the best use of the data [51].

The structure of a graphical model has two important properties. The first is that it defines the decomposition the probability distribution of **X**, called the *global distribution*, into a set of *local distributions*. For practical reasons, each local distribution should involve only a small number of variables when applying graphical modelling to high dimensional problems. For Bayesian networks it is related to the chain rule of probability [41]; it takes the form

$$P(\mathbf{X}) = \prod_{i=1}^{p} P(X_i \mid \Pi_{X_i}) \tag{9.1}$$

so that each local distribution is associated with a single node X_i and depends only on the joint distribution of its parents Π_{X_i}. This decomposition holds for any Bayesian network, regardless of its graph structure. In Markov networks local distributions are associated with the *cliques* $\mathbf{C}_1, \mathbf{C}_2, \ldots, \mathbf{C}_k$, the maximal subsets of nodes in which each element is adjacent to all the others:

$$P(\mathbf{X}) = \prod_{i=1}^{k} \psi_i(\mathbf{C}_i). \tag{9.2}$$

The functions $\psi_1, \psi_2, \ldots, \psi_k$ are called *Gibbs' potentials* [56], *factor potentials* [12] or simply *potentials*, and are non-negative functions representing the relative mass of probability of each clique. They are proper probability or density functions only when the graph is *decomposable* or *triangulated*, that is, when it contains no induced cycles other than triangles. In this case the global distribution factorises again according to the chain rule and can be written as

$$P(\mathbf{X}) = \frac{\prod_{i=1}^{k} P(\mathbf{C}_i)}{\prod_{i=1}^{k} P(\mathbf{S}_i)} \tag{9.3}$$

where $\mathbf{S}_i$ are the nodes of $\mathbf{C}_i$ which are also part of any other clique up to $\mathbf{C}_{i-1}$ [56].

The second important property is that the *Markov blanket* of each node can be easily identified from the structure of the graph. For instance, in Bayesian networks the Markov blanket of a node X_i is the set consisting of the parents of X_i, the children of X_i and all the other nodes sharing a child with X_i [56]. Since the Markov blanket is defined as the set of nodes that makes the target node (*i.e.* X_i) independent from all the other nodes in $\mathbf{X}$, it provides a theoretically-sound solution to the *feature selection* problem [40].

9.2 Data and Models in Statistical Genetics and Systems Biology

In genetics and systems biology, graphical models are employed to describe and identify interdependencies among genes and gene products, with the eventual aim to better understand the molecular mechanisms linking them. Data made commonly available for this task by current technologies fall into three groups:

1. gene expression data [28, 65], which measure the intensity of the activity of a particular gene through the presence of *messenger RNA* (mRNA, for protein-coding genes) or other kinds of *non-coding RNA* (ncRNA, for non-coding genes);
2. protein signalling data [58], which measure the proteins produced as a result of each gene's activity;
3. sequence data [50], which provide the nucleotide sequence of each gene. For both biological and computational reasons, such data contain mostly *single-nucleotide polymorphisms* (SNPs) – genes which vary in only one nucleotide between individuals – having only two possible alleles, called *biallelic SNPs*.

In the case of gene expression and protein signalling data (Sects. 9.2.1 and 9.2.2), we are interested in grouping them into tempporal sequences determining some molecular process (the *functional pathways*). Bayesian networks are naturally suited to this task. If we assign each gene to one node in the network, edges represent the interplay between different genes. They can describe either direct interactions or indirect influences that are mediated by unobserved genes. This is a crucial property because it is impossible in practice to completely observe a complex molecular process: either we do not know all the genes involved or we may be unable to obtain reliable measurements of all their expression levels. Furthermore, under appropriate conditions [39, 55] edge directions may be indicative of the causal relationships in the underlying pathways. In that case, the Bayesian network reflects the ordering of connections between pathway components and the actual flow of the molecular process.

Similar considerations can be made when protein signalling data are used just to identify protein-protein interactions, limiting ourselves to the study of the cell's physiology.

On the other hand, in sequence data analysis (Sect. 9.2.3) we are interested in modelling the behaviour of one or more *phenotypic traits* (*e.g.* the presence of a disease in humans, yield in plants, milk production in cows, etc.) by capturing direct and indirect causal genetic effects. Unless some prior knowledge on the *genetic architecture* of a trait is available, a large set of genes spread over the whole genome is required for such effects to be detectable. If the focus is on identifying the genes that are strongly associated with a trait, the analysis is called a *genome-wide association study* (GWAS).

Applications of Bayesian networks to sequence data are more problematic than in the previous cases; some care must be taken in their interpretation as causal models. Edges linking genes to a trait can be considered direct associations. As was the case for gene expression data, under appropriate conditions such associations may actually be indicative of real causal effects. On the other hand, edges linking genes to other genes arise from the genetic structure of the individuals in the sample. It is expected, for example, that genes that are located near each other on a chromosome are more likely to be inherited together during meiosis, and are therefore said to be *genetically linked* [22]. Furthermore, even genes that are far apart in the genome can be in *linkage disequilibrium* (LD) if some of their configurations occur more often or less often than it would be expected from their marginal frequencies. Both these phenomena induce associations between the genes, but not cause-effects relationships. From a strictly causal point of view, a chain graph in which genes are linked by undirected edges and the only directed edges are the ones incident on the traits provides a better visual representation of the network structure.

9.2.1 Gene Expression Data

Gene expression data are typically composed of a set of *intensities* measuring the abundance of several RNA patterns, each meant to probe a particular gene. These

intensities are measured either radioactively or fluorescently, using labels that mark
the desired RNA patterns [20, 46, 48].

The measured abundances present several limitations. First of all, microarrays
measure abundances only in terms of relative probe intensities, not on an absolute
scale. As a result, comparing different studies or including them in a meta-analysis
is difficult in practice without the use of rank-based methods [8]. Furthermore, even
within a single study abundance measurements are systematically biased by *batch
effects* introduced by the instruments and the chemical reactions used in collecting
the data [61].

By their nature, gene expression data are modelled as continuous random variables and are investigated using Pearson's correlation, either assuming a Gaussian
distribution or applying results from robust statistics [34, 69]. The simplest graphical models used for gene expression data are *relevance networks* [9], also known in
statistics as *correlation graphs*. Relevance networks are constructed by estimating
the correlation matrix of the genes and thresholding its elements, so that weak correlations are set to zero. Finally, a graph is drawn in order to depict the remaining
strong correlations.

Covariance selection models [19], also known as *concentration graphs* or *graphical Gaussian models* [72], consider conditional rather than marginal dependencies;
the presence of an edge is determined by the value of the corresponding *partial correlation*. In the context of systems biology, the resulting graphs are often called *gene
association networks*, and are not trivial to estimate from high-dimensional genomic

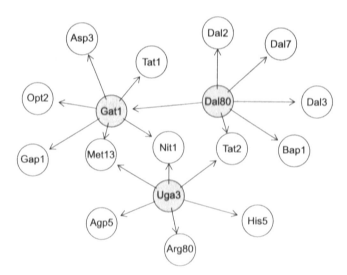

Fig. 9.1   A Bayesian network learned from gene expression data and used as an example in Friedman
[24]. Grey nodes correspond to the *regulators* of the network, the genes controlling the expression
of the other (*target*) genes involved in a molecular process.

data. Several solutions have been proposed in literature, based either on James-Stein regularisation [59, 60] or on different penalised maximum likelihood approaches [5, 23, 47].

Both gene relevance and gene association networks are undirected graphs. The application of Bayesian networks to learn large-scale directed graphs from microarray data was pioneered by Friedman *et al.* [30], and has also been reviewed more recently in Friedman [24] (see Fig. 9.1). The high dimensionality of the model, combined with low sample sizes, means that inference procedures are usually unable to identify a single best Bayesian network, settling instead on a set of equally well behaved models. For this reason, it is important to incorporate prior biological knowledge into the network through the use of informative priors [51] and to produce confidence scores in its graphical features [26, 35].

9.2.2 Protein Signalling Data

Protein signalling data are similar to gene expression data in many respects, and in fact are often used to indirectly investigate the expression of a set of genes. In general, the relationships between proteins are indicative of their physical location within the cell and of the development over time of the molecular processes they are involved in.

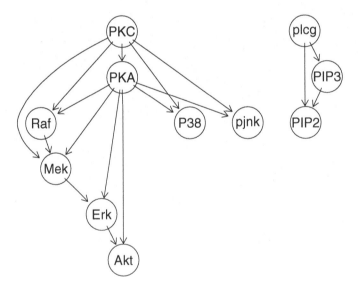

Fig. 9.2 The Bayesian network learned from the protein-signalling data in Sachs *et al.* [58] using model averaging and data from several experiments performed under different stimulatory and inhibitory cues.

From a modelling perspective, all the approaches covered in Sect. 9.2.1 can be applied to protein signalling data with little or no change. However, it is important to note that protein signalling data sometimes have sample sizes that are much larger than either gene expression or sequence data; an example is the study from Sachs et al. [58] on how to derive a causal Bayesian network from multi-parameter single-cell data (Fig. 9.2).

9.2.3 Sequence Data

Sequence data are fundamentally different from both gene expression and protein signalling data, for several reasons. First, sequence data provide direct access to the genome's information, without relying on indirect measurements. As a result, they provide a closer view of the genetic layout of an organism than other approaches. Second, sequence information is intrinsic to each individual, and does not vary over time; therefore, the inability of static Bayesian networks to model feedback loops is not a limitation in this case.

Furthermore, sequence data is naturally defined on a discrete rather than continuous domain. Each gene has a finite number of possible states, determined by the number of combinations of nucleotides differing between the individuals in the sample. In the case of biallelic SNPs, each SNP X_i differs at a single base-pair location and has only three possible variants. They are determined by the (unordered) combinations of the two nucleotides observed at that location, called the *alleles*, and are often denoted as "AA", "Aa", "aa". The "A" and "a" labels can be assigned to the nucleotides in several ways; for instance, "A" can be chosen as either the most common in the sample (which makes models easier to interpret) or by following the alphabetical order of the nucleotides (which makes the labelling independent from the sample). "AA" and "aa" individuals are said to be *homozygotes*, because both nucleotides in the pair have the same allele; "Aa" individuals are said to be *heterozygotes*.

From a graphical modelling perspective, modelling each SNP as a discrete variable is the most convenient option; multinomial models have received much more attention in literature than Gaussian or mixed ones. On the other hand, the standard approach in genetics is to recode the alleles as numeric variables, e.g.

$$X_i = \begin{cases} 1 \text{ if the SNP is "AA"} \\ 0 \text{ if the SNP is "Aa"} \\ -1 \text{ if the SNP is "aa"} \end{cases} \quad \text{or} \quad X_i = \begin{cases} 2 \text{ if the SNP is "AA"} \\ 1 \text{ if the SNP is "Aa"} \\ 0 \text{ if the SNP is "aa"} \end{cases} \quad (9.4)$$

In both cases, the recoded variables are typically modelled using an additive Bayesian linear regression model of the form

$$\mathbf{y} = \mu + \sum_{i=1}^{n} X_i g_i + \boldsymbol{\varepsilon}, \qquad\qquad g_i \sim \pi_{g_i}, \; \boldsymbol{\varepsilon} \sim N(\mathbf{0}, \Sigma) \qquad (9.5)$$

where g_i denotes the effect of gene X_i, $\mathbf{y}$ is the trait under study and μ is the population mean. The matrix Σ models the relatedness of the subjects, which is called *kinship* in genetics, and populations structure [4]. In human genetics, it is often assumed to be the identity matrix, which implies the assumptions that individuals are unrelated. Several implementations of Eq. 9.5 based on linear mixed models and penalised regressions have been proposed, mostly within the framework of Bayesian statistics. Some examples are the Genomic BLUP (GBLUP), BayesA and BayesB from Meuwissen et al. [49], the Bayesian LASSO from Park and Casella [54] and the BayesCπ from Habier et al. [18].

Graphical models, and Bayesian networks in particular, provide a systematic way to categorise and extend such models. Consider the four different models shown in Fig. 9.3. The classic additive model from Equation 9.5 is shown in the top-left panel; SNPs are independent from each other and all contribute in explaining the behaviour of the phenotypic trait. This is the case for BayesA and GBLUP. In the top-right panel, some SNPs are identified as non-significant and excluded from the additive model. Models of this kind include BayesB, BayesCπ and the Bayesian LASSO, which perform feature selection in the context of model estimation.

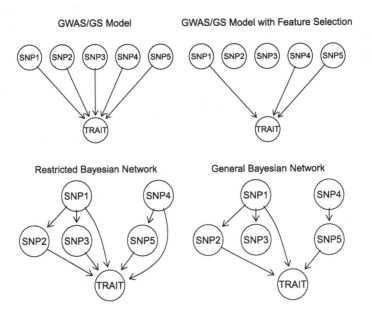

Fig. 9.3 Different approaches to GWAS. On the top, classic additive Bayesian linear regression models with and without feature selection. On the bottom, more complex models based on Bayesian networks.

A natural way to extend these models is to include interactions between the SNPs, as shown in the two bottom panels. A recent study by Morota *et al.* [50] has shown that assuming additive effects can only be justified on the grounds of computational efficiency, because interactions between the SNPs are so complex that even pairwise dependence measures are not able to capture them completely. On the other hand, Bayesian networks provide a more accurate picture of these dependencies and are more effective at capturing and displaying them. If the trait is discrete, Bayesian network classifiers [25] such as the Tree-Augmented Naïve Bayes (TAN) can also be used to implement GWAS models.

9.3 Challenges in Bayesian Network Modelling

Gene expression, protein signalling and sequence data are difficult to analyse in a rigorous and effective way regardless of the model used, as they present significant computational and statistical challenges. We review some of them in the following, concentrating on those that affect the earliest stages of model specification. Obviously, the quality of the models estimated from the data rests crucially on their structure and estimation; and the accuracy of subsequent inference may vary substantially depending on how model specification relates to the phenomena under investigation.

The combination of small sample sizes and large numbers of variables ($n \ll p$), often called the "curse of dimensionality", is perhaps the most evident problem in model specification and algorithm implementation. This is especially true for Bayesian networks, because both learning and inference are NP-hard [14, 15]. This may rise some concerns about the amount of information present in the data and in the computational complexity of model estimation (Sect. 9.3.1). The former can be tackled by effective distributional assumptions (Sect. 9.3.2), and the latter by the use of feature selection to reduce the dimensionality of the problem (Sect. 9.3.3).

9.3.1 Limits of the "$n \ll P$" Data Sets

The disparity between the available sample sizes and the number of genes or proteins under investigation is probably the most important limiting factor in genetics and systems biology. In a few cases, the underlying phenomenon is known to the extent that only the relevant variables are included in the model (Sachs *et al.* [58] is one such study). However, in general molecular processes are so complex that statistical modelling is used more as a tool for exploratory analysis than to provide mechanistic explanations. In the former case, we have that $n \gg p$, and we can use results from large-sample theory [44] and computationally-intensive techniques [6, 10] in selecting and estimating our models. In the latter, the limits of the model depend heavily on what knowledge is available on the phenomenon and on our ability to incorporate it in the prior.

Consider, following Bayes' theorem, the posterior distribution of the parameters in the model (say θ) given the data

$$p(\theta \mid \mathbf{X}) \propto p(\mathbf{X} \mid \theta) \cdot p(\theta) = L(\theta; \mathbf{X}) \cdot p(\theta) \tag{9.6}$$

or, equivalently,

$$\log p(\theta \mid \mathbf{X}) = c + \log L(\theta; \mathbf{X}) + \log p(\theta). \tag{9.7}$$

The log-likelihood, $\log L(\theta; \mathbf{X})$, is a function of the data and therefore scales with the sample size, while the prior density does not. For small sample sizes, there may not be enough data available to disprove the assumptions encoded in the prior. As a result, conclusions arising from model estimation and inference reflect our beliefs on the phenomenon (as encoded in the prior) more than the reality of the observed molecular processes. In this context, even the use of non-informative priors may result in posteriors with undesirable properties [7].

In that regard, Bayesian networks present considerable advantages. First, they are very flexible in specifying variable selection rates and interactions. In other words, the prior makes fewer assumptions on the probabilistic structure of the data and is therefore less likely to completely dominate the likelihood. Second, the effects of the values assigned to the parameters of a non-informative prior are well understood for both small and large samples [66, 67], and corrected posterior density functions are available in closed form.

Another important consideration is the ease of estimating the model. Models used in genetics and systems biology often require expensive Markov Chain Monte Carlo simulations; two such examples are BayesA and BayesB. On the other hand, many closed form results are available for both discrete and Gaussian Bayesian networks. For networks up to 100 variables, exact structure learning algorithms are available [38] and exact inference algorithms such as Variable Elimination and Clique Trees [39] are feasible to use. For larger networks, efficient structure learning heuristics such as the Semi-Interleaved Hiton-PC from Aliferis et al. [2, 3] and approximate inference algorithms such as the Adaptive Importance Sampling for Bayesian Networks (AIS-BN) from Cheng and Druzdel [13] are feasible up to several thousand variables.

9.3.2 Discrete or Continuous Variables?

All the data types covered in Sect. 9.2 are often modelled using Gaussian Bayesian networks, which represent the natural evolution of the linear regression models used in literature. In the case of gene expression and protein signalling data, sometimes [32, 58] the data are discretised into intervals and a discrete Bayesian network is used instead. As for gene expression data, both Gaussian and discrete Bayesian networks can be used depending on whether we use the numeric coding in Eq. 9.4 or not.

Clearly, both distributional assumptions present important limitations. Gaussian Bayesian networks assume that the global distribution is multivariate normal. This is unreasonable in the case of sequence data, which can only assume a finite, discrete set of values. Gene expression and protein signalling data, while continuous, are in general significantly skewed unless preprocessed with a Box-Cox transformation [73]. Furthermore, Gaussian Bayesian networks are only able to capture linear dependencies, and have a low power in detecting non-linear ones. On the other hand, using discrete Bayesian networks and assuming a multinomial distribution disregards useful information present in the data and may result in models with a very large number of parameters. If the ordering of the intervals (in discretised gene expression and protein signalling data) or of the alleles (in sequence data) is ignored, both learning and subsequent inference are not aware that dependencies are likely to take the form of stochastic trends. This is true, in particular, for sequence data, as the effect of the heterozygous allele is necessarily comprised between the effect of the two heterozygous alleles.

An approach that has the potential to outperform both discrete and Gaussian assumptions has been recently proposed by Musella [52] with Bayesian networks learned from ordinal data. Structure learning is performed with a constraint-based approach (in particular, the PC algorithm from Sprites *et al.* [64]) using the Jonckheere-Terpstra test for trend among ordered alternatives [36, 68]. Consider a conditional independence test for $X_1 \perp\!\!\!\perp X_3 \mid X_2$, where X_1, X_2 and X_3 have T, L and C levels respectively. The test statistic is defined as

$$JT = \sum_{k=1}^{L} \sum_{i=2}^{T} \sum_{j=1}^{i-1} \left[\sum_{s=1}^{C} w_{ijsk} n_{isk} - \frac{n_{i+k}(n_{i+k}+1)}{2} \right] \tag{9.8}$$

where the w_{ijsk} are Wilcoxon scores, defined as

$$w_{ijsk} = \sum_{t=1}^{s-1} \left[n_{itk} + n_{jtk} + \frac{n_{isk} + n_{jsk} + 1}{2} \right], \tag{9.9}$$

and has an asymptotic normal distribution with mean and variance defined in Lehmann [45] and Pirie [57]. The null hypothesis is that of homogeneity; if we denote with $F_{i,k}(x_3)$ the distribution function of $X_3 \mid X_1 = i, X_2 = k$,

$$H_0 : F_{1,k}(x_3) = F_{2,k}(x_3) = \ldots = F_{T,k}(x_3) \qquad \text{for } \forall x_3 \text{ and } \forall k.$$

The alternative hypothesis $H_1 = H_{1,1} \cup H_{1,2}$ is that of stochastic ordering, either increasing

$$H_{1,1} : F_{i,k}(x_3) \geqslant F_{j,k}(x_3) \qquad \text{with } i < j \text{ for } \forall x_3 \text{ and } \forall k$$

or decreasing

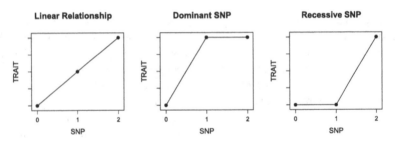

Fig. 9.4 Three patterns of SNP effects on a phenotypic trait: linear association (left), a dominant SNP (centre), a recessive SNP (right).

$$H_{1,2} : F_{i,k}(x_3) \leqslant F_{j,k}(x_3) \qquad \text{with } i < j \text{ for } \forall x_3 \text{ and } \forall k.$$

The advantages of the Jonckheere-Terpstra test compared to linear association can be illustrated, for example, by considering the different patterns of dominance of a single SNP shown in Fig. 9.4. Due to the way SNPs are recoded as numeric variables, assuming that dependence relationships are linear (left panel) forces the effect of heterozygotes to be the mean of the effects of the respective homozygotes. This is not always the case, as SNPs can be *dominant* (centre) or *recessive* (right) for a trait, either singly or in groups [22]. Tests for linear association have very low power against such nonlinear alternative hypotheses. On the other hand, the alternative hypothesis of the Jonckheere-Terpstra test characterises correctly both dominant and recessive SNPs. Furthermore, the Jonckheere-Terpstra test exhibits more power than the independence tests used in discrete Bayesian networks because of the more specific alternative hypothesis (*e.g.* stochastic ordering is just one particular case of stochastic dependence).

9.3.3 Feature Selection as a Data Pre-Processing Step

It is not possible, nor expected, for all genes in modern, genome-wide data sets to be relevant for the trait or the molecular process under study. In part, this is because of the curse of dimensionality, but it is also because different genes may provide essentially the same information due to linkage disequilibrium. Furthermore, the effects of some genes on a trait may be mediated by other genes, thus making them redundant. For this reason, in practice statistical models in systems biology and genetics require a feature selection to be performed, either during the learning process or as a separate data pre-processing step.

In the context of GWAS models, we aim to find the subset of genes $S \subset X$ such that

$$P(y \mid X) = P(y \mid S, X \setminus S) \approx P(y \mid S), \tag{9.10}$$

that is, the subset of genes (**S**) that makes all other markers (**X** \ **S**) redundant as far as the trait **y** we are studying is concerned. Markov blankets identify such a subset in the framework of graphical models; several algorithms have been proposed in literature for their learning [2, 70]. After the set **S** has been identified, we can either fit one of the Bayesian linear regression models from Sect. 9.2.3 or learn a Bayesian network from **y** and **S**. In both cases, the smaller number of variables included in the model reduces the effects of the curse of dimensionality [63]. On the other hand, the conditional independence tests used by Markov blanket learning algorithms do not take kinship into account. Therefore, interpreting edges from **S** to **y** as direct causal influences may lead to spurious results, even when the model shows good predictive power [2].

As far as gene expression and protein signalling data are concerned, the problem of feature selection is more complicated. In many cases, we are interested in a complex molecular process, as opposed to a single trait. If we don't know a priori at least some of the genes involved in the molecular process, performing feature selection as a data pre-processing step is impossible; we have to identify the pathways we are interested in from the structure of the Bayesian network learned from **X**. At most we can enforce sparsity in the network by using shrinkage tests [62] or non-uniform structural priors [27].

Even if we know which genes are involved, using Markov blankets for feature selection presents significant drawbacks. The Markov blanket of each gene must be learned separately because almost all algorithms in literature accept only one target node. If no information is shared between different runs of the learning algorithm, this task is embarrassingly parallel but still computationally intensive. If, on the other hand, we use backtracking and other optimisations to share information between different runs, significant speed-ups are possible at the cost of an increased error rate (*i.e.* false positives and false negatives among the nodes included in each Markov blanket). In both cases, merging the Markov blankets of each gene into a single set requires the use of *symmetry corrections* [2, 71] that violate the proofs of correctness of the learning algorithms.

9.4 Conclusions

Data sets in genetics and systems biology often contain several thousand variables and only a few tens or hundreds of observations. This raises problems in both computational complexity and the statistical significance of the resulting networks, which are collectively known as the "curse of dimensionality". Furthermore, the data themselves are difficult to model correctly due to the limited understanding of the underlying molecular mechanisms. Bayesian networks provide a very flexible framework to model such data, extending, complementing or replacing classic models present in literature. Their flexibility in incorporating prior knowledge, different parametric assumptions and different dependence structures makes them a suitable choice for the analysis of gene expression, protein signalling and sequence data.

References

1. Abramson, B., et al.: Hailfinder: a Bayesian system for forecasting severe weather. Int. J. Forecast. **12**(1), 57–71 (1996)
2. Aliferis, C.F., et al.: Local causal and Markov Blanket induction for causal discovery and feature selection for classification part i: algorithms and empirical evaluation. J. Mach. Learn. Res. **11**, 171–234 (2010)
3. Aliferis, C.F., et al.: Local causal and Markov Blanket induction for causal discovery and feature selection for classification part II: analysis and extensions. J. Mach. Learn. Res. **11**, 235–284 (2010)
4. Astle, W., Balding, D.J.: Population structure and cryptic relatedness in genetic association studies. Stat. Sci. **24**(4), 451–471 (2009)
5. Banerjee, O., El Ghaoui, L., d'Aspremont, A.: Model selection through sparse maximum likelihood estimation for multivariate Gaussian or binary data. J. Mach. Learn. Res. **9**, 485–516 (2008)
6. Baragona, R., Battaglia, F., Poli, I.: Evolutionary Statistical Procedures: An Evolutionary Computation Approach to Statistical Procedures Designs and Applications. Springer, Heidelberg (2011)
7. Bernardo, J.M., Smith, A.F.M.: Bayesian Theory. Wiley, Chichester (2000)
8. Breitling, R., et al.: Rank Products: a simple, yet powerful, new method to detect differentially regulated genes in replicated microarray experiments. FEBS Lett. **573**(1–3), 83–92 (2004)
9. A. J. Butte et al. "Discovering Functional Relationships Between RNA Expression and Chemotherapeutic Susceptibility Using Relevance Networks". In: PNAS 97 (2000), pp. 12182–12186. 9 Graphical Modelling in Systems Biology 165
10. Cappé, O., Moulines, E., Rydén, T.: Inference in Hidden Markov Models. Springer, Heidelberg (2005)
11. Castelo, R., Roverato, A.: A robust procedure for Gaussian graphical model search from microarray data with p larger than n. J. Mach. Learn. Res. **7**, 2621–2650 (2006)
12. Castillo, E., Gutiérrez, J.M., Hadi, A.S.: Expert Systems and Probabilistic Network Models. Springer, Heidelberg (1997)
13. Cheng, J., Druzdel, M.J.: AIS-BN: An adaptive importance sampling algorithm for evidential reasoning in large Bayesian networks. J. Artif. Intell. Res. **13**, 155–188 (2000)
14. Chickering, D.M.: Learning Bayesian Networks is NP-Complete. In: Fisher, D., Lenz, H.J. (eds.) Learning from Data: Artificial Intelligence and Statistics V Part III. LNS, pp. 121–130. Springer-Verlag, Heidelberg (1996)
15. Cooper, G.F.: The computational complexity of probabilistic inference using Bayesian belief networks. Artif. Intell. **42**(2–3), 393–405 (1990)
16. Cowell, R.G., et al.: Probabilistic Networks and Expert Systems. Springer, Heidelberg (2007)
17. Cox, D.R., Wermuth, N.: Linear dependencies represented by chain graphs. Stat. Sci. **8**(3), 204–218 (1993)
18. Fernando, R.L., Habier, D., Kizilkaya, K., Garrick, D.J.: Extension of the Bayesian alphabet for genomic selection. BMC Bioinform. **12**(186), 1–12 (2011)
19. Dempster, A.P.: Covariance selection. Biometrics **28**, 157–175 (1972)
20. Duggan, D.J., et al.: Expression profiling using cDNA microarrays. Nature Genetics **21**, pp. 10–14 (1999). (Suppl. 1)
21. Edwards, D.I.: Introduction to Graphical Modelling, 2nd edn. Springer, Heidelberg (2000)
22. Falconer, D.S., Mackay, T.F.C.: Introduction to Quantitative Genetics, 4th edn. Longman, Harlow (1996)
23. Friedman, J., Hastie, T., Tibshirani, R.: Sparse inverse covariance estimation with the graphical lasso. Biostatistics **9**, 432–441 (2008)
24. Friedman, N.: Inferring cellular networks using probabilistic graphical models. Science **303**, 799–805 (2004)
25. Friedman, N., Geiger, D., Goldszmidt, M.: Bayesian Network Classifiers. Mach. Learn. **29**(2–3), 131–163 (1997)

26. Friedman, N., Goldszmidt, M., Wyner, A.: Data analysis with Bayesian networks: a bootstrap approach. In: Laskey, K.B., Prade, H. (eds.) Proceedings of the 15th Annual Conference on Uncertainty in Artificial Intelligence (UAI), pp. 206–215. Morgan Kaufmann, San Francisco (1999)
27. Friedman, N., Koller, D.: Being Bayesian about Bayesian network structure: A Bayesian approach to structure discovery in Bayesian networks. Mach. Learn. **50**(1–2), 95–126 (2003)
28. Friedman, N., Linial, M., Nachman, I.: Using Bayesian networks to analyze expression data. J. Comput. Biol. **7**, 601–620 (2000)
29. Friedman, N., Pe'er, D., Nachman, I.: "Learning Bayesian network structure from massive datasets: the "Sparse Candidate" algorithm". In: Proceedings of 15th Conference on Uncertainty in Artificial Intelligence (UAI), pp. 206–221. Morgan Kaufmann (1999)
30. Friedman, N., et al.: Using Bayesian networks to analyze gene expression data. J. Comput. Biol. **7**, 601–620 (2000)
31. Geiger, D., Heckerman, D.: Learning Gaussian networks. Technical report Available as Technical Report MSR-TR-94-10. Redmond, Washington: Microsoft Research (1994)
32. Hartemink, A.J.: Principled computational methods for the validation and discovery of genetic regulatory networks. PhD thesis. School of Electrical Engineering and Computer Science, Massachusetts Institute of Technology (2001)
33. Heckerman, D., Geiger, D., Chickering, D.M.: Learning Bayesian networks: the combination of knowledge and statistical data. Mach. Learn. **20**(3), 197–243 (1995). Available as Technical Report MSR-TR-94-09
34. Huber, W., et al.: Variance stabilization applied to microarray data calibration and to the quantification of differential expression. Bioinformatics **18**(Suppl. 1), S96–S104 (2002)
35. Imoto, S., et al.: Bootstrap analysis of gene networks based on Bayesian networks and nonparametric regression. Genome Inform. **13**, 369–370 (2002)
36. Jonckheere, A.: A Distribution-Free k-Sample test against ordered alternatives. Biometrika **41**, 133–145 (1954)
37. Kennet, R.S., Perruca, G., Salini, S.: In: Kennet, R.S., Salini, S. (eds.) Modern Analysis of Customer Surveys: with Applications Using R. Wiley, Chichester (2012). (Chap. 11)
38. Koivisto, M., Sood, K.: Exact Bayesian structure discovery in Bayesian networks. J. Mach. Learn. Res. **5**, 549–573 (2004)
39. Koller, D., Friedman, N.: Probabilistic Graphical Models: Principles and Techniques. MIT Press, Cambridge (2009)
40. Koller, D., Sahami, M.: Toward optimal feature selection. In: Proceedings of the 13th International Conference on Machine Learning (ICML), pp. 284–292 (1996)
41. Korb, K., Nicholson, A.: Bayesian Artificial Intelligence, 2nd edn. Chapman and Hall, Boca Raton (2010)
42. Larranaga, P., et al.: Learning Bayesian Networks by Genetic Algorithms: ACase Study in the Prediction of Survival in Malignant Skin Melanoma. In: Keravnou, E., Garbay, C., Baud, R., Wyatt, J. (eds.) AIME 1997. LNCS(LNAI), pp. 261–272. Springer, Heidelberg (1997)
43. Lauritzen, S.L., Wermuth, N.: Graphical models for associations between variables, some of which are qualitative and some quantitative. Ann. Stat. **17**(1), 31–57 (1989)
44. Lehmann, E.L.: Elements of Large Sample Theory, 3rd edn. Springer, Heidelberg (2004)
45. Lehmann, E.L.: Nonparametrics: Statistical Methods Based on Ranks. Springer, Heidelberg (2006)
46. Lennon, G.G., Lehrach, H.: Hybridization analyses of arrayed cDNA libraries. Trends Genet. **10**, 314–317 (1991)
47. Li, H., Gui, J.: Gradient directed regularization for sparse Gaussian concentration graphs, with applications to inference of genetic networks. Biostatistics **7**, 302–317 (2006)
48. Lipshutz, R.J., et al.: High density synthetic oligonucleotide arrays. Nat. Genet. **21**(Suppl. 1), 20–24 (1999)
49. Meuwissen, T.H.E., Hayes, B.J., Goddard, M.E.: Prediction of totalgenetic value using genome-wide dense marker maps. Genetics **157**, 1819–1829 (2001)

50. Morota, G., et al.: An assessment of linkage disequilibrium in Holstein Cattle Using a Bayesian Network. Journal of Animal Breeding and Genetics **129**, 474–487 (2012)
51. Mukherjee, S., Speed, T.P.: Network inference using informative priors. PNAS **105**, 14313–14318 (2008)
52. Musella, F.: Learning a Bayesian network from ordinal data. Working Paper 139. Dipartimento di Economia, Università degli Studi "Roma Tre" (2011)
53. Neapolitan, R.E.: Learning Bayesian Networks. Prentice Hall, New York (2003)
54. Park, T., Casella, G.: The Bayesian lasso. J. Am. Stat. Assoc. **103**(482), 681–686 (2008)
55. Pearl, J.: Causality: Models, Reasoning and Inference, 2nd edn. Cambridge University Press, Cambridge (2009)
56. Pearl, J.: Probabilistic Reasoning in Intelligent Systems: Networks of Plausible Inference. Morgan Kaufmann, San Francisco (1988)
57. Pirie, W.: Jonckheere Tests for Ordered Alternatives. In: Encyclopaedia of Statistical Sciences, pp. 315–318. Wiley (1983)
58. Sachs, K., et al.: Causal protein-signaling networks derived from multiparameter single-cell data. Science **308**(5721), 523–529 (2005)
59. Schäfer, J., Strimmer, K.: A Shrinkage approach to large-scale covariance matrix estimation and implications for functional genomics. Stat. Appl. Genet. Mol. Biol. **4**, 32 (2005)
60. Schäfer, J., Strimmer, K.: An Empirical bayes approach to inferring large-scale gene association networks. Bioinformatics **21**, 754–764 (2005)
61. Schuchhardt, J., et al.: Normalization strategies for cDNA microarrays. Nucleic Acids Res. **28**, e47 (2000)
62. Scutari, M., Brogini, A.: Bayesian network structure learning with permutation tests. Commun. Stat. Theory Methods **41**(16–17), 3233–3243 (2012)
63. Scutari, M., Mackay, I., Balding, D.J.: Improving the efficiency of genomic selection. Stat. Appl. Genet. Mol. Biol. **12**(4), 517–527 (2013)
64. Spirtes, P., Glymour, C., Scheines, R.: Causation, Prediction, and Search. MIT Press, Cambridge (2000)
65. Spirtes, P., et al.: Constructing Bayesian network models of gene expression networks from microarray data. In: Proceedings of the Atlantic Symposium on Computational Biology, Genome Information Systems and Technology (2001)
66. Steck, H.: "Learning the Bayesian network structure: Dirichlet prior versus data." In: Proceedings of the 24th Conference Annual Conference on Uncertainty in Artificial Intelligence (UAI 2008), pp. 511–518 (2008)
67. Steck, H., Jaakkola, T.: On the Dirichlet prior and Bayesian regularization. In: Advances in Neural Information Processing Systems (NIPS), pp. 697–704 (2002)
68. Terpstra, T.J.: The asymptotic normality and consistency of Kendall's test against trend when the ties are present in one ranking. indagationes mathematicae **14**, 327–333 (1952)
69. Thomas, J.G., et al.: An efficient and robust statistical modeling approach to discover differentially expressed genes using genomic expression profiles. Genome Res. **11**, 1227–1236 (2001)
70. Tsamardinos, I., Aliferis, C.F., Statnikov, A.: "Algorithms for large scale Markov blanket discovery". In: Proceedings of the 16th International Florida Artificial Intelligence Research Society Conference, pp. 376–381 (2003)
71. Tsamardinos, I., Brown, L.E., Aliferis, C.F.: The max-min hill-climbing Bayesian network structure learning algorithm. Mach. Learn. **65**(1), 31–78 (2006)
72. Whittaker, J.: Graphical Models in Applied Multivariate Statistics. Wiley, New York (1990)
73. Yeung, K.Y., et al.: Model-based clustering and data transformations for gene expression data. Bioinformatics **17**(10), 977–987 (2001)

Chapter 10
Chain Graphs and Gene Networks

Dag Sonntag and Jose M. Peña

Abstract Chain graphs are graphs with possibly directed and undirected edges, and no semidirected cycle. They have been extensively studied as a formalism to represent probabilistic independence models, because they can model symmetric and asymmetric relationships between random variables. This allows chain graphs to represent a wider range of systems than Bayesian networks. This in turn allows for a more correct representation of systems that may contain both causal and non-causal relationships between its variables, like for example biological systems. In this chapter we give an overview of how to use chain graphs and what research exists on them today. We also give examples on how chain graphs can be used to model advanced systems, that are not well understood, such as gene networks.

10.1 Introduction

In the previous chapter we saw how we could model advanced systems as Bayesian networks (BNs) by representing the causal relations between the variables in the system as directed edges. These models are widely used today but as noted in the previous chapter they do have certain shortcomings. In this chapter we will discuss one such shortcoming, namely the inability to model non-causal relations, and how this can be solved using more expressive probabilistic graphical model (PGM) classes such as chain graphs (CGs).

When an expert is modelling a system it is often relatively easy to find causal relations between the variables in the system and thereby model it as a BN. This is especially true for well known systems where all relevant factors are included as variables in the model. However, for more advanced systems some relations between directly correlated variables might not have such a clear causal structure. This can be for many reasons, such as that a hidden common cause exists between the variables or that there exist selection bias between them. Modelling these relations with directed edges is then incorrect from the perspective of interpretation and can cause incorrect reasoning subsequently.

© Springer International Publishing Switzerland 2015

A. Hommersom and P.J.F. Lucas (eds.), *Biomedical Knowledge Representation*, LNAI 9521, DOI 10.1007/978-3-319-28007-3_10

CGs solve this problem by extending the ideas of BNs with an additional type of edge representing non-causal relations between variables. Representing variables as nodes, causal relations with directed edges and non-causal relations with non-directed edges these models can therefore represent a larger set of models than BNs. At the same time CGs keep key features of BNs such as their interpretability and efficiency when it comes to inference and structure learning.

CGs are also interesting because they correctly can represent a much larger set of independence models, and thereby probability distributions, than BNs, Markov networks (MNs) or covariance graphs (covGs). BNs, MNs and covGs are the PGM classes most commonly used today when modelling bioinformatics systems. This means that for a probability distribution p there may be no BN G able to represent only and all independences in p when a CG F can. A BN can represent any probability distribution, but only by including fewer independences, and thereby additional dependences, than what actually exist in the underlying probability distribution. These spurious, additional, dependences can then later be "removed" by the correct parametrization, but this is still problematic for several reasons. Firstly, the advantage of using PGMs, such as the speed of inference, is larger the sparser the graph is. By having more edges than necessary this advantage is lost. Secondly, some of these edges might not make sense from a biological point of view. This is problematic for practitioners trying to understand the system through its graph, since the edges obscure the true (in)dependences between the variables.

A problem with CGs is however that there exists multiple types of non-causal relations as described above. This means that depending on what kind of non-causal relation we mean with the non-directed edge in our models we represent different systems and thereby independence models. To distinguish the different meanings of the non-directed edge we say that we have different CG interpretations, and that the non-directed edge is interpreted differently in different CG interpretations. Today there exists mainly three CG interpretations in research. These are the Lauritzen-Wermuth-Frydenberg (LWF) interpretation [7, 13], the Andersson-Madigan-Perlman (AMP) interpretation [1] and the multivariate regression (MVR) interpretation [3, 4].

One question that can be asked is how much more expressive CGs are compared to BNs? If the advantage is small the additional complexity might not translate into significantly better models. It has however been shown that as the number of variables increases CGs can express exponentially many more independence models compared to BNs. So for only 20 variables any CG interpretation can express approximate 1000 times more independence models, and thereby systems, compared to BNs [25, 26]. Hence for large domains with hundreds of variables the number of independence models representable by BNs is incredibly small compared the number of independence models representable by CGs. Therefore, CGs are much more likely to provide a realistic graph structure instead of obscuring the true relations in the system [25, 26].

In the rest of this chapter we will cover how these different CG interpretations work and what systems they can represent. First, in the next section, we will however describe the notation we use. In Sect. 10.3 we then describe the background and meaning of the different CG interpretations, while in Sect. 10.4 we describe how such a CG can be learnt from a probability distribution. After a short conclusion and summary in Sect. 10.5, we provide an alternative illustration of CGs as systems of linear equations in the Appendix. For simplicity we limit our discussion to continuous variables but most results can also be generalised to systems with discrete or mixed variables.

10.2 Background and Notation

In this section, we review some concepts from PGMs that are used later in this chapter. All graphs and probability distributions are defined over a finite set of variables V represented as nodes in the graphs.

If a graph G contains an edge between two nodes V_1 and V_2, we denote with $V_1 \rightarrow V_2$ a *directed edge*, with $V_1 \leftrightarrow V_2$ a *bidirected edge* (sometimes also called a *dashed edge*), and with $V_1 - V_2$ an *undirected edge*. With a *non-directed* edge we mean either a bidirected edge or undirected edge. A set of nodes is said to be *complete* if there exists edges between all pairs of nodes in the set. A complete set of nodes is said to be a *clique* if there exists no superset of it that is complete.

The *parents* of a set of nodes X of G is the set $pa_G(X) = \{V_1 | V_1 \rightarrow V_2$ is in G, $V_1 \notin X$ and $V_2 \in X\}$. The *children* of X is the set $ch_G(X) = \{V_1 | V_2 \rightarrow V_1$ is in G, $V_1 \notin X$ and $V_2 \in X\}$. The *spouses* of X is the set $sp_G(X) = \{V_1 | V_1 \leftrightarrow V_2$ is in G, $V_1 \notin X$ and $V_2 \in X\}$. The *neighbours* of X is the set $nb_G(X) = \{V_1 | V_1 - V_2$ is in G, $V_1 \notin X$ and $V_2 \in X\}$. The *boundary* of X is the set $bd_G(X) = pa_G(X) \cup nb_G(X) \cup sp_G(X)$. The *adjacents* of X is the set $ad_G(X) = \{V_1 | V_1 \rightarrow V_2, V_1 \leftarrow V_2, V_1 \leftrightarrow V_2$ or $V_1 - V_2$ is in G, $V_1 \notin X$ and $V_2 \in X\}$.

To exemplify these concepts we can study the graph G with five nodes shown in Fig. 10.1a. In the graph we can see two bidirected edges, one between B and D and one between D and E. Hence we know the spouses of D are B and E. G also contains two directed edges from A to B and from B to E and we can see that E is the only child of B and B is the only child of A. Finally G also contains one undirected edge between C and D and hence C is a neighbour of D. All and all this means that the boundary of B is A and D while the adjacents of B also contains E in addition to A and D.

A *route* from a node V_1 to a node V_n in G is a sequence of nodes $V_1, \ldots, V_n$ such that $V_i \in ad_G(V_{i+1})$ for all $1 \leq i < n$. A *path* is a route containing only distinct nodes. The length of a path is the number of edges in the path. A path is called a *cycle* if $V_n = V_1$. A path is *descending* if $V_i \in pa_G(V_{i+1}) \cup sp_G(V_{i+1}) \cup nb_G(V_{i+1})$ for all $1 \leq i < n$. The *descendants* of a set of nodes X of G is the set $de_G(X) = \{V_n |$ there is a descending path from V_1 to V_n in G, $V_1 \in X$ and $V_n \notin X\}$. A path is *strictly descending* if $V_i \in pa_G(V_{i+1})$ for all $1 \leq i < n$. The *strict descendants* of a set of nodes X of G is the set $sde_G(X) = \{V_n |$ there is a strictly descending path from V_1 to V_n in G, $V_1 \in X$ and $V_n \notin X\}$. The *ancestors* (resp. *strict ancestors*) of X is the set $an_G(X) = \{V_1 | V_n \in de_G(V_1), V_1 \notin X, V_n \in X\}$ (resp. $san_G(X) = \{V_1 | V_n \in sde_G(V_1), V_1 \notin X, V_n \in X\}$). Note that the definition for strict descendants given here coincides to the definition of descendants given by Richardson [21].

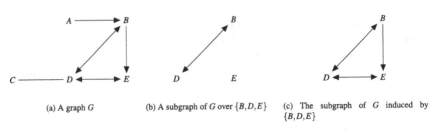

(a) A graph G   (b) A subgraph of G over {B,D,E}   (c) The subgraph of G induced by {B,D,E}

Fig. 10.1 Three different graphs

A cycle is called a *semi-directed cycle* if it is descending and $V_i \rightarrow V_{i+1}$ is in G for some $1 \leq i < n$.

To exemplify these concepts we can once again look at the graph G in Fig. 10.1a. We can here see two paths between B and C, $B \leftrightarrow D - C$ and $B \rightarrow E \leftrightarrow D - C$, and that the latter of these is descending while the former is not. An example of a route between B and C that is not a path is $B \leftrightarrow D \leftrightarrow E \leftarrow B \leftrightarrow D - C$. We can see that G contains one cycle $B \leftrightarrow D \leftrightarrow E \leftarrow B$ that is semi-directed. Moreover we can see that E is a strict descendant of A due to the strictly descending path $A \rightarrow B \rightarrow E$, while D is not. D is however in the descendants of A together with B, C and E. A is therefore an ancestor of all variables except itself.

A Markov network (MN) (resp. covariance graph (covG)) contains only undirected (resp. bidirected) edges while a BN only contains directed edges and no semi-directed cycles. A CG under the Lauritzen-Wermuth-Frydenberg (LWF) interpretation, denoted *LWF CG*, contains only directed and undirected edges but no semi-directed cycles. Likewise a CG under the Andersson-Madigan-Perlman (AMP) interpretation, denoted *AMP CG*, is a graph containing only directed and undirected edges but no semi-directed cycles. A CG under the multivariate regression (MVR) interpretation, denoted *MVR CG*, is a graph containing only directed and bidirected edges but no semi-directed cycles. A *chain component* C of a LWF CG or an AMP CG (resp. MVR CG) is a maximal set of nodes such that there exists a path between every pair of nodes in C containing only undirected edges (resp. bidirected edges). A *subgraph* of G is a subset of nodes and edges in G. A subgraph of G induced by a set of its nodes X is the graph over X that has all and only the edges in G whose both ends are in X.

If we go back to our example in Fig. 10.1 we can see that the graph in Fig. 10.1b is a subgraph of G over the variables B, D and E while the graph in Fig. 10.1c is a subgraph induced by the same variables. We can also see that G is not a CG of any of the interpretations since it contains a semi-directed cycle. An example of a LWF CG or an AMP CG is instead shown in Fig. 10.2a while an example of a MVR CG is shown in Fig. 10.2b. We can here see that H contains three connectivity components $\{A\}$, $\{B\}$ and $\{C, D\}$ and that F contains two connectivity components $\{A\}$ and $\{B, C, D\}$.

Let X, Y and Z denote three disjoint subsets of V. We say that X is *conditionally independent* from Y given Z if the value of X does not influence the value of Y when

Fig. 10.2 Two different CGs

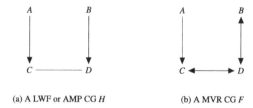

(a) A LWF or AMP CG H (b) A MVR CG F

the values of the variables in Z are known, i.e. $p(X, Y|Z) = p(X|Z)p(Y|Z)$ holds and $p(Z) > 0$. We denote this by $X \perp_p Y|Z$ if it holds in a probability distribution p while we with $X \not\perp_p Y|Z$ mean that it does not hold in p. Moreover we say that X is separated from Y given Z in a graph G if the separation criterion of G represents that X is conditionally independent of Y given Z. We denote the this by $X \perp_G Y|Z$ and we will discuss different separation criteria for CGs later in this chapter. Similarly we denote with $X \not\perp_G Y|Z$ that the separation criterion of G does not represent the conditional independence. A probability distribution p is said to fulfill the *global Markov property* with respect to a graph G, if for any $X \perp_G Y|Z$, given the separation criterion for the PGM class to which G belongs, $X \perp_p Y|Z$ holds. The *independence model M* induced by a probability distribution p (resp. a graph G), denoted as $I(p)$ (resp. $I(G)$), is the set of statements $X \perp_p Y|Z$ (resp. $X \perp_G Y|Z$) that holds in p (resp. G). Given two independence models M and N, we say that N includes M ($M \subseteq N$), iff $X \perp_M Y|Z$ implies that $X \perp_N Y|Z$ for every X, Y and Z.

We say that a probability distribution p is *faithful* to a graph G when $X \perp_p Y|Z$ iff $X \perp_G Y|Z$ for all X, Y and Z. We say that two graphs G and H are *Markov equivalent* or that they are in the same *Markov equivalence class* iff $I(G) = I(H)$. A graph G is *inclusion optimal* for a probability distribution p if $I(G) \subseteq I(p)$ and if there exists no other graph H in the PGM class of G such that $I(G) \subset I(H) \subseteq I(p)$.

To illustrate the last concepts we can look at the MVR CG J and the independence models in Fig. 10.3. In Fig. 10.3b we can see the independences that hold in J and hence the independence model of J. Finally we can also see another independence model in Fig. 10.3c such that $I(J) \subseteq M$ and hence that M includes the independence model represented by J.

10.3 CG Interpretations

The research on CGs started in the late 1980s with the Lauritzen-Wermuth-Frydenberg (LWF) interpretation in order to combine BNs and MNs into more expressive models. Subsequently, the Andersson-Madigan-Perlman (AMP) interpretation and the multivariate regression (MVR) interpretation, both in common use in recent literature, were proposed. Each interpretation is based on a different separation criterion and a different interpretation of the edges. No interpretation subsumes another [5, 23], and no interpretation is generally better than any other. LWF, AMP and MVR interpretations are

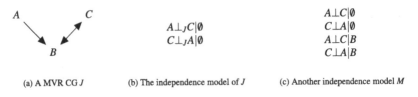

| (a) A MVR CG J | (b) The independence model of J | (c) Another independence model M |

Fig. 10.3 Example of independence models

just different from each other, similarly as BNs and MNs are different from each other, and are suited to different problems. We will in this chapter present each interpretation in three different ways. First in the classical sense, i.e. in terms of their separation criteria as in Drton [5], secondly in terms of systems of linear equations and third with some intuitive meaning behind the edges in the CGs. Finally we will also give examples of how they can be used. Moreover, in the next section we will discuss how to decide which interpretation to use when modelling a system with CGs.

First we will however see how BNs are presented in these three ways. For BNs the separation criterion is as follows. Given three disjoint sets of nodes X, Y and Z in a BN G, $X \perp_G Y | Z$ iff there exists no path between X and Y such that:

1. every non-collider on the path is not in Z and
2. every collider on the path is in Z or $san_G(Z)$.

A node B is said to be a *collider* between two nodes A and C on a path if the following configuration exists in the path: $A \rightarrow B \leftarrow C$. For any other configuration the node B is a non-collider on the path. In addition, the interpretation in terms of a system of linear equations is as follows. The probability distribution of every node in a BN depends only on its parents. This means that every node X_i is modelled by the equation $X_i = \beta_i * pa_G(X_i) + \epsilon^i$ in the associated system of linear equations, where β_i is a weight vector measuring the influence of the individual parents and the noise $\epsilon^i \sim \mathcal{N}(0, \sigma_i)$ is independent of any other node's noise. The intuitive meaning is simply that the parent nodes are the cause of the children nodes.

For CGs the different interpretations have different separation criteria. As noted in the introduction, the feature all CGs share is that they contain subgraphs, called chain components, that are connected to each other by directed edges. Within each chain component the type of edges varies depending on the interpretation: LWF CGs and AMP CGs contain undirected edges while MVR CGs contain bidirected edges. Even though the intuitive meaning of a CG is not as simple as for a BN, there are similarities between the two PGM classes. For example, the separation statements encoded by a CG correspond to the non-existence of routes with certain features, as in BNs. Moreover, in terms of linear equations each component of a CG can be seen as a supernode, with the corresponding probability distribution determined only by its parents. If we let K_i be the component i in a CG G, then G has an associated system of linear equations with normally distributed errors as follows:

$$K_i = \beta_i \, pa_G(K_i) + \epsilon^i \qquad \text{where} \qquad \epsilon^i \sim \mathcal{N}(0, \Lambda^i).$$

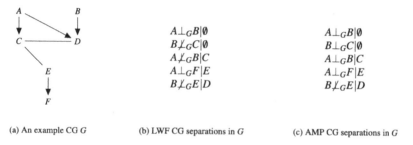

| (a) An example CG G | (b) LWF CG separations in G | (c) AMP CG separations in G |

Fig. 10.4 An example CG G and some corresponding separations according to the LWF and AMP interpretations.

ϵ^i represents the noise, or influence, between the nodes in the same component. How this noise and the β_i-vector are modelled varies between the different interpretations, and gives them different intuitive meanings.

10.3.1 The LWF Interpretation

The LWF interpretation was introduced by Lauritzen, Wermuth and Frydenberg in 1989 [7, 13] and is the most well researched CG interpretation. As noted above, LWF CGs contain components that are connected to each other by directed edges. The separation criterion is the following. Given three disjoint subsets of nodes X, Y and Z in a LWF CG G, $X \perp_G Y | Z$ iff there exists no route between X and Y such that:

1. every node in a non-collider section on the route is not in Z and
2. some node in every collider section on the route is in Z.

A *section* of a route is a maximal non-empty set of nodes $B_1 \ldots B_n$ such that the route contains the subroute $B_1 - B_2 - \ldots - B_n$. It is called a *collider section* if $B_1 \ldots B_n$ together with the two neighbouring nodes in the route, A and C (note that A and C might be the same node), form the subroute $A \rightarrow B_1 - B_2 - \ldots - B_n \leftarrow C$ in the route. For any other configuration the section is a non-collider section.

A simple example of a CG is shown in Fig. 10.4a. Here the CG has four chain components: A, B, $\{C, D, E\}$ and F. If the graph is interpreted as a LWF CG the separations and non-separations shown in Fig. 10.4b hold. Note that these are not all the separations that hold in G.

When reasoning in terms of linear equations, the parents of a component can be interpreted as the causes of the nodes in that component, and directed edges have the same meaning as in a BN. So the linear equation of a node X_j in a LWF CG is $X_j = \beta_j \, pa_G(K_i) + \epsilon^j$ where K_i is the component to which X_j. As shown in the Appendix, the k-th element of β_j can be interpreted as the sum of the weights of all the paths in G between the parent X_k of K_i and the node X_j of K_i such that the nodes in these paths are all in $X_k \cup K_i$, and where the path weight itself is the product of the weight of its edges. The noise ϵ^j is then determined by the associated inverse covariance matrix of that component. Furthermore, the corresponding entry in the inverse covariance matrix for two nodes X_j and X_m can be non-zero iff there exists an undirected edge $X_j - X_m$ in G (see the Appendix for details). For example, we can see from Fig. 10.4a that the influence from node B onto node D is direct since there only exists one path between them. However, the influence from node A onto node E is determined by the path $A \rightarrow C - E$ as well as $A \rightarrow D - C - E$ (see the Appendix for details).

This characterisation of the influence of a parent of K_i means that parents influence all the nodes in K_i, as influence propagates to all of K_i through its undirected edges. We can see, for example, that in the second example above the influence from A onto E is the same as A onto C except for the last path between C and E. This makes LWF CGs similar to module networks, another PGM class that has shown promising results for gene networks [22]. In module networks every node in a module, which is similar to a component, has the same parents and parameters. In a LWF CG, every node in the same component have the same parents when the LWF CG is seen as a system of linear equations. However, the influence of the parents on a node depends on the paths between them and, thus, it may be different for different nodes in the component.

An example of a situation when LWF CGs are useful is when we want to model a system with knowledge obtained from several experts, each with his or her own exclusive field of competence. Each expert then gives information about the structural relationships between the variables within his or her domain given outside factors that affect the variables in his or her domain of expertise. The expert does this by providing a MN over the variables in the domain and their outside factors. Moreover, since the expert only knows about his or her domain and not how the outside factors are related, he or she must assume that all outside factors are adjacent when creating the MN. The subgraph of the MN induced by the variables in the experts domain can then be seen as a component in a resulting LWF CG while the outside factors are added as parents to their previous neighbours in the component. The internal structure of the outside factors will be defined by some other expert, who is expert over that domain. If a strict causal ordering is kept between the variables, putting the different chain components together into a single graph then results in LWF CG [28]. An example of this in medicine can be if we have three experts, one expert modelling the probability that a person have certain gene-expressions in his or her DNA, one that models the probability of different protein signalling data occurring in blood samples given these gene-expressions and one that models the occurrence of different traits, such as diseases, given the gene-expressions.

Other settings in which LWF CGs are appropriate is for modelling the equilibrium state of a system containing feedback loops [12] or when variables of a system only can be measured in an aggregated state [6]. It can also be noted that if a LWF CG only contains directed edges it can be read as a BN while if it only contains undirected edges it can be read as a MN.

10.3.2 The AMP Interpretation

The AMP CG interpretation was introduced by Andersson, Madigan and Perlman [1] as an alternative to the LWF interpretation because it preserves the recursive characteristics of BNs. Similarly to LWF CGs, AMP CGs also contain components connected to each other by directed edges, whereas each component internally only contains undirected edges. As a result, an AMP CG containing only directed edges can be read as a BN and an AMP CG containing only undirected edges can be read as a MN similarly as a LWF CG. However, the separation criterion is different compared to LWF CGs. Given three disjoint subsets of nodes X, Y and Z in an AMP CG G, $X \perp_G Y|Z$ iff there exists no route between X and Y such that:

1. every non-collider on the route is not in Z and
2. every collider on the route is in Z or $san_G(Z)$.

A node B is said to be a *collider* in an AMP CG G between two nodes A and C on a route if one of the following configurations exists in G: $A \rightarrow B \leftarrow C$, $A \rightarrow B - C$ or $A - B \leftarrow C$. For any other configuration the node B is a non-collider. In the case of the CG shown in Fig. 10.4a, we can see that the separations and non-separations in Fig. 10.4c hold if we interpret it as an AMP CG. Note that these are not all the separations and non-separations that hold in G.

The modelling of the noise also differs from LWF CGs. In the Appendix it is shown that the associated linear equation of a node X_j in an AMP CG G is $X_j = \beta_j \, pa_G(X_j) + \epsilon^j$. The node depends only on its parents and not on the parents of the whole component, as it does in the case of LWF CGs. The noise ϵ^j is then controlled by the inverse covariance matrix of that component. Furthermore, the corresponding entry in the inverse covariance matrix for two nodes X_j and X_k can be non-zero iff there exists an undirected edge $X_j - X_k$ in G (see the Appendix for details). Intuitively, a small set of nodes works as an interface between other nodes in the component and its parents. For example, we can see that C and D in Fig. 10.4a block the influence from the parents A and B onto E if the graph is interpreted as an AMP CG.

AMP CGs are useful when we have a set of variables for which the internal relations has no causal ordering, so the relations should be modelled as a MN, but also a second set of variables which can be seen as causes for some of these variables in the first set. The internal structure of the first set of variables can then be modelled as a MN, creating a chain component in an AMP CG, and the causes as parents of some of the variables in the chain component. Note that for AMP CGs the parents only affects the direct children in the chain component, not all the nodes in the chain component such as in the case of LWF CGs. An example in medicine when such a model might be appropriate is when we are modelling pain levels on different areas on the body of a patient. The pain levels can then be seen as correlated "geographically" over the body, and hence be modelled as a MN. Certain other factors do however exist that alters the pain levels locally at some of these areas, such as the type of body part the area is located on or if local anaesthetic has been administered in that area and so on. These outside factors can then be modelled as parents affecting the pain levels locally.

While both LWF CGs and AMP CGs consist of MNs as chain components they differ in the way the parents of the component affect the variables in the component. In a LWF CG each parent affects all the variables in the component, i.e. the information travels through the children, while in an AMP CG the parents only affects the actual children, i.e. the information does not travel to the other variables in the chain component. Hence when we have a system for which some parts best are modelled as MNs and some parts as BNs we can use either a LWF CG or AMP CG, depending on which type fits the independence model of the system best.

10.3.3 The MVR Interpretation

MVR CGs were originally introduced by Cox and Wermuth [3, 4], and are equivalent to the acyclic directed mixed graphs without semi-directed cycles presented by Richardson [21]. Cox and Wermuth represented these graphs using directed edges and dashed edges, but we follow Richardson [21] as we feel that the notation is closer to that of BNs when it comes to the separation criterion.

The most important difference between the MVR CGs compared to AMP CGs and LWF CGs is that MVR CG components contains bidirected instead of undirected edges. As a result, MVR CGs is a superclass of BNs and covGs instead of BNs and MNs as in the case of AMP and LWF CGs [4]. MVR CGs also have the following separation criterion: Given three disjoint subsets of nodes X, Y and Z in a MVR CG G, $X \perp_G Y | Z$ iff there exists no path between X and Y such that:

1. every non-collider on the path is not in Z and
2. every collider on the path is in Z or $san_G(Z)$.

A node B is said to be a *collider* in a MVR CG G between two nodes A and C on a path iff one of the following configurations exists in the path: $A \rightarrow B \leftarrow C$, $A \rightarrow B \leftrightarrow C$, $A \leftrightarrow B \leftarrow C$ or $A \leftrightarrow B \leftrightarrow C$. For any other configuration the node B is said to be a non-collider. An example of a MVR CG is shown in Fig. 10.5c, with some of the corresponding separations and non-separations in Fig. 10.5b.

The associated system of linear equations is similar to that of the AMP CGs: each node depends only on its parents and not on the parents of the whole component.

Fig. 10.5 A MVR CG and some corresponding separations.

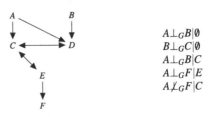

$A \perp_G B | \emptyset$
$B \perp_G C | \emptyset$
$A \perp_G B | C$
$A \perp_G F | E$
$A \not\perp_G F | C$

(a) Example CG G (b) MVR CG separations in G

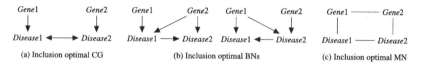

Fig. 10.6 A gene and disease example with MVR CG representation, BN representation and MN representation

The associated linear equation for a node X_j can therefore be written as $X_j = \beta_j\, pa(X_j) + \epsilon^j$, where ϵ^j is dependent on the other nodes in the same component. Unlike AMP CGs, MVR CGs can contain non-zero values in the corresponding covariance matrix (not the inverse covariance matrix as for AMP CGs) only for nodes that are spouses (see the Appendix for details). The intuitive meaning behind the MVR CGs is therefore very close to that of AMP CGs, differing only in the noise modelling.

A typical situation that gives rise to a MVR CG is in the presence of hidden variables, i.e. unobserved variables that are parents of at least two observed variables in the data. An example of a situation for which a MVR CG is useful is if we have a system containing two genes and two diseases caused by these such that *Gene1* is the cause of *Disease1* and *Gene2* is the cause of *Disease2* but where we also can see that the diseases are correlated. In this case we might suspect the presence of an unknown factor inducing the correlation between *Disease1* and *Disease2*, such as being exposed to a stressful environment. Having such a hidden variable results in the independence model described in the information above. We can now choose whether we would like to model this hidden variable in our model, but due to difficulties of measurement let us assume we do not. The MVR CG representing the information above is shown in Fig. 10.6a while the inclusion optimal BNs and MN are shown in Fig. 10.6b and 10.6c, respectively. We can now see that it is only the MVR CG that describes the relations in the system correctly.

10.4 CG Learning

As is the case with BNs, the graph structure of a CG can be learnt either from expert knowledge on the system or from data. The process of creating a CG from expert knowledge is very similar to that of a BN but where the non-directed edges can be used to model the variable correlations described in the previous section. An example of this process is given in Subsect. 10.4.1. In Subsects. 10.4.2 and 10.4.3 we then cover the structure learning algorithms that exist today that allow a CG to be learnt from a probability distribution p. First in the special case where we assume p is faithful to some CG and then the more general case where we do not. Finally, in Subsect. 10.4.4, we also discuss the current research on how CGs can be factorized and how the parameters can be learnt.

10.4.1 Learning CGs by Expert Knowledge

The process of creating a CG from expert knowledge of a domain is very similar to that of creating a BN from expert knowledge. Some important parts do however differ, such as choosing which CG interpretation to use. In this subsection we will therefore give an example of how this process can be performed.

The example we will be using was introduced by Lappenschaar et al. [10] and concerns the interaction between two diseases, *diabetes mellitus* and *lipid disorder*, along with typical blood measurements, two risk factors and a possible treatment. The blood measurements we are considering are *elevated blood cholesterol levels* and *elevated blood glucose levels* while the risk factors are *familial hypercholes-terolaemia* and *obesity* and the possible treatment *antidiabetic therapy*. In this case we know that familial hypercholesterolaemia increases the chance for lipid disorder and that lipid disorder in turn causes the blood cholesterol levels to be elevated. Similarly we know that antidiabetic therapy decreases the chance of having diabetes mellitus while having diabetes mellitus increases the blood glucose levels. Obesity is also known to cause both lipid disorder and diabetes mellitus. These are all causal relations and hence can be represented as directed edges in our CG. Finally we also know that there exists a correlation between diabetes mellitus and lipid disorder that cannot be explained only by the common parent obesity. I.e. if a person has diabetes mellitus he or she is more likely to also have lipid disorder than another person that does not have diabetes mellitus, even if they have the same level obesity. This correlation is not causal since it would be wrong to say that diabetes mellitus causes lipid disorder or vice versa and hence we represent the correlation with a non-directed edge. The resulting CG can be seen in Fig. 10.7.

As noted above the process so far corresponds well to that of BNs. The difficulty now is to choose which interpretation to use and thereafter to check that the CG can represent the dependences that exist in the system according to our expert knowledge. In some cases this might be easy and we might identify the non-causal correlation as a relation typically represented by a certain CG interpretation. This can for example be if we know that there exists some hidden common cause between variables that has non-directed edges between them (MVR CG) or if these relations are better described as feedback relations (LWF CG). In many cases we might however not have this information and we are then left to study the represented independence model. The first thing one can consider is whether or not information should "flow" through from parents of a component to all nodes in the component. In our case this would for example be whether familial hypercholesterolaemia increases the probability of having diabetes mellitus, given that no other information is known. If this is the case, then we know that the LWF CG interpretation is the only CG interpretation representing this dependency. If it is not the case, then we will have to consider both AMP and MVR CGs. To see the difference between these interpretations we need three nodes X, Y and Z in the same component such that X is adjacent of Y and Y is adjacent of Z while X and Z are non-adjacent. Then, if $X \perp Z | pa(X)$, we know that the relation is best represented by a MVR CG, while if $X \not\perp Z | pa(X)$, it

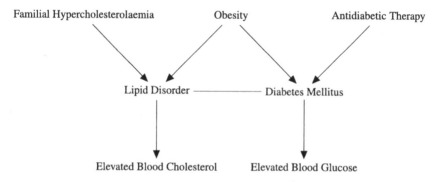

Fig. 10.7 The CG corresponding to the lipid disorder-diabetes mellitus example with a non-directed edge between lipid disorder and diabetes mellitus

is best represented by an AMP CG. Finding the best interpretation becomes even more problematic if multiple types of non-causal relations have been included in the model, corresponding to different CG interpretations. In such a case one either has to choose the interpretation that fits most of the relations or choose an even more general PGM class than CGs. In our example we can note that familial hypercholes- terolaemia does in fact increase the probability of having diabetes mellitus, given no other information, and hence we want to use the LWF CG interpretation. This also corresponds well with the authors choice, even though their choice is based on that lipid disorder and diabetes mellitus have a feedback relation between them and that the diseases almost always are in some kind of equilibrium [10].

Once a CG interpretation have been chosen it is also important to make sure that the model can represent all desired (conditional) dependences. If a (conditional) dependency is not represented an extra edge will have to be added. This is of course undesirable since it obscures the "true" relations in the system but as always in PGM modelling we want a model accurately representing all dependences in the underlying system while still representing as many independences as possible. This last step is especially important if the non-causal relation modelled does not perfectly correspond to a CG interpretation or if multiple types of non-causal relations exist in the modelled system.

10.4.2 Learning CGs Under the Faithfulness Assumption

All structure learning algorithms that exist for CGs today are constraint based and assume that the data comes in the form of a probability distribution p. Such a dis- tribution can for example be found through a set of samples of the system. In this subsection we will cover the case where we assume that p is faithful to some CG while we in the next subsection relax that assumption. We say that a probability distribution p is faithful to some CG G iff G have the same separations and non-separations as independences and dependences in p, i.e. that G can perfectly represent the independence model of p. This means that a probability distribution p that is faithful to some LWF CG G not necessarily is faithful to some AMP CG H, and hence that faithfulness is dependent on the PGM class we have in mind [23].

It is important to stress that this is a strong assumption. However, faithfulness allows for very fast and efficient algorithms since the reasoning in the algorithms can be made in the space of all CG models, instead of in the much larger space of all independence models. Today there exist structure learning algorithms for all three interpretations under the faithfulness assumption. Three of these are based on the PC algorithm [15, 27] used for BNs and contain three phases. In the first phase they learn the adjacencies of the CG; in the second they orient some of the edges according to simple rules; and in the third the remaining edges are oriented to avoid semi-directed cycles. This allows for an efficient way of learning the structure where no step has to be backtracked. For a comprehensive treatment of these algorithms we refer the reader to Studený's work [29] for LWF CGs, Peña's work for AMP CGs [19] and Sonntag and Peña's work [24] for MVR CGs. Finally there also exists a second, decomposition-based algorithm for learning LWF CGs developed by Ma et al. that has been shown to be of lower complexity than the PC variant algorithm [14]. It should be noted that since all structure learning algorithms are constraint based they will only find a CG with the correct independence model. Finding the CG with the correct causal explanation requires additional expert knowledge or experiments. However, having a CG with the correct independence model allows us find all possible causal explanations and their corresponding CGs.

10.4.3   Weakening the Faithfulness Assumption

It has been argued that it is unlikely that a randomly generated probability distribution that factorizes according to a BN is unfaithful to the BN [16]. While this is true if every parameter in a BN is generated randomly, the argument may not hold if the parameters have been hand picked (e.g. by a designer or by nature through evolution). Needless to say these are the systems we are mostly interested in modelling.

If one would apply the learning algorithms described in the previous subsection on a probability distribution that is not faithful to a CG of the appropriate interpretation it can no longer be guaranteed that the learnt CG can factorize the probability distribution properly. This means that the learnt CG might represent independences that do not exist in the underlying system which the probability distribution represents. Hence there might exist relations between variables in the underlying system that are not represented in the CG model. Moreover this means that no matter how the CG is parametrized it can never represent the original probability distribution perfectly. This is of course a problem since we would like to learn an inclusion optimal CG, i.e. a CG that can factorize the probability distribution, but contains as many separations as possible [20].

Unfortunately, learning a CG without assuming faithfulness is very complex and computationally demanding. The only algorithm for this task in the current literature is the CKES algorithm for LWF CGs presented by Peña et al. [20], which is based on a similar algorithm for BNs called KES [17]. The algorithm works by iteratively adding (resp. removing) separations between variables in the CG that are independent (resp. dependent) in the probability distribution given their boundary in the CG of that iteration. This is performed by removing (resp. adding) the appropriate edges in the CG. Moreover, to ensure that an inclusion optimal CG is reached at the end of the algorithm all CGs in the Markov equivalence class of the CG in any iteration may have to be searched for improvements. Like all efficient learning algorithms certain assumptions do however have to be made about the probability distribution. These are that the independence model induced by it fulfills the graphoid properties as well as the composition property [20]. The graphoid properties are satisfied for all strictly positive probability distributions, while the composition property is satisfied for every Gaussian probability distribution.

10.4.4   Factorisation and Parameter Learning

Hitherto very little research has been done on CG parameter learning and hence it is one of the weak points of CGs. Although parametrizations exist for all three CG interpretations for continuous variables [1, 3, 18, 31] it exists no efficient way of learning these parameters from a probability distribution. Instead iterative algorithms have to be used similarly as for MNs. We will here show an example of how this is done for LWF CGs.

The factorisation of a probability distribution p with variables $X_1, \ldots, X_n$ according to a LWF CG G with components $K_1, \ldots, K_m$ is

$$p(X_1, \ldots, X_n) = \prod_{i=1}^{m} p(K_i | pa_G(K_i)). \qquad (10.1)$$

Each component K_i can then be factorized clique-wise as follows

$$p(K_i | pa_G(K_i)) = \frac{1}{Z_i} \prod_{M \in M_C} \phi_M, \qquad (10.2)$$

where M_C are the complete subsets in the closure graph of K_i, i.e. the induced subgraph $G_{K_i \cup pa_G(K_i)}$ where each directed edge is replaced by an undirected edge and each pair of vertices in $pa_G(K_i)$ also are connected by an undirected edge. Each ϕ_M is then a potential over the variables in M and Z_i is a normalization constant. In other words, the probability distribution of the closure graph of each component can be seen as a MN. To parametrize these products and potentials we can then simply parametrize the system of linear equations since there exists a one to one relation between it and the probability distribution.

Another way to parametrize LWF CGs have been introduced by Lappenschaar et al. [10]. They proposed a qualitative approach to LWF CGs in which it is only calculated whether two variables adjacent in the graph have positive, negative or ambiguous influence on each other, and not the actual parameter value. In the article Lappenschaar et al. describes how these parameters can be learnt from data and uses the approach for modelling the interaction between diabetes and lipid disorder given the relevant factors. Their results show that one of the advantages of using qualitative LWF CGs compared to qualitative BNs is the ability to capture equilibrium models.

10.5 Summary

In this chapter we have shown how CGs can be used to model complex system such as gene networks. We have also shown some advantages of using CGs compared to using BNs, MNs or covGs, which are more commonly used in real-world applications today. The main advantage is that CGs are more flexible since they can represent both causal and non-causal relations and thereby represent a larger set of independence models compared to BNs, MNs or covGs. This means that CGs can express a model that is closer, or at least as close, to the real system as any BN, MN or covG. At the same time, they are still easy to interpret and one can relate their structure to the underlying molecular processes.

We have also discussed structure learning algorithms for all of the CG interpretations. Using these algorithms on samples from an advanced system like a gene network will result in a CG which may give good insight into how the variables in the system interact, even if it contains non-causal relations between its variables.

10.6 Appendix, System of Linear Equations for CGs

In this appendix we derive and present how the separation criteria of the different interpretations translate into systems of linear equations.

10.6.1 LWF CGs

Let G be a LWF CG with connectivity components $K_1, \ldots, K_n$. Let $\mathcal{N}(G)$ denote the set of regular Gaussian distributions that factorize with respect to G, which coincide with the set of distributions that satisfy the LWF global Markov property with respect to G [11, Theorems 3.34 and 3.36]. Let $p \in \mathcal{N}(G)$. Assume without loss of generality that p has mean 0. Let $\Omega^i_{K_i, K_i}$ and $\Omega^i_{K_i, pa_G(K_i)}$ denote submatrices of the precision matrix Ω^i of $p(K_i, pa_G(K_i))$. Then, as shown in [2, Sect. 2.3.1],

$$K_i | pa_G(K_i) \sim \mathcal{N}(\beta^i \, pa_G(K_i), \Lambda^i) \tag{10.3}$$

where

$$\beta^i = -(\Omega^i_{K_i, K_i})^{-1} \Omega^i_{K_i, pa_G(K_i)} \tag{10.4}$$

and

$$(\Lambda^i)^{-1} = \Omega^i_{K_i, K_i}. \tag{10.5}$$

Then, as shown in [18, Sect. 3], G has associated a system of linear equations with normally distributed errors as follows. For every K_i,

$$K_i = \beta^i \, pa_G(K_i) + \epsilon^i \tag{10.6}$$

where

$$\epsilon^i \sim \mathcal{N}(0, \Lambda^i) \tag{10.7}$$

and

$$(\Omega^i_{K_i, K_i})_{j,k} = 0 \text{ for all } j, k \in K_i \text{ such that } j - k \text{ is not in } G \tag{10.8}$$

and

$$(\Omega^i_{K_i, pa_G(K_i)})_{j,k} = 0 \text{ for all } j \in K_i \text{ and } k \in pa_G(K_i) \text{ such that } j \leftarrow k \text{ is not in } G. \tag{10.9}$$

It is worth mentioning that the mapping above between the probability distributions in $\mathcal{N}(G)$ and the systems of linear equations is bijective [18, Lemma 1]. Moreover, an alternative (but equivalent) parameterization of the probability distributions in $\mathcal{N}(G)$ is presented in [30].

Then, G has associated a system of linear equations with correlated errors as follows. For every $X_j \in K_i$,

$$X_j = \beta_j \, pa_G(K_i) + \epsilon^j \tag{10.10}$$

where

$$\beta_j \text{ is the } j - \text{th row of } \beta^i \tag{10.11}$$

and

$$Cov(\epsilon^j, \epsilon^k) = (\Lambda^i)_{j,k}. \tag{10.12}$$

Note that X_j is a linear combination of $pa_G(K_i)$ and not of $pa_G(X_j)$. Note also that, as shown in [32, Propositon 5.7.3],

$$(\Omega^i_{K_i, K_i})^{-1} = \Sigma_{K_i \cdot pa_G(K_i)} \tag{10.13}$$

where $\Sigma_{K_i \cdot pa_G(K_i)}$ represents the partial covariance matrix of K_i given $pa_G(K_i)$.

Then, as shown in [8, Theorem 1], the element (A, B) of $(\Omega^i_{K_i,K_i})^{-1}$ can be written as a sum of path weights over all the paths in G between A and B through nodes in K_i. Specifically,

$$((\Omega^i_{K_i,K_i})^{-1})_{A,B} = (\Sigma_{K_i \cdot pa_G(K_i)})_{A,B} = \sum_{\rho \in \rho_{A,B}} (-1)^{|\rho|+1} \frac{|(\Omega^i_{K_i,K_i})_{\backslash \rho}|}{|\Omega^i_{K_i,K_i}|} \prod_{l=1}^{|\rho|-1} (\Omega^i_{K_i,K_i})_{\rho_l,\rho_{l+1}}$$

(10.14)

where $\rho_{A,B}$ denotes the set of paths in G between A and B through nodes in K_i, $|\rho|$ denotes the number of nodes in a path ρ, ρ_l denotes the l-th node in ρ, and $(\Omega^i_{K_i,K_i})_{\backslash \rho}$ is the matrix with the rows and columns corresponding to the nodes in ρ omitted. Moreover, the determinant of a zero-dimensional matrix is taken to be 1. This leads to the following interpretation of β_j: By Eqs. 10.4, 10.11 and 10.14, the k-th element of β_j can be written as sum of path weights over all the paths in G between X_k and X_j trough nodes in K_i.

10.6.2 AMP CGs

Let G be an AMP CG with connectivity components $K_1, \ldots, K_n$. Let $\mathcal{N}(G)$ denote the set of regular Gaussian distributions that satisfy the AMP global Markov property with respect to G. Let $p \in \mathcal{N}(G)$. Assume without loss of generality that p has mean 0. Then, as shown above, $K_i | pa_G(K_i) \sim \mathcal{N}(\beta^i pa_G(K_i), \Lambda^i)$. Then, as shown in [1, Sect. 5], G has associated a system of linear equations with normally distributed errors as follows. For every K_i,

$$K_i = \beta^i \, pa_G(K_i) + \epsilon^i$$

(10.15)

where

$$\epsilon^i \sim \mathcal{N}(0, \Lambda^i)$$

(10.16)

and

$$((\Lambda^i)^{-1})_{j,k} = 0 \text{ for all } j, k \in K_i \text{ such that } j - k \text{ is not in } G$$

(10.17)

and

$$(\beta^i)_{j,k} = 0 \text{ for all } j \in K_i \text{ and } k \in pa_G(K_i) \text{ such that } j \leftarrow k \text{ is not in } G. \quad (10.18)$$

It is worth mentioning that the mapping above between the probability distributions in $\mathcal{N}(G)$ and the systems of linear equations is bijective [1, Sect. 5]. Moreover, the first constraint here coincides with the first constraint in the previous section.

Then, G has associated a system of linear equations with correlated errors as follows. For every $X_j \in K_i$,

$$X_j = \beta_j \, pa_G(X_j) + \epsilon^j \tag{10.19}$$

where

$$\beta_j \text{ contains the nonzero elements of } (\beta^i)_j. \tag{10.20}$$

and

$$Cov(\epsilon^j, \epsilon^k) = (\Lambda^i)_{j,k}. \tag{10.21}$$

Note that, unlike in the previous section, X_j is here a linear combination of $pa_G(X_j)$ and not of $pa_G(K_i)$.

10.6.3   MVR CGs

Let G be a MVR CG with connectivity components $K_1, \ldots, K_n$. Then, G has associated a system of linear equations with normally distributed errors as shown in the previous section except for two differences. First, $\mathcal{N}(G)$ now denotes the set of regular Gaussian distributions that satisfy the MVR global Markov property with respect to G. Second, we now replace Eq. 10.17 with

$$(\Lambda^i)_{j,k} = 0 \text{ for all } j, k \in K_i \text{ such that } j \longleftrightarrow k \text{ is not in } G. \tag{10.22}$$

See also [9].

Acknowledgements. This work is funded by the Center for Industrial Information Technology (CENIIT) and a so-called career contract at Linköping University, and by the Swedish Research Council (ref. 2010-4808).

References

1. Andersson, S.A., Madigan, D., Perlman, M.D.: An alternative Markov property for chain graphs. Scand. J. Stat. **28**, 33–85 (2001)
2. Bishop, C.M.: Pattern Recognition and Machine Learning. Springer, New York (2006)
3. Cox, D.R., Wermuth, N.: Linear dependencies represented by chain graphs. Stat. Sci. **8**, 204–218 (1993)
4. Cox, D.R., Wermuth, N.: Multivariate Dependencies: Models, Analysis and Interpretation. Chapman and Hall, London (1996)
5. Drton, M.: Discrete chain graph models. Bernoulli **15**, 736–753 (2009)
6. Ferráandiz, J., Castillo, E.F., Snamartín, P.: Temporal aggregation in chain graph models. J. Stat. Plann. Infer. **133**, 69–93 (2005)
7. Frydenberg, M.: The chain graph Markov property. Scand. J. Stat. **17**, 333–353 (1990)
8. Jones, B., West, M.: Covariance decomposition in undirected Gaussian graphical models. Biometrika **92**, 779–786 (2005)
9. Kang, C., Tian, J.: Markov properties for linear causal models with correlated errors. J. Mach. Learn. Res. **10**, 41–70 (2009)

10. Lappenschaar, M., Hommersom, A., Lucas, P.J.F.: Qualatitive chain graphs and their application. Int. J. Approximate Reasoning **55**, 957–976 (2014)
11. Lauritzen, S.L.: Graphical Models. Clarendon Press, Oxford (1996)
12. Lauritzen, S.L., Richardson, T.S.: Chain graph models and their causal interpretations. J. Roy. Stat. Soc. B **64**, 321–361 (2002)
13. Lauritzen, S.L., Wermuth, N.: Graphical models for association between variables, some of which are qualitative and some quantitative. Ann. Stat. **17**, 31–57 (1989)
14. Ma, Z., Xie, X., Geng, Z.: Structural learning of chain graphs via decomposition. J. Mach. Learn. Res. **9**, 2847–2880 (2008)
15. Meek, C.: Causal inference and causal explanation with background knowledge. In: Proceedings of Eleventh Conference on Uncertainty in Artificial Intelligence, pp. 403–410 (1995)
16. Meek, C.: Strong completeness and faithfulness in Bayesian networks. In: Proceedings of Eleventh Conference on Uncertainty in Artificial Intelligence, pp. 411–418 (1995)
17. Nielsen, J.D., Kočka, T., Peña, J.M.: On local optima in learning Bayesian networks. In: Proceedings of the 19th Conference on Uncertainty in Artificial Intelligence, pp. 435–442 (2003)
18. Peña, J.M.: Faithfulness in chain graphs: the Gaussian case. In: Proceedings of the 14th International Conference on Artificial Intelligence and Statistics, pp. 588–599 (2011)
19. Peña, J.M.: Learning AMP chain graphs under faithfulness. In: Proceedings of the 6th European Workshop on Probabilistic Graphical Models, pp. 251–258 (2012)
20. Peña, J.M., Sonntag, D., Nielsen, J.: An inclusion optimal algorithm for chain graph structure learning. In: Proceedings of the 17th International Conference on Artificial Intelligence and Statistics, pp. 778–786 (2014)
21. Richardson, T.S.: Markov properties for acyclic directed mixed graphs. Scand. J. Stat. **30**, 145–157 (2003)
22. Segal, E., et al.: Learning module networks. J. Mach. Learn. Res. **6**, 557–588 (2005)
23. Sonntag, D., Peña, J.M.: Chain graph interpretations and their relations. In: van der Gaag, L.C. (ed.) ECSQARU 2013. LNCS, vol. 7958, pp. 510–521. Springer, Heidelberg (2013)
24. Sonntag, D., Peña, J.M.: Learning multivariate regression chain graphs under faithfulness. In: Proceedings of the 6th European Workshop on Probabilistic Graphical Models, pp. 299–306 (2012)
25. Sonntag, D.: On expressiveness of the AMP chain graph interpretation. In: van der Gaag, L.C., Feelders, A.J. (eds.) PGM 2014. LNCS, vol. 8754, pp. 458–470. Springer, Heidelberg (2014)
26. Sonntag, D., Peñna, J.M., Gómez-Olmedo, M.: Approximate counting of graphical models via MCMC revisited. Int. J. Intell. Syst. **30**, 384–420 (2015)
27. Spirtes, P., Glymour, C., Scheines, R.: Causation, Prediction, and Search. Springer, New York (1993)
28. Studený, M.: Bayesian networks from the point of view of chain graphs. In: Proceedings of the 14th Conference on Uncertainty in Artificial Intelligence, pp. 496–503 (1998)
29. Studený, M.: On recovery algorithms for chain graphs. Int. J. Approximate Reasoning **17**, 265–293 (1997)
30. Wermuth, N.: On block-recursive linear regression equations (with discussion). Braz. J. Probab. Stat. **6**, 1–56 (1992)
31. Wermuth, N., Wiedenbeck, M., Cox, D.R.: Partial inversion for linear systems and partial closure of independence graphs. BIT Numer. Math. **46**, 883–901 (2006)
32. Whittaker, J.: Graphical Models in Applied Multivariate Statistics. Wiley, New York (1990)

Prediction and Prognosis of Health and Disease

Chapter 11
Prediction and Prognosis of Health and Disease

Agnieszka Onisko, Allan Tucker and Marek J. Druzdzel

11.1 Introduction

Medical prognosis is defined as the prediction of the probable course and outcome of a disease. This prediction should facilitate understanding patterns of disease progression as well as its management. Medical prognosis is closely related to other medical tasks, such as diagnosis, treatment, and therapy planning [15, 23].

Various methodologies have been applied to medical prognosis [1, 4, 19]. These methodologies can be divided into three classes: (1) statistical predictive models, such as logistic regression, Cox regression models, state-space models, or Box-Jenkins method, (2) data mining approaches, such as decision tree classifiers, genetic algorithms, or artificial neural networks, and (3) mixed approaches, such as those based on probabilistic graphical models. Two review papers, by Augusto [3] and Adlassnig et al. [2] discuss various applications of temporal models in medicine, in which prognosis takes a prominent place.

Some of these approaches do not model time explicitly, others include time as one of the model variables. *Cross-sectional studies* record attributes (such as clinical test results and demographics) across a sample of the population, thus providing a snapshot of a particular process but without any measurement of progression of the process over time [6]. An advantage of cross sectional studies is that they capture the diversity of a sample of the population and, therefore, the degree of variation in the symptoms. They are also relatively cheap compared to longitudinal studies that involve extensive follow up (see below). The main disadvantage of such studies is that the progression of many biological and medical processes, such as the development of a disease, are inherently temporal in nature and the time dimension is not captured.

Longitudinal studies [7] measure clinical variables from a number of people over time. Often, the results of multiple tests are recorded, generating multivariate time-series data. This is common for patients who have high risk indicators of disease and who are monitored regularly prior to diagnosis. The main advantage of longitudinal data is that they capture the temporal details of the disease progression. However, the data are often limited in terms of the cohort size due to the expensive nature of the

© Springer International Publishing Switzerland 2015
A. Hommersom and P.J.F. Lucas (eds.), *Biomedical Knowledge Representation*, LNAI 9521, DOI 10.1007/978-3-319-28007-3_11

studies. *Panel analysis* [16] involves trying to build models along both the temporal dimension and the population dimension, though similar issues with longitudinal studies arise (such as biased samples and lack of diversity in the sample). For both longitudinal and panel analysis, the patients are usually already identified as being at risk and, therefore, controls are usually not available. As a result, the early stages of the disease may be missed.

11.2 Temporal Models of Disease Progression

Degenerative diseases such as Parkinson's disease, glaucoma, or cancer are charac-terised by a continuing deterioration to organs or tissues over time. This monotonic increase in severity of symptoms is not always straightforward, however. The rate can vary within patients during the course of their disease so that sometimes rapid deterioration is observed and other times the symptoms of the disease may stabilise (or even improve — for example, when medication is used). Figure 11.1 shows several plots of visual field sensitivity data over a number of visits to clinic at approximately 6 month intervals for five patients who suffer from high Intra Ocular Pressure (IOP), a risk factor in the development of glaucoma. Please note the variation in both degree and rate between the individual cases. Interventions, such as medication or surgery, can make a huge difference to the quality of life and slow the process of disease pro-gression and, sometimes, change the long term prognosis. In degenerative diseases, a prognostic model shows a general transition from healthy to early onset and to advanced stages.

When time stamps (discrete or continuous) are available, such as is the case with longitudinal data, we can build temporal models. These models can be used to try and predict future values of the data or the disease outcome. In the rest of this section we will list briefly several approaches that belong to one of the three

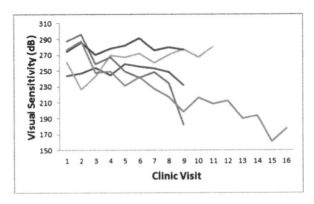

Fig. 11.1 Examples of the visual field sensitivity of five glaucoma sufferers, highlighting the variation in rates of progression

groups: (1) statistical predictive models, (2) data mining approaches, and (3) mixed approaches. In our description we will elaborate on mixed approaches which include probabilistic graphical models. Our focus on probabilistic graphical models refers to three applications of dynamic Bayesian networks that we explore later in this chapter.

11.2.1   Statistical Predictive Models

There are a number of popular statistical approaches to modelling time-series. For example, regression techniques that fit a model (linear or polynomial) through the data where time is used to predict the rate of change in some set of clinical variables [26]. However, care must be taken as each observation may not be independent of other observations (e.g., symptoms at time t are typically dependent on the symptoms at $t - 1$). As a result, standard residual error analysis cannot be carried out in this context.

Another very common time-series modelling approach is the Box-Jenkins method [5]. It is also known as the Autoregressive Integrated Moving Average (ARIMA) as it combines the autoregressive and moving average processes to model current and past observations and errors. It handles trends and cycles through differencing the data. Fitting an ARIMA involves identifying an initial model (which includes determining seasonality and stationarity), estimating the parameters, and verifying the assumptions of the model through residual analysis. The approach is attractive due to its ability to capture a diverse set of time-series behaviours. However, as a result of its flexibility, it risks overfitting data.

State space models [9] are powerful techniques in that they capture uncertainty in the development of underlying processes by using a transition equation, and uncertainty in the observation of a system through the use of a measurement equation.

11.2.2   Data Mining Approaches

When no time stamps are available, as is the case with cross sectional data, we can attempt to reconstruct sequences. This involves trying to find the best order for a particular set of data. The principal curve algorithm [17] essentially tries to fit curves through (potentially cross-sectional) data points in order to build a model of some temporal process. More recently the use of PQ-Trees has been explored to encode partial orderings in order to account for uncertainty in the data due to elements such as noise [20]. A PQ-Tree can be converted into a single ordering, using a hill-climb method to further minimise the distance within the PQ-Tree constraints. In [25], the algorithm was extended to also constrain the search to find paths with a fixed, user-defined start and end point representing the most extreme healthy and diseased cases in cross-sectional data.

11.2.3 Mixed Approaches

Statistical approaches can be data intensive and rely on good quality data with relatively large samples. Probabilistic graphical models, however, allow for combining data with expert knowledge or, in case there are no data, drawing entirely on expert knowledge. This makes probabilistic graphical models, such as Markov chains, hidden Markov models (HMMs) [21], Markov decision processes (MDPs and POMDPs), and dynamic Bayesian networks particularly attractive and popular in practice.

Dynamic Bayesian networks (DBNs) offer a framework for explicit modelling of temporal relationships and are useful as both prognostic and diagnostic tools. DBNs are more general than Hidden Markov Models, which assume a single discrete variable representing a hidden state and possibly multiple observation variables. Figure 11.2[1] captures an example of a dynamic Bayesian network model, modelling the effect of three risk factors on breast cancer. Each arc in this graph represents a probabilistic relationship (strictly speaking, lack of arcs between nodes represents conditional independence assumptions), which is usually, although not always, thought of as a causal relationship, and it is quantified by a conditional probability distribution. Some of the arcs, marked by a square with a single digit number, represent temporal influences between variables. The number denotes the temporal delay of influence. Arcs without a mark denote instantaneous influence. An arc labelled as *1* between the variables *Lesion (L)* and *Breast Cancer (BC)*, for example, denotes an influence that takes one time step, while an arc labelled as *2* originating and terminating at *Breast Cancer (BC)* denotes an influence that takes two time steps. Effectively, the model encodes the following conditional probability distribution over the variable *Breast Cancer (BC)*:

$$P(BC_t | A_t, FH, L_{t-1}, BC_{t-2}).$$

In other words, the conditional probability distribution over the variable *Breast Cancer (BC)* depends on the patient *Age (A)* and *Family History (FH)*. Furthermore, it depends on *Lesion (L)* result in previous time step, and also on *Breast Cancer* result two time steps ago. The duration of the time step is a design choice and could be, for example, a second, a day, a month, or a year.

There are three different conditional probability tables that quantify the variable *Breast Cancer*. Equations 11.1, 11.2, and 11.3 below correspond respectively to these three conditional probability tables, i.e., regular arcs: ($t = 0$), temporal arcs labelled as *1*: ($t = 1$), and temporal arcs labelled as *2*: ($t = 2$):

$$P(BC_{t=0} | A_t, FH) \tag{11.1}$$

$$P(BC_{t=1} | A_t, L_{t=0}) \tag{11.2}$$

$$P(BC_{t=2} | A_t, L_{t=1}, BC_{t=0}) \tag{11.3}$$

---

[1]This and other images are created by means of GeNIe software [8] developed at the University of Pittsburgh and available at http://genie.sis.pitt.edu/.

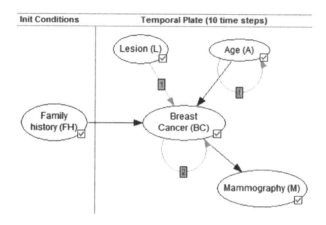

Fig. 11.2 Example of a DBN model

Age (A)		age_below_55					age_55_65	
Lesion (L) [t-1]		present		absent			present	
(Self) [t-2]	yes	no	yes	no		yes	no	yes
yes	0.1	0.08	0.1	0.08		0.03	0.012	[
no	0.9	0.92	0.9	0.92		0.97	0.988	[

Fig. 11.3 Fragment of a conditional probability table for the variable *Breast Cancer*

The parameters encoded in the tables can be learned from the time series data. Typically, the parameters are learned from data by maximizing the posterior probability of the parameters given the data [14]. When the structure is fixed and the prior probability distribution over the parameters is uniform, this corresponds to maximizing the likelihood function.

Figure 11.3 shows a fragment of the conditional probability table for the variable *Breast Cancer* for the time step $t \geq 2$ (see also Eq. 11.3). In this case, the conditional probability distribution for *Breast Cancer* depends on the variables *Age* and *Lesion* in the previous time step $(t - 1)$. Furthermore, this conditional probability distribution depends on the variable *Breast Cancer* at time step $t - 2$ (denoted as *(Self)[t-2]* in Fig. 11.3). One way of interpreting a DBN is through the process of "unrolling" it.

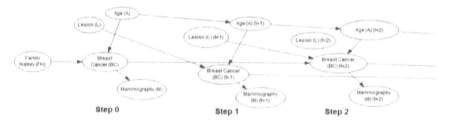

Fig. 11.4 Unrolled DBN model for the first 3 time steps

Fig. 11.5 Risk of a breast
cancer over time

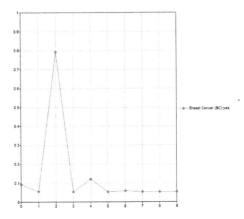

Figure 11.4 captures three time steps of the unrolled DBN model of Fig. 11.2. Five
out of six variables (*Age, Lesion, Breast Cancer*, and *Mammography*) are repeated at
each time step. The variable *Family History* is not repeated, because it was modelled
only as an initial condition and it is not changing over time. Evidence in a DBN
can be observed for any time step for which the model is defined. Given observed
dynamic evidence, the model can derive the probability distribution over a variable
under investigation (in this case, the variable *Breast Cancer*) as a function of time.
For example, the model may be used to calculate the following probability:

$$P(BC(present)|E) ,$$

where

$$E = A_{t=2}(55), L_{t=0}(present), M_{t=2}(abnormal) .$$

In this case, the model calculates the probability of breast cancer over 10 time steps
for a 55 old woman with an abnormal mammography result at time $(t = 2)$ that had
a lesion at $(t = 0)$. This result can be used to estimate the optimal time for follow-up
medical tests and procedures. DBN algorithms are more general than algorithms for
HMMs. The prominent representative of the latter, the *forward algorithm*, allows for
estimation of the probability of the hidden state from the previous and current values
of measured variables. This process is known as *filtering* and can be used to estimate
future probabilities of disease states from historical longitudinal data.

Although DBNs can capture the time-dependent nature of interactions among
variables, they are models for *stationary processes* meaning that parameters and
relations between variables cannot change over time. In many medical contexts,
however, dependency relations between variables can change over time. For example
in glaucoma, the Optic Nerve Head (ONH), which carries the visual functional signal,
changes during the progression of the disease, resulting in non-stationary series [28].
To overcome the non-stationarity in time series modelling with graphical models,
non-stationary DBNs, introduced recently [12, 22, 24], attempt to learn when the
changes in structure occur.

11.3 Summary

The above review is meant to provide a general introduction to the set of problems related to modelling dynamic systems by means of dynamic Bayesian networks. We introduced DBNs, learning of DBN parameters from data, the interpretation of DBNs, evidence and inference in DBNs, and hinted problems related to non-stationarity of the underlying model.

Several applications of DBNs have been proposed in medicine. Leong, Harmanec, Xiang, and colleagues [13, 18, 27], use a combination of graphical models with Markov chains to address different medical problems, including colorectal cancer management, neurosurgery ICU monitoring, and cleft lip and palate management. Galan et al. [10] describe NasoNet, a system for diagnosis and prognosis of nasopharyngeal cancer. van Gerven et al. [11] describe a DBN for management of patients suffering from a carcinoid tumour.

This chapter explores three applications of dynamic Bayesian networks to building models of health or disease progression from medical time series data. The focus is upon examples from visual field test non-stationary time series data, cervical cancer screening data spanning over up to eight years, and monitoring woman's monthly cycle. These models aim to predict the health of a patient or the onset and progression of a disease, although the difficulties encountered and the methodologies used are applicable in other settings.

References

1. Abu-Hanna, A., Lucas, P.J.F.: Prognostic models in medicine. Methods Inf. Med. **40**, 1–5 (2001)
2. Adlassnig, K.-P., et al.: Temporal representation and reasoning in medicine: research directions and challenges. Artif. Intell. Med. **38**, 101–113 (2006)
3. Augusto, J.: Temporal reasoning for decision support in medicine. Artif. Intell. Med. **33**, 1–24 (2005)
4. Bellazzi, R., Zupan, B.: Predictive data mining in clinical medicine: current issues and guidelines. Int. J. Med. Inform. **77**, 81–97 (2008)
5. Box, G.E.P., Jenkins, G.M.: Time Series Analysis: Forecasting and control. Holden-Day, San Francisco (1970)
6. Coggon, D., Rose, G., Barker, D.J.P.: Chapter 8: epidemiology for the uninitiated. Case-Control and Cross-Sectional Studies. BMJ (British Medical Journal) Publishing, Hoboken (1997)
7. Diggle, P.J., et al.: Analysis of Longitudinal Data. Oxford University Press, Oxford (2013)
8. Druzdzel, M.J.: SMILE: structural modeling, inference, and learning engine and GeNIe: a development environment for graphical decision- theoretic models. In: Proceedings of the Sixteenth National Conference on Artificial Intelligence (AAAI 1999). Orlando, FL, pp. 902–903 (1999)
9. Durbin, J., Koopman, S.J.: Time Series Analysis by State Space Methods. Oxford University Press (Sd), Oxford (2012)
10. Galan, S.F., et al.: NasoNet, modeling the spread of nasopharyngeal cancer with networks of probabilistic events in discrete time. Artif. Intell. Med. **25**, 247–264 (2002)
11. van Gerven, M.A.J., Taal, B.G., Lucas, P.J.F.: Dynamic Bayesian neworks as prognostic models for clinical patient management. J. Biomed. Inform. **41**, 515–529 (2008)

12. Grzegorczyk, M., Husmeier, D.: Non-stationary continuous dynamic Bayesian networks. In: Proceedings of the Twenty-Third Annual Conference on Neural Information Processing Systems (NIPS 2009), pp. 682–690. Curran Associates (2009)

13. Harmanec, D., et al.: Decision analytic approach to severe head injury management. In: Proceedings of the 1999 Annual Meeting of the American Medical Informatics Association (AMIA 1999). Washington, D.C., pp. 271–275 (1999)

14. Heckerman, D., Geiger, D., Chickering, D.: Learning Bayesian networks: the combination of knowledge and statistical data. In: KDD Workshop, pp. 85–96 (1994)

15. Hilden, J., Habbema, J.D.F.: Prognosis in medicine: an analysis of its meaning and roles. Theor. Med. **8**(3), 349–365 (1987)

16. Kasprzyk, D., et al.: Panel Surveys. Wiley, New York (1989)

17. Kegl, B., et al.: Learning and design of principal curves. IEEE Trans. Pattern Anal. Mach. Intell. **22**, 281–297 (2000)

18. Leong, T.-Y.: Multiple perspective dynamic decision making. Artif. Intell. **105**, 209–261 (1998)

19. Lucas, P.J.F., Abu-Hanna, A.: Prognostic methods in medicine. Artif. Intell. **15**(2), 105–119 (1999)

20. Magwene, P.M., Lizardi, P., Kim, J.: Reconstructing the temporal ordering of biological samples using microarray data. Bioinformatics **19**(7), 842–850 (2003)

21. Rabiner, L.R.: A tutorial on HMM and selected applications in speech recognition. Proc. IEEE **77**(2), 257–286 (1989)

22. Robinson, J.W., Hartemink, A.J.: Learning non-stationary dynamic Bayesian networks. J. Mach. Learn. Res. **11**, 3647–3680 (2010)

23. Schoolman, H.M., Bernstein, L.M.: Computer use in diagnosis, prognosis, and therapy. Science **200**(4344), 926–31 (1978)

24. Talih, N., Hengartner, N.: Structural learning with time-varying components: tracking the cross-section of financial time series. J. Roy. Stat. Soc. B **67**(3), 321–341 (2005)

25. Tucker, A., Garway-Heath, D.: The pseudotemporal bootstrap for predicting glaucoma from cross-sectional visual field data. IEEE Trans. Inf. Technol. Biomed. **14**(1), 79–85 (2010)

26. Viswanathan, A.C., Fitzke, F.W., Hitchings, R.A.: Early detection of visual field progression in glaucoma: a comparison of PROGRESSOR and STATPAC2. Br. J. Ophthalmol. **81**(12), 1037–1042 (1997)

27. Xiang, Y., Poh, K.-L.: Time-critical dynamic decision modeling in medicine. Comput. Biol. Med. **32**, 85–97 (2002)

28. Yanoff, M., Duker, J.S.: Ophthalmology, 2nd edn. Mosby, St. Louis (2003)

Chapter 12
Trajectories Through the Disease Process: Cross Sectional and Longitudinal Studies

Allan Tucker, Yuanxi Li, Stefano Ceccon and Stephen Swift

Abstract This paper explores the use of two different techniques for building models of disease progression from clinical data. Firstly, it explores the use of non-stationary dynamic Bayesian networks to model disease progression where the underlying model changes over time (as is common with many diseases where some tissue or organ becomes damaged throughout the duration of disease progression. Secondly, the fitting of trajectories through cross-sectional data in order to build models of progression from larger cohorts but without any stamps. The methods are applied to simulated data and real clinical data based on visual field tests from sufferers of glaucoma, the second largest cause of blindness in the world. Results demonstrate the importance of integrating cross-sectional and longitudinal data, both of which offer different advantages to understanding disease progression, and the use of models that account for changing underlying structures.

12.1 Introduction

This paper explores the use of two different techniques for building models of disease progression from different types of clinical data, longitudinal and cross-sectional. The focus is upon examples from glaucoma and visual field test data to predict the onset and progression of the disease, though the issues dealt with are far from unique to this disease. Glaucoma is a neuropathic disease of the eye and is the second largest cause of blindness in the world. In 2002, there were 4.5 million sufferers worldwide, and according to [23] and the WHO Vision 2020 [21], there will be about 80 million people with glaucoma by 2020, given the ageing of the World's population. While there is no definitive cure for glaucoma, clinical practice has shown that, like many diseases, early medication can slow its progression [14, 15]. However, early diagnosis is a very challenging task, because of the variability of the pathology and its overlap with the physiology of the subject. The Visual Field (VF) test assesses the sensitivity of the retina to light. It is typically measured by automated perimetry, a technique in which the subject views a dim background as brighter spots of light are shone onto

© Springer International Publishing Switzerland 2015
A. Hommersom and P.J.F. Lucas (eds.), *Biomedical Knowledge Representation*, LNAI 9521, DOI 10.1007/978-3-319-28007-3_12

Fig. 12.1 A typical VF test
from a glaucomatous eye
showing loss of visual
sensitivity as dark patches

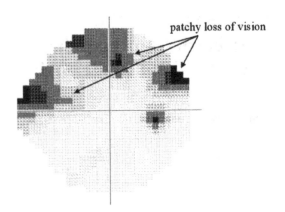

patchy loss of vision

the background at various locations in a regular grid pattern. The brightness at which
the subject sees the spots of light is related to the retinal sensitivity. See Fig. 12.1 for
an example of a VF test from a patient suffering from glaucoma.

Interventions such as medication or surgery can make a huge difference to quality
of life and slow the process of disease progression but they rarely change the long
term prognosis. The characteristics of many degenerative diseases, such as glaucoma,
is therefore a general transition from healthy to early onset to advanced stages. If we
look at some quantifiable set of symptoms (say the outcome of a set of clinical tests)
and plot them in two dimensions (using dimensionality reduction techniques) we can
see the general 'direction' of the disease process as a trend from an area of apparent
'healthy' individuals through to individuals with 'mild' symptoms and resulting in
an area representing advanced symptoms. Figure 12.2 shows two examples of this
'trend'. One is taken from breast cancer data that contains tumour descriptors and is
available from the UCI repository [8], and the other is from glaucoma patient data as
documented in [31]. Both are plotted using classical multidimensional scaling with
Euclidean distance [27].

Clearly these trends will depend upon a number of factors such as which clinical
variables are selected, how much data there is available in the sample, and whether
the disease process is generally monotonic. In order to infer the process of disease
progression, we must make an appropriate use of the available clinical data and in the
next section some different types of survey are discussed with their implications for
modelling. In the next Section we will explore some typical approaches to modelling
time-series from longitudinal studies before focussing in Sect. 12.2 on an approach to
model non-stationary time-series which is typical in clinical data such as the visual
field test data. Finally, in Sect. 12.3, we explore an approach at sequence reconstruction from cross-sectional data in order to build *pseudo time-series* of disease
progression, before concluding in Sect. 12.4.

Fig. 12.2 Trends in progression of degenerative diseases. An example from glaucoma (top) and breast cancer (bottom) where dots represent healthy individuals and crosses represent patients diagnosed with the respective disease. For many datasets there is generally a smooth transition as people move from healthy to early onset and then advanced disease.

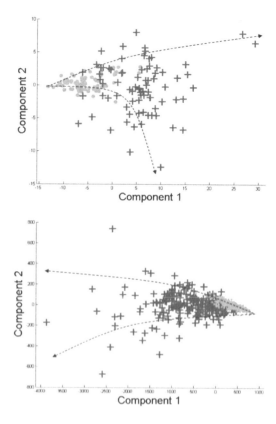

12.2 Fitting Trajectories Through Time-Stamped Data

When time stamps (discrete or continuous) are available, such as is the case with longitudinal data, we can build time-series models. These models can be used to try to predict future values of the data or the disease outcome.

12.2.1 Statistical and Machine Learning Models

There are a number of popular approaches to modelling time-series. For example, regression techniques that fit a model (linear or polynomial) through the data where time is used to predict the rate of change in some set of clinical variables [33]. However, care must be taken as each observation is not independent of one another (symptoms at time t are typically dependent on the symptoms at $t - 1$). As a result, standard residual error analysis cannot be carried out. Another very common time-series modelling approach is the Box-Jenkins method [3]. It is also known as the

Fig. 12.3 Architectures of
(a) A hidden Markov model
with a hidden node H, and
N observed variables X_i,
and (b) A dynamic Bayesian
network with N nodes
including various links
within the same time slice
and from nodes at $t-1$ to
nodes at t.

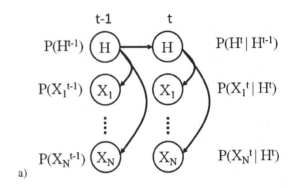

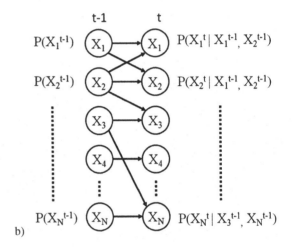

Autoregressive Integrated Moving Average (ARIMA) as it combines the autoregressive and moving average processes to model past observations and errors. It handles
trends and cycles through differencing the data. Fitting an ARIMA involves identifying an initial model (which includes determining seasonality and stationarity),
estimating the parameters, and verification through residual analysis. The approach is
attractive due to its ability to capture a diverse set of time-series behaviour. However,
as a result of its flexibility it can risk overfitting data.

A popular model for modelling sequential and time-series data is known as the
Hidden Markov Model (HMM) [24], which assumes a single discrete hidden state,
H and a continuous observed process, X. See Fig. 12.3 for the general architecture
where directed links determine conditional probability distributions. The transition
equation is modelled using a discrete distribution of the state H at time t, H^t con-
ditioned upon the state at $t-1$. This is written as $p(H^t|H^{t-1})$ (and gives rise to the
link $H^{t-1} \rightarrow H^t$ in Fig. 12.3). The measurement equation is captured using a distribution of each variable at time t conditioned upon the hidden state at time t, written

as $p(X^t|H^t)$ (giving rise to the links, $H^t \rightarrow X_1^t$, $H^t \rightarrow X_2^t$, ..., $H^t \rightarrow X_N^t$). The *forward algorithm* allows the probability of the hidden state at time, H^t to be estimated from the previous and current values of measured variables, $X^{1...t}$. In other words, to predict $p(H^t|X^{1...t})$, where H^t represents the hidden state at time t and X^t represents the variables in the time series. This process is known as *filtering* and can be used to estimate future probabilities of disease states from historical longitudinal data.

Linear Dynamic Systems (LDS) are a variant of the HMM that assume a linear normal Gaussian for the underlying process. The Kalman Filter [1] offers a way to perform filtering on this class of model. More recently, Dynamic Bayesian Networks (DBNs) [9, 10] have become popular for modelling disease [32] because they explicitly model temporal and non-temporal relationships and are flexible enough to model latent variables similar to the hidden process in HMMs. A simple example of a HMM and a DBN is shown in Fig. 12.3.

To build a DBN, the structure of the network and the parameters - the conditional probability distributions (CPDs) of all the variables must be obtained. Typically, the CPDs are learned from data by maximizing the posterior probability of the parameters given the data [13]. When the structure is fixed and the prior distribution of the parameters is uniform, this corresponds to maximizing the likelihood function.

12.2.2 Non Stationary Dynamic Bayesian Networks for Modelling Glaucoma

Although DBNs can capture the time-dependent nature of the relations in the data, they are models for *stationary processes* meaning that parameters and relations between variables cannot change over time. Once a set of time slices are created, the model is replicated over time. In many medical contexts, however, dependency relations between variables can change over time. For example in glaucoma, the Optic Nerve Head (ONH), which carries the visual functional signal, structurally changes during the progression of the disease, resulting in non-stationary series [35].

To overcome the stationarity in time series modelling with graphical models, Non-stationary DBNs have been recently introduced. In the learning process, both a model parameterisation and a segmentation process are performed. However, the search space is usually limited by constraining one or more degrees of freedom, i.e. the segmentation points of the time series, the parameters of the variables, the dependencies between the variables and the number of segments for the model. Among the most recent and complete work, Talin and Hengartner (2005) used a Monte Carlo Markov Chain approach to estimate the variance structure of the data, but the search space was limited to a fixed number of segments and for learning undirected edges only [29]. Xuan and Muphy (2007) proposed an approach to model changing dependency structures from multivariate time series, but also in this case the search was limited to undirected edges [34]. Robinson and Hartemink (2010) formalized the concept and proposed a solution that tackles all the degrees of freedom described except for the parameters [25]. Grzegorczyk and Husmeier (2009) instead retained the stationarity of the structure in favour of the parameters flexibility, arguing that structure changes lead almost certainly to over-flexibility of the model with short time-series [11]. While the first approach may only capture parameters changes that are strong enough to give rise to a structural change, the latter may not model correctly underlying conditional dependencies over the stages. The ability to both assess weak and strong changes in variable distributions and explicitly model the evolution of their relationships would be extremely useful from the informative point of view, especially in unknown processes such as glaucoma.

The issues involved with differing rates of progression that were highlighted earlier (in the introduction to this chapter) can be addressed to some degree by exploiting non-stationary DBNs. In [5] a form of DBN that clusters sections of time series whilst simultaneously learning DBN structure and parameters was used to model glaucoma patients. The Bayesian Information Criterion (BIC) [26] was used in conjunction with Simulated Annealing (SA) [17] for learning both the BNs and the clusters. BIC incorporates a penalizing factor that is proportional to the number of parameters in the model and the number of cases in the data, and helps to prevent overfitting.

The proposed algorithm in [5] is a 2-step SA technique that switches between 'warping' operations on the data and 'structural' operations on the model. The warping operation is carried out with probability p and performs the segmentation of the time series into the model stages. With probability $1 - p \ll 1$, a stage may also be added to or removed from the model. When no better solution is found for $L1$ search iterations, structural operations are carried out. This corresponds to adding or removing conditional dependencies from the model. When structural changes don't improve the model score for $L2$ iterations, the segmentation search is again performed. New solutions are accepted according to the current temperature t and the score improvement of the last operation. The function regulating the solution acceptance is an exponential function commonly used in SA-based algorithms. When a solution is accepted, the structure and the parameters of the model are updated and the old segmentation is replaced. The search stops when no better solutions are found for L total iterations. Intuitively, since the parameters depend on the segmentation of the data and the score of a new segmentation depends on the current parameters and the structure of the model, the algorithm tends to converge by grouping together similar data. Given that data is not forced to pass through all the stages, if clusters of data are present they will tend to aggregate into separate set of stages, forming clusters of temporal processes. The algorithm is described in detail in [5].

Figure 12.4 demonstrates the result of applying this model fitting process on simulated data with three different DBN structures at different points in the time-series. The original structures are shown in the top panel, labeled as TRUE. From each of these structures a set of data points was sampled and three time series were built by concatenating the data as showed in the lower section of the figure. Each of the time series corresponds to a temporal Cluster, being sampled only on two of the three original structures. Below each of the TRUE structures, the correspondent learnt structures are reported. The learnt number of stages was correct and all the relations

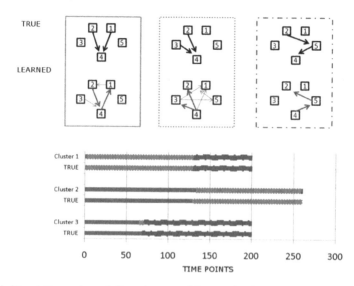

Fig. 12.4 Non stationary dynamic Bayesian network learnt using the non-stationary DBN approach from [5] on simulated data. TRUE networks represent the original networks used to generate the data and LEARNED networks represent those learnt from the data. The weight of the arrows represent the confidence in the links. The time-series plots illustrate which sections of time-series data are constructed using the three different underlying networks.

were captured by the algorithm, though there were numerous spurious relations also included. In the lower section of the figure, the TRUE and discovered distribution of data points is shown throughout each time-series. Essentially, this demonstrates that the three time-series were correctly clustered in the three groups, and data was segmented very closely to the original and in the correct sequence for all the clusters.

Figure 12.5 demonstrates the result of applying the model fitting on longitudinal data from two glaucoma sufferers. The plots are of visual sensitivity for differing sectors of the visual field. The dark lines represent the positions where changes in stages have been discovered. Below each plot, a simulation of the visual field sensitivity map was obtained from the learnt model. A bar chart of the number of visits for each stage is also reported. The first patient presents a general stable condition and a sudden drop in sensitivity, which was well captured as a switch from stage A (early stage) to F (final severe stage). The second patient presents slightly less clear disease progression, with higher fluctuation and brief improvement of conditions, captured by stage C. By breaking up the time-series for patients into these key stages not only improves predictive performance but also helps to explain the different phases of disease progression.

Fig. 12.5 Non stationary dynamic Bayesian network learnt using the non-stationary DBN approach from [31] on longitudinal Glaucoma data from 2 patients. The plots show sensitivity over different sectors of the visual field (t - temporal, n - nasal, s - superior, i - inferior). Vertical bars show the discovered changes in DBN structure (Labelled A - F). Also included are expected VF plots generated from the model and shown as greyscale images where Darker regions represent lower sensitivity.

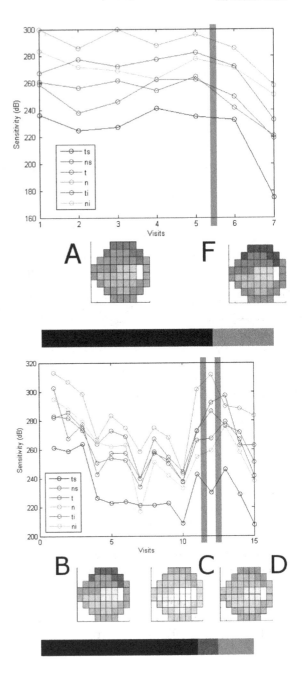

12.3   Fitting Trajectories Through Cross Sectional Data: Sequence Reconstruction

When no time stamps are available as is the case with cross sectional data, we can attempt to reconstruct sequences. This involves trying to find the best order for a particular set of data. Methods include the travelling salesman problem approach which aims minimise the distance between datapoints [28] and the calculation of the Minimum Spanning Tree (MST) [22] which efficiently identifies the shortest path through data coordinates. The principal curve algorithm [16] essentially tries to fit curves through (potentially cross-sectional) data points in order to build a model of some temporal process. More recently the use of PQ-Trees has been explored to encode partial orderings in order to account for uncertainty in the data due to elements such as noise [20].

PQ-Trees are a graph-structure device that can represent an ordering of points, and indicate which parts of the ordering are well-supported (Q-nodes) and which parts contain more uncertainty (P-nodes). Whilst the children of a P-node can be put into any order, children of a Q-node may be reversed in order but may not otherwise be reordered. A minimum spanning tree is generated from the distance matrix and the diameter path of this is used as the main Q-node of the PQ tree - the backbone of the reconstructed ordering. Branches of the diameter path are added as P and Q nodes to the main Q node. Therefore, the constructed PQ-tree represents a partial ordering of the data samples. Figure 12.6 illustrates an example minimum spanning tree and the subsequent PQ-Tree. A PQ-Tree can be converted into a single ordering, O using a hill-climb method to further minimise the distance within the PQ-Tree constraints. In [31], the algorithm was extended to also constrain the search to find paths with a fixed, user-defined, start and end point representing the most extreme healthy and diseased cases in cross-sectional data.

12.3.1   Pseudo Time-Series

A resampling approach known as the Pseudo Temporal Bootstrap (TBS) [31] aims to build multiple trajectories through cross sectional data in order to approximate genuine longitudinal data. These *Pseudo Time-Series* (PTS) can then be used to build approximate temporal models for prediction.

Definition: Let a dataset D be defined as a real valued matrix where m (rows) is the number of samples - here patients - and n (columns) is the number of variables - clinical test data. We define $D(i)$ as the ith row of matrix D. The vector $C = [c_1, c_2, ..., c_m]$ represents defined classes, where each $c_i \in \{0,1\}$ corresponds to the sample i, $c_i = 0$ represents that sample i is a healthy case, and $c_i = 1$ represents that sample i is a diseased case. These classifications are based upon the diagnoses made by experts.

Fig. 12.6 (a) shows an example minimum spanning tree and (b) shows the PQ-Tree generated from it

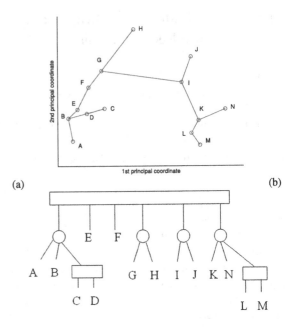

(a)   (b)

We define a time-series as a real valued T (row) by n (column) matrix where each row corresponds to an observation measured over T time points. We say that if $T(i)$ was observed before $T(j)$ then $i < j$.

We define a set of pseudo time-series indices as $P = \{p_1, p_2, \ldots p_k\}$ where each p_i is a T length vector where $T > 0$. We define p_{ij} as the jth element of p_i and each $p_{ij} \in \{1, \ldots, m\}$. We define the function $F(p_i) = [p_{i1}, \ldots, p_{iT}]$ as creating a T by n matrix where each row of $F(p_i) = D(p_{ij})$. A pseudo time-series can be constructed from each p_i using this operator. For example, if a pseudo time-series index vector $p_1 = [3, 7, 2]$ then $F(p_1)$ is a matrix where the first row is $D(3)$, the second row is $D(7)$ and the third row is $D(2)$. The corresponding class vector of each pseudo time-series generated by $F(p_i)$ is given by $G(p_i) = [C(p_{i1}), \ldots, C(P_{iT})]$.

12.3.2 The Pseudo Temporal Bootstrap

The elements of p_i are determined based upon a uniform random sampling procedure with replacement. The ordering of the elements in p_i is based upon randomly selecting a start and end in the p_i such that the associated classifications are $c_{start} = 0$ and $c_{end} = 1$. This means that the time-series will progress from a healthy state to a disease state. The ordering is then determined by the shortest path, calculated based upon the Floyd Warshall algorithm [7] applied to the Euclidean distance matrix between samples in $F(p_i)$. See [31] for the full algorithm.

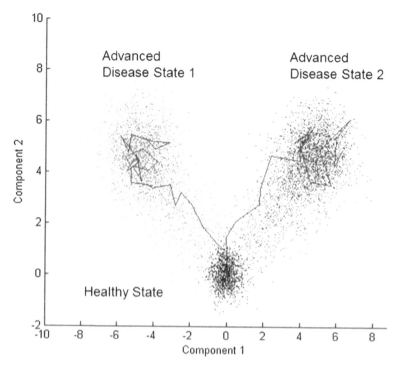

Fig. 12.7 Scatterplot of the first two components using multidimensional scaling on simulated data (generated from an ARHMM with 3 states, one representing healthy control patients, and two representing different disease symptoms). Two of the original MTS are plotted along with the full cross section (one sampled from each MTS).

As an example we can explore how well multivariate time-series models can be reverse-engineered from cross section data by simulating the cross sectional study process. Figure 12.7 shows the result of simulating a differing number of time-series from an AutoRegressive HMM (ARHMM) with two disease states and one healthy state. The data shown is a result of sampling a single point from each series randomly (essentially generating a cross section of the population of time-series). We can then use the temporal bootstrap to learn pseudo time-series prior to building a pseudo temporal model. The error rates (Table 12.1) and classification accuracy (Table 12.2) resulting from the pseudo time-series models are labelled (TBS) compared to the statistics generated from a model learnt from the original time-series (Full MTS).

Notice that the TBS results actually appear to be better than the model inferred from the full MTS. This is because the resampling process in the TBS procedure smooths the data and so also shown are the results of the full MTS after smoothing which are the most accurate (as would be expected - it is highly unlikely that the pseudo time-series will generate more accurate models). However as the sample size increases and approaches 500, the statistics appear to almost converge (results taken from [31]).

Table 12.1 Mean forecast sum squared error and 95% confidence for model learnt using the temporal bootstrap on cross-section data shown in Fig. 12.7 (TBS), the original time-series with smoothing (MTS smoothed) and without (MTS)

L	Full MTS	TBS	MTS smoothed
50	0.129 ± 0.039	0.251 ± 0.228	0.095 ± 0.055
100	0.125 ± 0.023	0.158 ± 0.121	0.086 ± 0.012
250	0.126 ± 0.013	0.079 ± 0.034	0.083 ± 0.012
500	0.125 ± 0.015	0.067 ± 0.023	0.084 ± 0.014

Table 12.2 Mean classification forecast accuracy and 95% confidence for model learnt using the temporal bootstrap on cross-section data shown in Fig. 12.7 (TBS), the original time-series with smoothing (MTS smoothed) and without (MTS)

L	Full MTS	TBS	MTS smoothed
50	0.907 ± 0.047	0.897 ± 0.092	0.903 ± 0.055
100	0.905 ± 0.045	0.912 ± 0.044	0.905 ± 0.048
250	0.905 ± 0.046	0.910 ± 0.046	0.905 ± 0.048
500	0.905 ± 0.046	0.912 ± 0.044	0.904 ± 0.049

Testing this approach on real VF cross sectional data, where we can validate using available longitudinal data, reveals similar results. Figure 12.8 illustrates some sample pseudo time-series generated from the cross sectional VF data and Fig. 12.9 shows the results of one step ahead forecasting using the TBS model and the model learnt from the longitudinal data. Also included are the Sum Squared Errors (SSE) scored using the previous sensitivity value as the forecast, *PrevDatum*, in order to provide a baseline - this is used as clinicians generally consider there to be slow progression between tests. The mean SSE over all patients is 0.4806 for the Full MTS data (longitudinal), 0.5392 for the TBS model (learnt from the sampled cross section), and 0.5701 for the *PrevDatum* approach. It appears that the TBS model captures some of the dynamics of the disease process in that it improves the accuracy of forecasts of the longitudinal data compared with the baseline *PrevDatum*. The TBS model seems to perform significantly better on some patients. This could be due to the TBS capturing two apparent distinct trajectories where the end states seem to sit in different regions of Fig. 12.8. Figure 12.9 shows the scatterplots of each predicted sensitivity for 6 sectors of the visual field against the actual measurement including individual SSE values. Firstly, this shows that some sectors are more easily predicted than others, possibly due to varying noise. It also seems that the accuracy is better for higher values of sensitivity which makes sense because as sensitivity decreases there is known to be increased noise within the visual field.

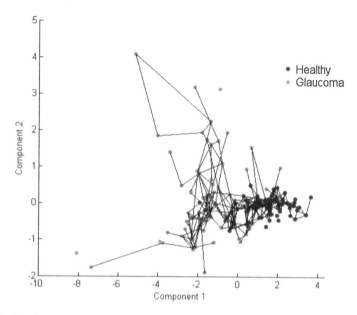

Fig. 12.8 Sample pseudo time-series generated using the temporal bootstrap on glaucoma cross-section data.

12.3.3   Identifying Key Areas in Trajectories Using EM

Assuming that a good approximation of a time-series model can be learnt from cross-sectional data by exploring sequence reconstruction approaches such as those presented in the previous section, methods can be explored to identify important stages in the trajectories using unsupervised methods on time-series models. For example, the Expectation Maximisation algorithm [2] can be used to cluster a sequence of data into different sections. By applying this approach different key stages can be identified in a disease process [19]. What is more, the ordering of the discovered sequences (i.e. the pseudo time-series) can lead to more informative clusters and transitions than simply clustering the unordered cross-sectional data (for example using standard clustering such as K-means [12]).

Figure 12.10 shows the results of clustering pseudo time-series generated from the glaucoma cross-sectional study using the EM algorithm. Panel A shows the mean values for a clinical test for glaucoma based upon retinal images of the rim area (*Diff_rim*) whilst Panel B shows the mean values of VF sensitivity for the pre-classified glaucomatous (marked with circles) and control patients (marked with crosses) for 6 different sectors of the eye. Notice that healthy people generally have high sensitivity values and low Diff_rim values, whereas the reverse is true for glaucomatous. Panel C shows the results of clustering using the EM algorithm on HMMs learnt from the pseudo time-series. The values represent the expected values of sensitivity and Diff_Rim for four different discovered clusters (or states). Notice that

Fig. 12.9 1 step ahead forecast scatterplots for each NFB - predicted with TBS vs actual. Individual SSE values are also shown.

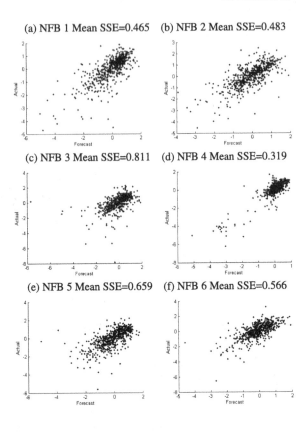

there are clearly two clusters that represent the healthy and glaucomatous (marked up with crosses and circles, respectively) but that there are also two other intermediate states. We can also explore the transition diagram for the states generated by the HMM to given an indication of where the states lie on the trajectory. This diagram (Panel E) supports the idea that two states are indeed intermediate states where glaucoma symptoms are either evident in the sensitivity values but not the Diff_Rim or vice versa (the states have been labelled accordingly). Simply using standard clustering of the cross-sectional data without exploiting the discovered trajectories shows less meaningful clusters are generated (Panel D).

12.4 Conclusions

In this paper, two different approaches to modelling trajectories through clinical data are explored. Firstly, some methods to infer time-series models from longitudinal studies are discussed. This includes statistical models such as Box-Jenkins and methods that can deal with uncertainty such as hidden Markov models and dynamic Bayesian

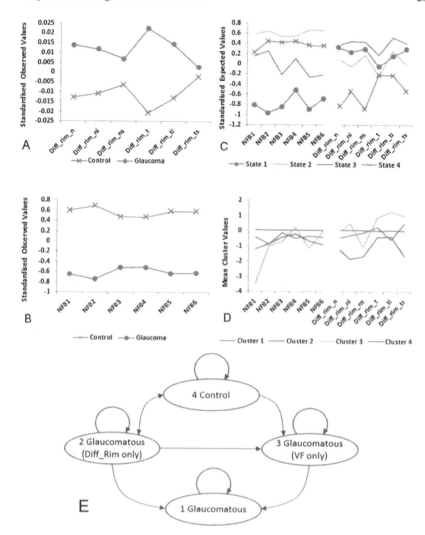

Fig. 12.10 Mean visual sensitivity (B) and other clinical test values (A) for different sectors of the eye. Also, included are the expected values for states discovered using EM temporal models trained on pseudo time-series (C) as compared to the profiles of clusters (using standard K-means) discovered from cross sectional data that does not exploit any trajectory information (D). The state transition diagram for the discovered states in (C) are shown in (E)

networks. Some of the ways to overcome the limitations of these techniques such as the non-stationarity of disease progression are explored in more detail with some examples. Secondly, some new techniques for building trajectories through cross-sectional data are explored with a focus on sequence reconstruction. Techniques for both types of data are demonstrated with examples from both simulated data and glaucoma studies. It is clear that many of the longstanding approaches to modelling disease progression are proving inadequate to dealing with issues of uncertainty in the dynamic and measurement processes, issues of non-stationarity in the dynamic processes, and the ability to integrate cross-sectional studies (which offer the advantages of diversity in the population and the inclusion of fully healthy controls) with longitudinal studies (which offer the ability to learn genuinely temporal models).

In economics *pooling* techniques attempt to combine longitudinal studies in order to create a greater cross section of individuals. There has been some exploration of integrating data by determining parameters from cross-sectional data and then using these to update the parameters of a time-series model [18]. Different variations on this general idea were developed including the balanced utilisation of pooled data, which assigns equal importance to both the cross-sectional and the longitudinal study by applying generalised least squares methods to both [30]. For a review of pooling see [6]. In fact, some of the methods described in this document can be extended to integrate the data. By adopting a Bayesian approach to integration, cross-sectional studies can be used to learn prior models [4]. This can be performed either directly from the data, resulting in static Bayesian networks, or via the pseudo time-series approach described in this document to give dynamic Bayesian network models. These priors can then be updated using longitudinal studies in order to 'calibrate' the temporal models. This overcomes some of the issues with the models generated from the sequence reconstruction models such as the lack of genuine temporal information. By integrating both types of data should offer the advantage of modelling a diverse population incorporating samples of all stages of disease whilst also encoding the genuine temporal characteristics of disease processes.

Acknowledgements. We would like to thank Professor David Garway-Heath of Moorfields Eye Hospital and the Institute of Ophthalmology, London for the availability of the Visual Field test data.

References

1. Anderson, B.D.O., Moore, J.B.: Optimal Filtering. Prentice-Hall, Englewood Cliffs (1979)
2. Bilmes, J.: A gentle tutorial on the em algorithm and its application to parameter estimation for gaussian mixture and hidden Markov models. Technical report TR-97-021, ICSI (1997)
3. Box, G.E.P., Jenkins, G.M.: Time Series Analysis: Forecasting and Control. Holden-Day, San Francisco (1970)
4. Castelo, R., Siebes, A.: Priors on network structures: biasing the search for Bayesian networks. Int. J. Approximate Reasoning **24**, 39–57 (2000)
5. Ceccon, S., Crabb, D., Garway-Heath, D., Tucker, A.: Non-stationary clustering Bayesian networks for Glaucoma. In: Proceedings of the Workshop on Machine Learning for Clincial Data Analysis, ICML 2012 (2012)
6. Fanfani, R.: Pooling time-series and cross-section data: a review. Eur. Rev. Agric. Econ. **2**(1), 63–85 (1974)
7. Floyd, R.W.: Algorithm 97: shortest path. Commun. ACM **5**(6), 345 (1962)
8. Frank, A., Asuncion, A.: UCI machine learning repository. University of California, School of Information and Computer Science, Irvine, CA (2010). http://archive.ics.uci.edu/ml. Accessed 11 October 2012

9. Friedman, N., Murphy, K.P., Russell, S.J.: Learning the structure of dynamic probabilistic networks. In: Proceedings of the 14th Annual Conference on Uncertainty in AI, pp. 139–147 (1998)
10. Ghahramani, Z.: Learning dynamic Bayesian networks. In: Giles, C.L., Gori, M. (eds.) IIASS-EMFCSC-School 1997. LNCS (LNAI), vol. 1387, pp. 168–197. Springer, Heidelberg (1998)
11. Grzegorczyk, M., Husmeier, D.: Non-stationary continuous dynamic Bayesian networks. In: Proceedings of the Twenty-Third Annual Conference on Neural Information Processing Systems (NIPS 2009), pp. 682–690. Curran Associates (2009)
12. Hartigan, J.A., Wong, M.A.: A k-means clustering algorithm. Appl. Stat. **28**, 100–108 (1979)
13. Heckerman, D., Geiger, D., Chickering, D.: Learning Bayesian networks: the combination of knowledge and statistical data. In: KDD Workshop (1994)
14. Heijl, A., et al.: Reduction of intraocular pressure and Glaucoma progression: results from the early manifest Glaucoma trial. Arch. Ophthalmol. **120**(10), 1268 (2002)
15. Kass, M.A., et al.: The ocular hypertension treatment study: a randomized trial determines that topical ocular hypotensive medication delays or prevents the onset of primary open-angle Glaucoma. Arch. Ophthalmol. **120**(6), 701 (2002)
16. Kegl, B., et al.: Learning and design of principal curves. IEEE Trans. Pattern Anal. Mach. Intell. **22**, 281–297 (2000)
17. Kirkpatrick, S., Gelatt, C.D., Vecchi, M.P.: Optimization by simulated annealing. Science **220**, 671–680 (1983)
18. Klein, L.R.: A Textbook of Econometrics. Row Peterson and Company, New York (1953)
19. Li, Y., Tucker, A.: Uncovering disease regions using pseudo time-series trajectories on clinical trial data. In: Proceedings of the 3rd IEEE International Conference on BioMedical Engineering and Informatics (BMEI 2010) (2009)
20. Magwene, P.M., Lizardi, P., Kim, J.: Reconstructing the temporal ordering of biological samples using microarray data. Bioinformatics **19**(7), 842–850 (2003)
21. Pizzarello, L., et al.: VISION 2020: the right to sight: a global initiative to eliminate avoidable blindness. Arch. Ophthalmol. **122**(4), 615 (2004)
22. Prim, R.C.: Shortest connection networks and some generalizations. Bell Syst. Tech. J. **36**, 1389–1401 (1957)
23. Quigley, H.A., Broman, A.T.: The number of people with Glaucoma worldwide in 2010 and 2020. Br. J. Ophthalmol. **90**(3), 262 (2006)
24. Rabiner, L.R.: A tutorial on HMM and selected applications in speech recognition. Proc. IEEE **77**(2), 257–286 (1989)
25. Robinson, J.W., Hartemink, A.J.: Learning non-stationary dynamic Bayesian networks. J. Mach. Learn. Res. **11**, 3647–3680 (2010)
26. Schwarz, G.E.: Estimating the dimension of a model. Ann. Stat. **6**(2), 461–464 (1978)
27. Seber, G.A.F.: Multivariate Observations. Wiley, Hoboken (1984)
28. Skiena, S.S.: Traveling salesman problem. In: The Algorithm Design Manual, pp. 319–322. Springer, New York (1997)
29. Talih, N., Hengartner, N.: Structural learning with time-varying components: tracking the cross-section of financial time series. J. Roy. Stat. Soc. B **67**(3), 321–341 (2005)
30. Theil, H., Goldberger, A.S.: On pure and mixed statistical estimation in economics. Int. Econ. Rev. **2**, 1 (1961)
31. Tucker, A., Garway-Heath, D.: The pseudotemporal bootstrap for predicting Glaucoma from cross-sectional visual field data. IEEE Trans. Inf. Technol. Biomed. **14**(1), 79–85 (2010)
32. Tucker, A., et al.: A spatio-temporal Bayesian network classifier for understanding visual field deterioration. Artif. Intell. Med. **34**, 163–177 (2005)
33. Viswanathan, A.C., Fitzke, F.W., Hitchings, R.A.: Early detection of visual field progression in Glaucoma: a comparison of PROGRESSOR and STATPAC 2. Br. J. Ophthalmol. **81**, 1037–1042 (1997)
34. Xuan, X., Murphy, K.: Modeling changing dependency structure in multivariate time series. In: Proceedings of the 24th Annual International Conference on Machine Learning (ICML 2007), pp. 1055–1062 (2007)
35. Yanoff, M., Duker, J.S.: Ophthalmology, 2nd edn. Mosby, St. Louis (2003)

Chapter 13
Dynamic Bayesian Network for Cervical Cancer Screening

Agnieszka Onisko and R. Marshall Austin

Abstract In this chapter we will present the application of dynamic Bayesian networks to cervical cancer screening. The main goal of this project was to create a multivariate model that would incorporate several variables in one framework and predict the risk of developing cervical precancer and invasive cervical cancer. We were interested in identifying those women that are at higher risk of developing cervical cancer and that should be screened differently than indicated in the guidelines.

13.1 Introduction

Cervical cancer is the fourth most deadly cancer in women worldwide.[1] The introduction of the Papanicolaou test (also known as a Pap smear or a Pap test) for cervical cancer screening has dramatically reduced the incidence and mortality of cervical cancer. According to Ries et al. [15], screening for cervical cancer with the Pap test led to a 70 % drop in incidence of cervical cancers between 1950 and 1970 and a 40 % drop between 1970 and 1999 in the USA. Despite this fact, cervical cancer has not been eradicated, even in countries where the programs for cervical cancer screening exist. Prophylaxis has reduced the incidence and mortality of cervical cancer, although there is still need for improving the management of cervical cancer screening, for example, by means of identifying groups of women that are at higher risk of developing cervical cancer and that should be screened differently than indicated in the guidelines.

There are several studies that addressed the management of cervical cancer. Cantor et al. [7] presented several decision-analytic and cost-effectiveness models that could be applied to guide cervical cancer screening, diagnosis, and treatment decisions. One of the decision-analytic models was a Markov model for the natural history of high-risk strain of human papillomavirus (hrHPV) infection and cervical carcinogenesis [14]. The model assesses life-time risk of cervical cancer as well as approximates the

---

[1] World Health Organization (http://globocan.iarc.fr/), accessed on July, 2014.

© Springer International Publishing Switzerland 2015
A. Hommersom and P.J.F. Lucas (eds.), *Biomedical Knowledge Representation*, LNAI 9521, DOI 10.1007/978-3-319-28007-3_13

age-specific incidence of cervical cancer. A similar model was built for the German population [18]. The model was a Markov model for evaluating a life-time risk and life-time mortality of cervical cancer. Another group of tools for cervical cancer screening are cost-effectiveness models. Most of these cost-effectiveness models refer to investigation of an optimal scenario for cervical cancer screening based on two tests: Pap test and testing for the presence of hrHPV, e.g., [5, 10, 13].

There are many published studies that report risk assessments for cervical cancer, e.g., [8, 11, 12]. All these approaches have a major weakness, i.e., to our knowledge, most of these studies assess the risk based on the current results of patient screening tests and usually do not include any patient history record such as previous results of screening and diagnostic tests, or other clinical findings. In our project we were interested in building a multivariate model that would incorporate several variables in one framework and that would predict the risk of developing cervical precancer and invasive cervical cancer over time. One of the approaches that can address these challenges are dynamic Bayesian networks that were described in the introduction of this part of the book.

13.2 Medical Domain

In this section we will present a few important facts about cervical cancer, its risk factors, symptoms, and causes. We will also discuss screening for cervical cancer and describe screening data that we have used to build a dynamic Bayesian network model for cervical cancer risk assessment.

13.2.1 Cervical Cancer

Cervical cancer is one of the few cancers for which we know the cause. The most important risk factor in the development of cervical cancer is an infection with a high-risk strain of DNA human papillomavirus. In fact, the HPV infection by itself is the most frequent sexually transmitted disease in the world and in most cases this infection does not cause any clinical symptoms. The hrHPV infection is responsible for all cervical cancer cases, however, the relationship between the hrHPV infection and a development of cervical cancer is not deterministic, and only a small percentage of women that are infected with hrHPV will develop a cervical cancer. Furthermore, most cervical cancers are caused by a persistent hrHPV infection. There is still unknown why some women are good hosts to the hrHPV virus and why the infection leads in their case to a development of cervical cancer. Other risks of developing cervical cancer include smoking, oral contraceptives, or chlamydia infection. Cervical cancer rarely causes any clinical symptoms until it reaches a late stage. One of the few late stage cervical cancer symptoms is a vaginal bleeding.

There are two types of cervical cancer [1]. The first type of cervical cancer involves these cases that develop over years and progress to larger precancerous lesions. This type of cancer is usually preventable by screening. By cervical precancer we mean an abnormal tissue on the cervical surface or in endocervical canal. These lesions can progress to invasive cervical cancer, therefore, if a lesion is detected during screening, it is usually removed by one of the surgical procedures that prevents the lesion from becoming cancerous and from a spread to other body organs. Unfortunately, the screening is less effective for the cancer type 2 and to be detected usually requires more frequent screening. The cancer type 2 includes rapidly progressing cancers, cervical cancers in younger and elderly women, and the cases of glandular cervical cancer that usually arise in endocervical canal.

13.2.2 Screening for Cervical Cancer

An important part of cervical cancer management is its screening. Most of the cervical cancers develop over years, therefore, screening can be effective even if the screening tests are not 100% sensitive or specific. There are two major cervical cancer screening tests: (1) the Pap test and (2) the hrHPV test. A primary screening test in the USA is the Pap test. The Pap test is based on the analysis of cells sampled from the surface of the cervix, thus, in some countries it is simply known as a cytology test. Abnormal Pap test result suggests the presence of potentially premalignant or malignant changes in the cervix. Therefore, a woman with an abnormal Pap test result usually is directed to a further examination and to a possible preventive treatment. Recommendations for how often a Pap test should be performed vary, depending on a screening program, between once a year and once every five years. The second screening test is the hrHPV testing and it is often used as a complementary to Pap testing. While the Pap test shows possible changes in the cervix, the hrHPV test shows whether there is an infection present. Unfortunately, the hrHPV test result by itself does not tell anything about any previous infections.

In the last few years the HPV vaccine was introduced to the public. Up to date there are two vaccines available and they cover two strains of the hrHPV viruses (HPV16 and HPV18) that can lead to the development of cervical cancer. It is important to notice that the current vaccine does not provide a complete prevention for a cervical cancer. There are around 15 strains of the hrHPV virus that can lead to cervical cancer. Also, the vaccine is not effective if it is used in women infected already with the hrHPV virus [6].

13.2.3 Screening Data

The cervical cancer screening data available to us were collected during 8 years (2005–2012) at Magee-Womens Hospital, University of Pittsburgh Medical Center, USA. The data contained 791,092 Pap test results while 24.7% of these results were accompanied by hrHPV test results. Our data contained mainly the results of screening tests. Thus, diagnostic tests were recorded only for around 10% of

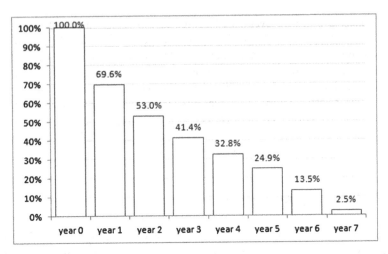

Fig. 13.1 The percentage of follow-up cases (Pap test results) available for each year in the Magee-Womens Hospital population.

screening tests, i.e., around 10 % of Pap test results were followed by a histopathological examination. The data were collected by means of advanced technologies such as liquid-based cytology (a new Pap test with a higher sensitivity than the conventional Pap smear test) and testing for the presence of the hrHPV virus. Furthermore, Pap test interpretations were assisted with a computer-based system that identifies abnormal cells [20]. The data contained also some clinical information such as the history of infections, cancers, or use of contraceptives. Our database registered also HPV vaccine status, although there were only 2,040 patient cases with HPV vaccine status recorded. Furthermore, histopathological examination results in our database were in a free text format. Therefore, these data entries required additional pre-processing, i.e., we had to convert these findings into dictionary entries.

While building any model based on time series data, the follow-up becomes a crucial issue. Our model focuses on assessing the prediction for cervical precancer and cervical invasive cancer, therefore, in our analysis we excluded vaginal Pap test results. The reason for this was that majority of women with vaginal Pap test results are those who had hysterectomy procedure performed in the past and had their cervix removed. We also excluded these patients that have only one Pap test performed and did not have any follow-up data recorded. This led us to the analysis of 575,936 cytology test results belonging to 170,560 patients. Figure 13.1 captures additional information on the follow-up data. *Year 0* in the figure indicates the year when a patient for the first time showed up for a screening test. Of all patients who appear in *year 0*, 69.6 % appeared for follow-up screening in *year 1*, while 53.0 % appeared in *year 2*, etc. Only 2.5 % of all patients appeared in *year 7* (this corresponds to 4,285 patients).

13.3   Pittsburgh Cervical Cancer Screening Model

We have built the Pittsburgh Cervical Cancer Screening Model (PCCSM) [2, 4]. The main goal of this project was to create a model that would incorporate several variables in one framework and predict the risk of cervical precancer and invasive cervical cancer. We were interested in identifying those women that are at higher risk of developing cervical cancer and that need more frequent screening or a reference to a diagnostic procedure such as a colposcopy. The PCCSM model is a dynamic Bayesian network, its structure was built based on textbooks and the expert knowledge[2] and then parameterized by means of the cervical cancer screening data collected at Magee-Womens Hospital.

13.3.1   Graphical Structure

The current version of the PCCSM model consists of 15 nodes that belong to four groups: (1) screening tests: Pap test and hrHPV test; (2) diagnostic or therapeutic procedures such as biopsy, cone biopsy, leep procedure, endocervical curettage, or hysterectomy; (3) patient history findings: menstrual history, cancer history, a use of contraception, HPV vaccine status; and (4) demographic variables: age and race. These variables has been chosen by the expert, although a procedure of selecting the model's variables was mainly driven by a set of medical finding recorded in the Magee-Womens Hospital electronic record system.

All variables were categorical, thus, we represented them in the model as the nodes with discrete values. The variable *Age* was discretized into three intervals: *below 30*, *between 30 and 50*, and *50 and up*. This discretization was suggested by our expert and it corresponds to three different cervical cancer risk groups. While modeling the node representing the Pap test we have distinguished 9 states. Our data on Pap test interpretations follow the Bethesda classification[3] and, in fact, the number of possible interpretations for the Pap test is even higher than modelled in the PCCSM. However, we grouped and merged some of the interpretations. For example, *Suspicious Malignant Cells, Positive Malignant Cells, Squamous Cell Carcinoma,* and *Adenocarcinoma* were merged into one state *SUSP/POS Malignant Cells.* This merge was performed mainly because of the lack of sufficient data for these categories. Similarly, we merged several interpretations of histopathologically verified diagnoses of cervix, for example, different types of cervical cancers: *Squamous Carcinoma, Adenocarcinoma,* or *Adenosquamous Carcinoma* were represented as one state and named as *Cervical Cancer.*

---

[2]The second author of this article is the expert of the PCCSM model.

[3]The Bethesda classification is a system for reporting Pap test interpretations. It was developed during the American Society for Colposcopy and Cervical Pathology Consensus Conference that took place in Bethesda, MD, USA [19]. The main goal of this meeting was to establish a standardized terminology in cytology diagnostic reports.

Table 13.1 Selected nodes of the PCCSM model along with their states

Node	States
Pap test	*Negative, ASCUS, LSIL, AGC, ASC-H, HSIL,* *SUSP/POS Malignant Cells, No Primary Interpretation, NA*
hrHPV test	*Negative, Positive, NA*
Cervix	*Benign, CIN1, CIN2, CIN3/AIS, Cervical Cancer,* *Metastatic Cancer in Cervix, NA*
HPV vaccine status	*Complete, Incomplete, NA*

Table 13.1 presents a list of possible results for two screening tests (Pap and hrHPV), a cervix status represented by the node *Cervix*, and a clinical finding describing HPV vaccine status. For example, the Pap test is described by 9 possible states: one state indicating a negative result, 6 states representing abnormal results, one state modeling the unsatisfactory result (*No Primary Interpretation*), and one state describing the result that is not available (*NA*).

A dynamic Bayesian network approach allows us to model a medical knowledge in the framework of a directed graph. While modelling the knowledge of cervical cancer screening we distinguished two types of relationships:

$$riskfactor \rightarrow disease \rightarrow screening test$$
$$riskfactor \rightarrow disease \rightarrow diagnostic test$$

$$cervix_t \rightarrow cervix_{t+1}$$
$$cervix_t \rightarrow cervix_{t+2}$$

While the first type of a relationship captures a static knowledge, the second type of a relationship shows a temporal knowledge. Figure 13.2 presents the graphical structure of the current version of the PCCSM model. The graphical structure of the model consists of two types of arcs: (1) regular arcs that model a static knowledge by means of probabilistic relationships between the variables in the same time step and (2) temporal arcs that model the relationships between the variables in different time steps. For example, the relationships between *Age*, *Cervix*, and *Pap test* capture a static knowledge and take place in the same time step. While a temporal relationship is represented by an arc with a label. For example, a label *2* in the node *Cervix* indicates a delay of an influence that takes two time steps.

Nine nodes out of 15 are temporal variables, i.e., they are repeated for each time step. In the GeNIe interface,[4] such nodes are placed within so called *Temporal Plate* (see Fig. 13.2). Five nodes were modeled as initial conditions and they represent patient clinical history record such as *History of contraception*, *History of Cancer*,

---

[4]The introduction to this part of the book contains a brief description of dynamic Bayesian networks with the examples presented in the GeNIe software.

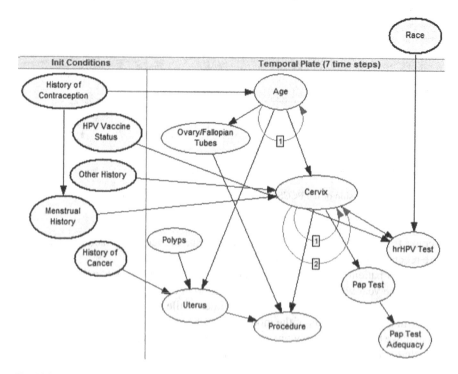

Fig. 13.2 Pittsburgh Cervical Cancer Screening Model

Menstrual History, the HPV *Vaccine Status*, and *Other History* (see the panel *Init Conditions* in Fig. 13.2). Another variable that does not change over time is *Race*. These static nodes are indicated in Fig. 13.2 by a bold border.

Most of the relationships modeled in the PCCSM model are causal, however, we also learned some of the relations from the data. For example, the relationship between *History of contraception* and *Age* was learned from the data. The average number of parents per node is 1.1, while the average number of states per node is 5.9. The node with the highest number of states is the one representing the *Pap test* and it consists of 9 states.

Figure 13.3 shows a version of the PCCSM model that is unfold for three time steps. To demonstrate the relationships between the variables in different time steps, we limited the model to four temporal nodes and five static nodes.

13.3.2   Time Granularity

The time step that we had chosen in the PCCSM model was one year. This is a consequence of cervical cancer screening guidelines in USA, recommending a woman

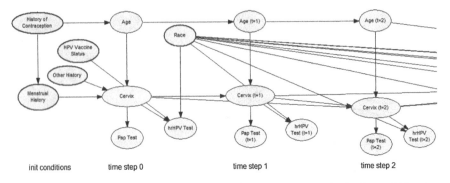

Fig. 13.3 Unfold version of the PCCSM model; a simplified version limited to 9 out of 15 nodes

to come for her Pap test examination once a year. In fact, these recommendations were recently changed to less frequent screening [17].

For each patient in the data set we defined the initial time as $t = 0$. Initial time indicates the year when the woman got registered in our database, i.e., usually when she showed up for the Pap test for the first time. While preparing the screening data for learning the parameters of the model, for each woman and for a particular model variable, we have chosen only one result per time step. For example, if a woman had more than one Pap test performed during a period of one year, we have chosen the most abnormal interpretation of this test.

13.3.3 Numerical Parameters

One of the feature of real world data is their incompleteness. Especially, in medical data collected over time we can expect missing entries. This is also a characteristic of our data. Figure 13.1 confirms that we do not have a complete follow-up data. In the PCCSM, we treated a missing value as an additional state and we modeled it explicitly as a possible state of a node. For example, if there was no Pap test result, we have modelled it as the state *not available* (*NA*). Please, note that each of the three nodes listed in Table 13.1 has the state *NA*. Similarly, if there was no diagnostic test result associated with a particular screening test result, we associated it with the value *not available*. Our data are screening data and 82 % of all screening test results are negative, i.e., they usually correspond to healthy women.

Another characteristic of our data is that they do not contain many cases of invasive cervical cancer. The reason for this is that if a woman is screened frequently enough, usually she will not develop an invasive cervical cancer due to treatment procedures that would be conducted if the presence of any precancerous cells will be detected on screening test results. Around 50 % of all women with cervical cancer in our database were not screened and did not have any previously recorded data.

We have learned the numerical parameters of the PCCSM model from the cervical cancer screening data collected at Magee-Womens Hospital. To learn the numerical parameters of the model we have applied the EM algorithm implemented in the SMILE library [9]. The resulting model has 2,414 independent numerical parameters.

13.4 Application of PCCSM

In this section we will present two applications of the PCCSM model: (1) the PCCSM as cervical cancer risk assessment tool and (2) the PCCSM as personalized aid for follow-up decision making.

13.4.1 Cervical Precancer and Invasive Cervical Cancer Predictions

The main outcome measure of the PCCSM model is the risk of developing cervical precancer or invasive cervical cancer. This risk is expressed by a posteriori probability calculated by the PCCSM model. The important advantage of dynamic Bayesian network approach is that it allows for looking at risk predictions for cervical precancer and invasive cervical cancer from different perspectives. Figure 13.4 presents the impact of patient history record on the cervical cancer risk assessments.

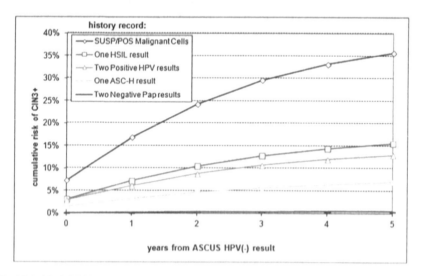

Fig. 13.4 The PCCSM risk assessments for cervical precancer and invasive cervical cancer (*CIN3+*) given history record

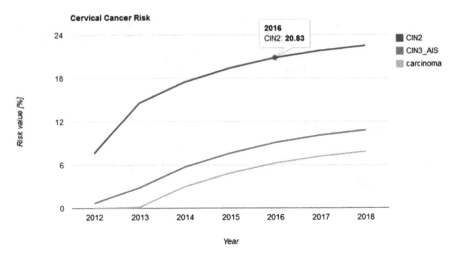

Fig. 13.5 A web-based interface of the PCCSM model: Risk assessments for cervical precancer (CIN2, CIN3/AIS) and invasive cervical cancer (carcinoma) over time

The figure captures quantitative risk predictions of precancer and invasive cervical cancer *(CIN3+)*[5] over the time period of five years for patients that in *year 0* had an abnormal Pap test result *(ASCUS)*[6] and a negative hrHPV test result. The five curves represent five groups of women with different history record. The PCCSM model allowed for identifying those risk categories that are crucial for follow-up planning, e.g., patients that are at higher risk of developing cervical cancer should be screened more often than patients that are at lower risk. For example, women with two negative Pap test results in the past (represented by a bottom curve in Fig. 13.4) are in a different risk category than women that had suspicious or positive malignant cells in the past (represented by a top curve in Fig. 13.4) even if they have the same screening test results in *year 0* (i.e., the *ASCUS* result for a Pap test and negative hrHPV test result).

13.4.2   Personalized Aid in Clinical Management and Follow-Up Decision Making

The PCCSM model allows for individualized management of patients and computes patient-specific risk based on the patients characteristics such as history data, demographics, and current screening test results. We have built a prototype web-based

---

[5]*CIN3+* stands for Cervical Intraepithelial Neoplasia grade 3 and indicates a severe dysplasia and worse including invasive cervical cancer.

[6]*ASCUS* stands for Atypical Squamous Cells of Undetermined Significance and indicates mild cellular abnormality in the cervix.

interface that helps to interact with the model [16]. This interface allows for entering patient data and saving them in patient data repository. The user of this tool can upload patient data and assess the risk prediction for cervical precancer and invasive cervical cancer. Figure 13.5 depicts one of the screen shots of this interface. The figure presents cumulative values of risk of developing cervical precancers ($CIN2^7$, $CIN3/AIS$) and invasive cervical cancer (*carcinoma*) over time. These results were calculated for a specific patient: a woman that at the beginning of the follow-up was 29, there were two years of follow-up data available: double ASCUS results for Pap test and double positive results for the hrHPV test. The PCCSM model shows that this woman will have a 20 % risk of developing $CIN2$ within four years.

13.5 Conclusions

In this chapter we have introduced the PCCSM model for cervical cancer screening. The PCCSM model allows for calculating the predictions of cervical precancer and invasive cervical cancer. It incorporates various variables in one framework and allows for looking at these predictions from different perspectives, including the perspective of patient history record. The model is capable of identifying groups of patients that are at higher risk of developing a disease. These quantitative predictions can be helpful in establishing the optimal timing of a follow-up screening.

We plan to use the PCCSM model in a routine medical practice as a quality control tool in high risk case selection for rescreening [3]. This can have a noticeable effect on the quality of medical care in our laboratory. Under the Clinical Laboratory Improvement Amendments of 1988 (CLIA 88), laboratories in USA are required to rescreen negative Pap test results. The challenge here is how to select negative Pap test slides for targeted high risk quality control rescreening. The process of high risk case selection at Magee-Womens Hospital is currently based on a simple identification of cases with an abnormal prior history, e.g., if a woman had a positive hrHPV test result or abnormal tissue result in the past, she is considered to be a high risk case and is selected for rescreening. We believe, that this process could be further improved by the PCCSM model.

Acknowledgments. We would like to thank Karen Lassige for her help in retrieving the data from the hospital database. We also acknowledge Magee-Womens Hospital cytology manager Nancy Mauser for her assistance in reviewing individual cytology reports and the lead cytotechnologist Jonee Matsko for her assistance in identifying cytology-histology correlates. Our study was approved by the Institutional Review Board, Magee-Womens Hospital, University of Pittsburgh (IRB#: PRO09070454).

Bayesian network models were created and tested using SMILE, an inference engine, and GeNIe, a development environment for reasoning in graphical probabilistic models, both developed at the Decision Systems Laboratory and available at https://dslpitt.org/genie/.

---

[7] $CIN2$ stands for Cervical Intraepithelial Neoplasia grade 2 and indicates moderate dysplasia that usually regresses.

References

1. Austin, R.M., Zhao, C.: Type 1 and type 2 cervical carcinomas: some cervical cancers are more difficult to prevent with screening. Cytopathology **23**(1), 6–12 (2012)
2. Marshall Austin, R., Oniśko, A., Druzdzel, M.J.: The pittsburgh cervical cancer screening model. a risk assessment tool. Arch. Pathol. Lab. Med. **134**, 744–750 (2010)
3. Austin, R.M., Oniśko, A., Druzdzel, M.J.: Bayesian network model analysis as a quality control and risk assessment tool in cervical cancer screening. J. Lower Genital Tract Dis. **12**(2), 153–179 (2008)
4. Austin, R.M., Oniśko, A., Druzdzel, M.J.: Patient history dependent risk assessments for cervical pre-cancer and invasive cancer using the pittsburgh cervical cancer screening model. J. Am. Soc. Cytopathol. **1**(1), S3–S4 (2012)
5. Bidus, M.A., et al.: Cost-effectiveness analysis of liquid-based cytology and human papillomavirus testing in cervical cancer screening. Obstetricians Gynecologists **107**(5), 997–1005 (2006)
6. Brotherton, J.M., et al.: Early effect of the HPV vaccination programme on cervical abnormalities in Victoria, Australia: an ecological study. Lancet **377**, 2085–2092 (2011)
7. Cantor, S.B., et al.: Decision science and cervical cancer. Cancer **98**(9), 2003–2008 (2003)
8. Castle, P.E., et al.: Risk assessmenmt to guide the prevention of cervical cancer. Am. J. Obstet. Gynecol. **197**, 356.e1–356.e6 (2007)
9. Decision Systems Laboratory, University of Pittsburgh, GeNIe and SMILE Software. https://dslpitt.org/genie/
10. Goldie, S.J., Kim, J.J., Wright, T.C.: Cost-Effectiveness of Human Papillomavirus DNA testing for Cervical Cancer Screening in women aged 30 years or more. Obstetricians Gynecologists **103**(4), 619–631 (2004)
11. Katki, H.A.: Cervical cancer risk for women undergoing concurrent testing for human papillomavirus and cervical cytology: a population-based study in routine clinical practice. Lancet Oncol. **12**(7), 663–672 (2011)
12. Khan, M.J., et al.: The Elevated 10-Year Risk of Cervical Precancer and Cancer in women with Human Papillomavirus (HPV) Type 16 or 18 and the Possible Utility of Type-Specific HPV Testing in Clinical Practice. J. Natl. Cancer Inst. **97**(14), 1072–1079 (2005)
13. Kim, J.J., Wright, T.C., Goldie, S.J.: Cost-effectiveness of alternative triage strategies for atypical squamous cells of undetermined significance. JAMA **287**, 2382–2390 (2002)
14. Myers, E.R., et al.: Mathematical model for the natural history of Human Papillomavirus infection and Cervical Carcinogenesis. Am. J. Epidemiol. **151**, 1158–1171 (2000)
15. Ries, L.A., Eisner, M.P., Kosary, C.: SEER Cancer Statistics Review, 1973–1999. National Cancer Institute, Bethesda (2002)
16. Sadkowski. J.A.: Computer-based system for cervical cancer risk assessment (in Polish). MA thesis. Bialystok, Poland, Faculty of Computer Science, Bialystok University of Technology, October 2011
17. Saslow, D., et al.: American Cancer Society, American Society for Colposcopy and Cervical Pathology, and American Society for Clinical Pathology screening guidelines for the prevention and early detection of cervical cancer. CA Cancer J. Clin. **62**(3), 147–172 (2012)
18. Siebert, U., et al.: The German Cervical Cancer Screening Model: development and validation of a decision-analytic model for cervical cancer screening in Germany. Eur. J. Public Health **16**(2), 185–192 (2006)
19. Solomon, D., et al.: The 2001 Bethesda system: terminology for reporting results of cervical cytology. JAMA **287**(16), 2114–2119 (2002)
20. ThinPrep imaging system product insert. Marlborough, MA: Cytyc Corporation. http://www.thinprep.com/pdfs/thinprep_package_insert_imaging.pdf. Accessed 31 October 2013

Chapter 14
Modeling Dynamic Processes with Memory by Higher Order Temporal Models

Anna Łupińska-Dubicka and Marek J. Druzdzel

Abstract Most practical uses of Dynamic Bayesian Networks (DBNs) involve temporal influences of the first order, i.e., influences between neighboring time steps. This choice is a convenient approximation influenced by the existence of efficient algorithms for first order models and limitations of available tools. In this paper, we focus on the question whether constructing higher time-order models is worth the effort when the underlying system's memory goes beyond the current state. We present the results of an experiment in which we successively introduce higher order DBN models monitoring woman's monthly cycle and measure the accuracy of these models in estimating the fertile period around the day of ovulation. We show that higher order models are more accurate than first order models. However, we have also observed over-fitting and a resulting decrease in accuracy when the time order chosen is too high.

14.1   Introduction

While all real world systems change over time, modeling their equilibrium states or ignoring change altogether, when it is sufficiently slow, is sufficient for solving a wide spectrum of practical problems. In some cases, however, it is necessary to follow the change that the system is undergoing and introduce time as one of the model variables.

We concentrate in this chapter on models that belong to the class of probabilistic graphical models, with their two prominent members: Bayesian networks (BNs) [7] and dynamic Bayesian networks (DBNs) [3]. BNs are widely used practical tools for knowledge representation and reasoning under uncertainty in equilibrium systems. DBNs extend them to time-dependent domains by introducing an explicit notion of time and influences that span over time. Most practical uses of DBNs involve temporal influences of the first order, i.e., influences between neighboring time steps. This choice is a convenient approximation influenced by existence of efficient algorithms for first order models and limitations of available tools. After all, introducing higher

© Springer International Publishing Switzerland 2015
A. Hommersom and P.J.F. Lucas (eds.), *Biomedical Knowledge Representation*, LNAI 9521, DOI 10.1007/978-3-319-28007-3_14

order temporal influences may be costly in terms of the resulting computational complexity of inference, which is NP-hard even for static models. Limiting temporal influences to influences between neighboring time periods is equivalent to assuming that the only thing that matters in the future trajectory of the system is its current state. Many real world systems, however, have memory that spans beyond their current state.

The question that we pose in this chapter is whether introducing higher order influences, i.e., influences that span over multiple steps, is worth the effort in the sense of improving the accuracy of the model. The idea of increasing modeling accuracy by means of increasing the time order of a dynamic model was beautifully illustrated by Shannon. In his seminal paper [11], outlining the principles of theory of information, he shows sentences in the English language, generated by a series of Markov chain models of increasing time order, trained by means of the same corpus of text. The following sentence was generated by a first order model:

```
OCRO HLI RGWR NMIELWIS EU LL NBNESEBYA TH
EEI ALHENHTTPA OOBTTVA NAH BRL.
```

Compare this with the following sentence generated by a sixth order model:

```
THE HEAD AND IN FRONTAL ATTACK ON AN ENGLISH
WRITER THAT THE CHARACTER OF THIS POINT IS
THEREFORE ANOTHER METHOD FOR THE LETTERS
THAT THE TIME OF WHO EVER TOLD THE PROBLEM
FOR AN UNEXPECTED.
```

The resemblance of the latter sentence to ordinary English text, an informal measure of the model's accuracy, has increased dramatically between the first and the sixth orders. A first order model was essentially impotent in its ability to learn and model the language.

While generation of English sentences may be too hard of a problem, the vehicle for our experiments with varying time order is the problem of monitoring the woman's monthly cycle, a problem central to human fertility. Every couple seeking help in a fertility clinic is asked to monitor the monthly cycle before any medical intervention is undertaken. An accurate monitoring model can be a great aid in natural family planning, indicating optimal days for sexual intercourse. There exist methods for fairly precise determining of the day of ovulation (e.g., blood hormone level tests or ultrasonographic analysis of the ovaries), but they either require laboratory visits or expensive testing kits. What is important from the perspective of the question posed in this chapter is that woman's monthly cycle is a system with memory going most certainly beyond one day and probably spanning over a period of roughly a month.

We report the results of an experiment in which we successively introduce higher order DBNs modeling the monthly cycle and measure the accuracy of these models in estimating the fertile period around the day of ovulation. We train our models on real time series data obtained from a longitudinal study of fecundability conducted in several European centers [2]. We show that increasing the time order of the model greatly improves its accuracy but only up to a certain point. Too high order of a model decreases accuracy, probably though over-fitting the training data.

The remainder of the chapter is structured as follows. Section 14.3 reviews what we know about woman's monthly cycle. Section 14.5 describes the data that we used in training our models. Section 14.4 describes our DBN models, Sect. 14.6 describes our experiments, and Sect. 14.7 summarizes the results of our experiments with the models. Finally, Sect. 14.8 offers some advice to knowledge engineers building DBN models in practice.

14.2 Bayesian Networks

Bayesian networks (BNs) are probabilistic graphical models that offer a compact representation of the joint probability distribution over a set of random variables $X = x_1, \ldots, x_n$. Formally, a Bayesian network is a pair (G, Θ), where G is a acyclic directed graph (ADG) in which nodes represent random variables $x_1, i \ldots, x_n$ and edges represent direct dependencies between pairs of variables. The second component of a Bayesian network, Θ, represents the set of parameters that describes a conditional distribution for each node x_i in G, given its parents in G, i.e., $P(x_i|Pa(x_i))$. Very often, the structure of the graph is given a causal interpretation, convenient from the point of view of knowledge engineering and user interfaces. Bayesian networks allow for computing probability distributions over subsets of their variables conditional on other subsets of observed variables. This can be given the interpretation of computing the probability of a hypothesis in light of evidence. BNs are widely applied in decision support systems, where they typically form the central inferential engine.

Consider the simple Bayesian network shown in Fig. 14.1. This is a simplified example, illustrating various causes of allergy in children. The tendency to develop allergies is often hereditary. Allergic parents are more likely to have allergic chil-

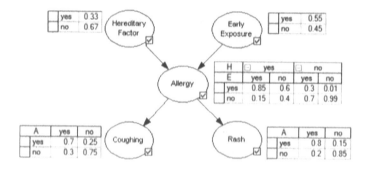

Fig. 14.1 A simple Bayesian network illustrating selected causes and effects of allergy in children.

dren, and their allergies are likely to be more severe than those from non-allergic parents. Exposure to allergens, especially in early life, is also an important risk factor for allergy. When an allergen enters the body of an allergic child, the child can cough or develop a rash. Figure 14.1 shows the dependency structure among the variables and the conditional probability distributions for each of the variables. All variables in this example are Boolean. At the roots, we have the prior probabilities (e.g., that one or both of the parents suffer from allergies or a child had a contact with allergen in early life). The conditional probabilities for the non-root nodes give the probability distributions over the nodes conditional on various outcomes of the direct predecessors in the graph (e.g., probability distribution over the variable coughing given that a child has allergy).

Dynamic Bayesian networks (DBNs) are an extension of Bayesian networks for modeling dynamic systems. In a DBN, the state of a system at time t is represented by a set of random variables $X_t = (X_{1,t}, \ldots, X_{n,t})$. The state at time t generally dependents on the states at previous time steps. Typically, we assume that each state only depends on the immediately preceding state (i.e., the system is first-order Markov), and thus we represent the transition distribution $P(X_t|X_{t-1})$. This can be done using a two-slice Bayesian network fragment (2TBN) B_t, which contains variables from X_t whose parents are variables from X_{t-1} and/or X_t, and variables from X_{t-1} without their parents. The term *dynamic* means that we model the state of a system over time, not that the model structure and its parameters change over time (even though the latter is theoretically possible). A DBN is typically defined as a pair of Bayesian networks $(B_0, B_\rightarrow)$, where B_0 represents the initial distribution $P(X_0$, and $B_\rightarrow$ is a two time slice Bayesian netwok, which defines the transition distribution $P(X_t|Xt - 1)$ as follows [3]:

$$P(X_t|X_{t-1}) = \prod_{i=1}^{N} P(X_{i,t}|Pa(X_{i,t}))$$

Consider a two years old child whose parents suffer from allergy and who has been exposed to some allergens. We know that this child has not developed any symptoms of allergy in the previous year. Suppose that we want to know the probability that allergy appears in the third year. If we use the BN pictured in Fig. 14.1, we omit all historical information except for the previous year. Figure 14.2 (a) shows a DBN of first temporal order, which means that we take into consideration not only present observations but also these from the previous year.

As we mentioned above, one often assumes in practice that each state depends only on the immediately preceding state. In most cases, taking into consideration only the first-order dependence is probably sufficient. However, in general, we can specify layers from $t - n$ to n. There is a possibility that some phenomena could be modeled with higher efficiency if they also take account of the influence of states earlier than immediately preceding the current state of the model. To our knowledge, the question whether such simplification of dynamic models leads to incomplete and even erroneous results has never been studied systematically.

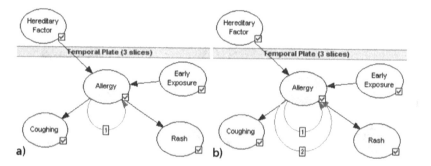

Fig. 14.2 Dynamic Bayesian networks modeling causes and effects an allergy in children: (a) first order DBN, (b) second order DBN. Number of slices is the number of steps for which we perform the inference. In this example, one step means one year. Temporal plate is the part of dynamic network that contains the temporal nodes. Hereditary Factor is time independent; the values of remaining the nodes can change over time.

Figure 14.2(b) shows a second order dynamic network, i.e., in which there are two temporal arcs from node *Allergy*, the first order takes the information from one step before, the second from two steps before. Typically, the older the child the lower the probability of allergy appearing. And, generally, the child that has not developed allergy two years in a row, has a lower chance of developing allergy in the third year.

14.3   Woman's Monthly Cycle

Woman's monthly cycle is driven by a highly complex interaction among hormones produced by three organs of the body: the hypothalamus, the pituitary gland, and the ovaries. There are five main hormones involved in the menstrual cycle process: estrogen, progesterone, gonadotropin releasing hormone (GnRH), follicle stimulating hormone (FSH), and luteinizing hormone (LH).

Estrogen refers to a group of hormones that stimulate growth and strengthen tissues. It is needed to build up the lining of the uterus so that it may nourish and sustain a fertilized egg. Progesterone is produced by the follicle from which the mature egg has been released (the follicle that has released an egg is called *corpus luteum*). Progesterone helps make the endometrial lining ready for implantation if an egg is fertilized during the cycle. It also prevents the egg follicles from developing any further. GnRH, produced by the hypothalamus in the brain, is responsible for the production and levels of estrogen in the body. FSH is secreted by the pituitary gland, which is stimulated by the hypothalamus' production of GnRH. Increased levels of FSH help to stimulate egg follicles. LH, produced by the pituitary gland, is needed to trigger the ovulation.

The woman's monthly cycle consists of four phases (Fig. 14.3 shows these four phases along with the associated hormone levels): (1) menstruation, (2) the follicular phase, (3) ovulation, and (4) the luteal phase. Counting from the first day of the

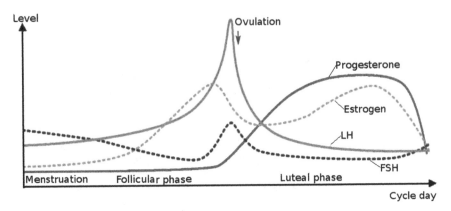

Fig. 14.3 Levels of hormones during the phases of the woman's monthly cycle [13]

menstrual flow, the length of each phase may vary from woman to woman and from cycle to cycle, although the entire cycle takes typically between 24 and 32 days.

Menstruation begins with the first day of bleeding. Contraction of the muscle layer occurs, expelling blood and endometrial cells through the vagina. During the follicular phase (or the proliferative phase), the follicles in the ovary mature. The main hormone controlling this stage is estrogen. Just before the ovulation, the level of estrogen is high enough to cause an increased release of luteinizing hormone and, as a result, the egg is released from the ovary. The luteal (or the secretory) phase is the latter phase of the menstrual cycle. The main hormone associated with this stage is progesterone, which occurs at significantly higher levels during the luteal phase than during the other phases of the cycle.

In addition to measurable blood hormone levels, there are several readily accessible indicators of the phase of the cycle, two of which we will use in our models. The basal body temperature (BBT) is defined as the body temperature measured immediately after awakening and before any physical activity has been undertaken. It should be measured every day at the same time. Before ovulation, BBT is relatively low. Following the ovulation, as a result of an increased level of progesterone in the body, women typically experience an increase in the basal body temperature (BBT) of at least 0.2 °C. This shift indicates that ovulation has occurred. The BBT charting may provide valuable information about woman's monthly cycle, such as duration of the cycle, length of the follicular and luteal phases, and the pattern of the timing of ovulation. Sometimes BBT can rise due to causes other than ovulation. This atypical rise is treated as disturbance and can be caused by a change in conditions around the measurement, such as later measurement time, lack of sleep, different thermometer, high stress, travel, or illness. As the cycle progresses, due to hormonal fluctuations, the cervical mucus increases in volume and changes texture. When there is no mucus or the mucus discharge is small, the day is considered infertile. There can be also a feeling of dryness around the vulva. Around the ovulation, mucus is the thinnest, clearest, and most abundant, resembling egg white. In the luteal phase, it returns to the sticky stage. During the monthly cycle, the cervix changes its position, firmness, and openness, in response to the same hormones that cause cervical mucus to be produced and to dry up. At the beginning of the cycle, cervix is located low in the vaginal canal and the os (the orifice of the uterus) is relatively small or closed. As ovulation approaches, cervix moves up the vaginal canal and becomes softer, with the os opening up. After ovulation cervix moves down and closes.

The menstrual cycle is a fairly noisy temporal process with memory spanning over the entire cycle. This means that the current state is not only influenced by the previous state but also by prior days, going back even to the beginning of the phase.

14.4 The Model

Accurate prediction of the fertile phase of the menstrual cycle is crucial for couples who want to conceive or couples who want to avoid pregnancy using natural methods. The fertile phase of the menstrual cycle is defined as the time when an intercourse has a non–zero probability of resulting in conception. Because the fertile period starts roughly five days before ovulation (this is essentially due to the fact that sperm can live up to five and fertilize the egg when ovulation happens, prediction has to be made in advance and, hence, asks for models that include an explicit notion of time.

Our model (Fig. 14.4), combines information retrieved from BBT charting with observations of the cervical mucus secretions. It contains a variable *Phase* with four states: *menstruation, follicular, ovulation,* and *luteal.* We included three observation variables: *Basal Body Temperature (BBT), Bleeding* and *Mucus observation.* All variables are discrete. *BBT* has two possible values: lower range and higher range, representing temperature before and after the BBT shift respectively. *Bleeding* describes whether on a particular day the woman had menses or not. *Mucus observation* can be in one of four states (*s1* through *s4*), described in detail in [4]. We modeled time explicitly as n time steps, where n is the number of days of the longest monthly cycle of the modeled woman. The model is of k-order, i.e., it contains temporal influences between 1 and k. Figure 14.4 shows an example DBN of 3rd order. Furthermore, while any DBN model should contain at least one first order influence, a model of order k does not need to include influences of all orders between 1 and $k - 1$.

To train a complex model we need a large number of observations. Learning models from data is based on strong theoretical foundations. Having sufficient amount of data, we can reliably learn numerical parameters of the model. In practice, however, the number of data records is often limited and generally making it challenging to learn reliable estimates of the parameters. Collecting data in case of a woman's monthly cycle problem will never result in sufficiently large data sets. Assuming that a woman is fertile during 40 years of her life, with roughly 13 cycles each year, she can collect at most 520 records. When these 520 records have been accrued, they are useless, as the woman is no longer fertile. In practice a woman will have not more than a couple of years worth of reliable data, i.e., roughly twenty-something records.

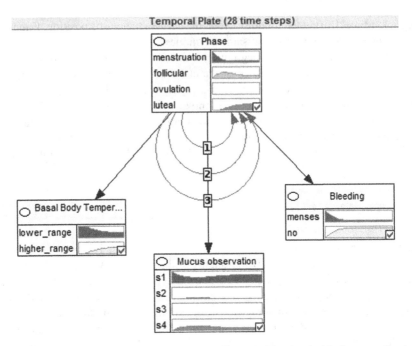

Fig. 14.4 A 3rd order DBN model of woman's monthly cycle. The plots inside the rectangles show the marginal probability distributions over the variables that they represent.

Typically, a model that aids in conception or in avoiding pregnancy, needs to rest on a handful of records.

Learning conditional probability distribution tables amounts essentially to counting data records for different conditions encoded in the network. The number of parameters required to specify a CPT for a node grows exponentially in the number of its parents, and thus the higher the order the more complex its structure and the more data are needed to learn parameters. In case of a fifth order DBN network of woman's monthly cycle for the node *Phase*, we need to estimate 1, 024 parameters. Even if we take into consideration that due to the specifics of the domain many columns of the CPTs represent unlikely cases, we are still dealing with a problem of insufficient amount of data. Please note, that most practical fertility awareness methods advise to consider charting at least six cycles to become familiar with a method. This means two problems: (1) Constant struggle against over-fitting the model to the data, and (2) Necessity to use prior knowledge, as a handful of records will never be enough to learn a complex probabilistic model.

When we learn the network parameters from such a small amount of data, some of the CPT entries might be learned from an insufficient number of records or there might even be no data records to learn distributions for some combination of the outcomes of the parents in a node. In order to provide more meaningful results and to compensate for the small amount data, we have based the initial structure of a model and its parameters on the domain knowledge. This procedure can be described as follows. We randomly divided all women into five equal subsets. For each woman the training data set was the sum of four subsets, excluding this which the woman belonged to. We learned the initial model parameters based on the population of women. Then we applied these population–based model as the *a priori* parameters in all woman–specific models. And as our intention was to simulate usage of a model by woman who wants to become pregnant or wants to avoid pregnancy, we adjusted the initial model to each woman using data for her first six cycles.

14.5 The Training Data

Our training data are drawn from an Italian study of daily fecundability [2], which enrolled women from seven European centers (Milan, Verona, Lugano, Düsseldorf, Paris, London and Brussels) and from Auckland, New Zealand. To our knowledge, this is one of the most comprehensive data sets describing woman's monthly cycle. Between the years 1992 and 1996, 881 women recorded a total of over seven thousand monthly cycles. Women participating in the study satisfied the following five entry criteria: (1) experienced in use of a Natural Family Planning method, (2) married or in a stable relationship, (3) between 18th and 40th birthday at admission, (4) had at least one menses after cessation of breastfeeding or after delivery, (5) not taking hormonal medication or drugs affecting fertility. In addition, neither partner could be permanently infertile and both had to be free from any illness that could affect fertility.

In each menstrual cycle, the woman was asked to record the days of her period, her basal body temperature, and any disturbances such as illness, disruption of sleep, or travel. She was also asked to observe and chart her cervical mucus symptoms daily during the cycle and to record every episode of coitus, with specification whether the couple used contraceptives or not.

A menstrual cycle was defined as the interval in days between the first day of menstrual bleeding in two neighboring cycles, where day 1 was the first day of fresh red bleeding, excluding any preceding days with spotting. The day of ovulation was identified in each cycle from records of basal body temperature and mucus symptoms. The daily mucus observations were classified into four classes; ranging from a score of 1 (no discharge and dry) to 4 (transparent, stretchy, slippery) [4]. The cervical mucus peak day was defined as the last day with best quality mucus, in a specific cycle of the woman. If there were different mucus observations on one day, the most fertile characteristic of the mucus observed determined the classification. To determine the BBT shift, the "three over six" rule (popular among fertility awareness methods or FAMs) was used: The first time in the menstrual cycle when three consecutive temperatures were registered, all of which were above the average temperature of the last six proceeding days.

In our analysis, we included only 3, 432 (of 7, 017) cycles from 236 (of 881) women. We excluded all women who collected fewer than seven cycles, because a woman needs at least six cycles to become familiar with a chosen fertility awareness method. We also excluded cycles with no uniquely identified mucus peak or the BBT shift days, because our model uses these values to determine the beginning of the post–ovulatory infertility. We also excluded women with very long cycles (longer than 40 days).

14.6 Experiments

For each woman, we created seven DBNs of temporal orders ranging from 1 to 7. Additionally, for each woman we created a model, with a structure that can change after each cycle. We changed the structure of that model by adding or removing temporal arcs, bearing in mind that first order arc is necessary and cannot be removed. For the last 12 cycles, we calculated the minimal and most frequent day of the ovulation. Dividing these values by two we received the order of temporal arcs that should appear in the model. Typically these orders were between six and nine. We determined the initial parameters of all models based on domain knowledge. We personalized each model using data for the first six cycles. After each cycle we re-evaluated the model's parameters based on previous cycles of the woman. Because a woman's body can also change over time and with it the characteristics of the cycle, we updated the structure and parameters using not more than the last 12 monthly cycles.

In case of monitoring a woman's monthly cycle, the main goal is to predict the day of ovulation and based on it to determine the fertile window. The number of fertile days during a menstrual cycle is difficult to specify, as it depends on the life span of the ovum and sperm, which varies from person to person and from cycle to cycle. Most menstrual cycles start with infertile days (pre–ovulatory infertility), a period of fertility and then several infertile days until the next menstruation (post–ovulatory infertility). It is generally believed that an ovum can be fertilized only within the first 24 h after ovulation [10]. Many authors agree that the start of the fertile interval is strictly connected with changes in vaginal discharge and, in particular, estrogenic–type cervical mucus secretions. However, they differ in their estimates of the length of the fertile window. Potter [8] calculated that there are only two days during the menstrual cycle when a woman can become pregnant. Wilcox *et al.* [14] found that the maximum sperm life span equals approximately five days (in presence of sufficient level of estrogenic–type mucus), which comes down to a fertile period of six days, including the day of the ovulation. The results of a multi–center study conducted by the World Health Organization [6] estimate the fertile period to be as many as 10 days before ovulation. Some of the fertility awareness methods assume this interval to be as long as 13 days or even longer [1, 5, 9, 12].

Our intention was to simulate the usage of DBN model by women who want to become pregnant or want to avoid pregnancy. At every time step (i.e., every day of the cycle), our model computed the most probable day of ovulation. If a time interval between the current day and the day with the highest probability of the ovulation was shorter than seven days, we marked the current day as fertile. To find the beginning

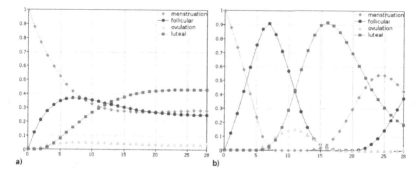

Fig. 14.5 Probabilities of each phase during the monthly cycle: (a) order 1, and (b) order 7 DBNs

of the post–ovulatory phase, our model used the BBT shift: We considered the third day after the BBT shift as infertile.

Just to give an idea of the capability of such models to reproduce the monthly cycle, we present the probabilities of the four phases of the monthly cycle as a function of time in Fig. 14.5. These probabilities were generated by DBNs models of (a) first and (b) seventh order DBNs, trained on monthly charts of one of the women in the data set. We entered no observation into the models, except for anchoring the first time step to the first day of menses, i.e., first day of the monthly cycle. Please note the increased similarity of the shape of the curves to that of the hormone levels in Fig. 14.3, which are direct indications of phases of the monthly cycle.

To compare the accuracy of different models, we used two measures: (1) the percentage length of the infertile period (the union of the pre–ovulatory and the post–ovulatory phase), and (2) the percentage length of the fertile window. We determined the number of fertile and infertile days in all cycles and divided this number by the total length of the cycle for each woman and for each cycle. Effectively, we obtained the percentage of all days that were classified as infertile and percentage of all days that were classified as fertile. In our opinion, these two numbers (they add up to 100 %) are a good indication of the precision of each model.

From the practical perspective, for a model of a monthly cycle to be useful, it has to predict the day of ovulation and, ultimately, to determine the fertile window. Days inside the fertile window that were classified as infertile are false negatives. Please note that because of a possible application of a model like this in natural family planning, false negatives may be much more serious than false positives, so the model should minimize its false negative rate to zero. This is essentially the case with all fertility awareness methods. Days that were marked as fertile and were outside the fertile window are false positives. The smaller the false positive rate, the closer the predicted day of ovulation is to the real day of ovulation, which can be helpful for couples seeking pregnancy. In our experiment, as the gold standard, we followed Wilcox et al. [14], who define the fertile window as the period between day of ovulation minus five days and day of ovulation plus one day.

14.7 Results

Table 14.1 and Fig. 14.6 show the average percentage of fertile and infertile days during a woman's monthly cycle sorted in the descending order (i.e., the longest to the shortest infertile period). The number of days in which a woman should abstain from intercourse to prevent unplanned pregnancy is larger for lower order models. The smaller the false positive rate, the closer the predicted day of ovulation is to the real day of ovulation, which can be helpful for couples seeking pregnancy. The higher the order of the model, the lower the percentage of the false positives. The 7–th order DBN model was most precise and indicated the longest infertile periods and the shortest fertile periods.

False negatives (Table 14.1 and Fig. 14.7) are an important measure of accuracy of a FAM, because on one hand they may lead to unplanned pregnancy and on the other hand to less likely conception in case of couples seeking pregnancy.

Table 14.1 Average percentage of fertile and infertile days and false negatives/false positives during the monthly cycle for each of the compared DBN models.

Method	% infertile days	% fertile days	% false negatives	% false positives
SEL orders	0.52 %	0.48 %	0.0000 %	22.84 %
1st order	0.53 %	0.47 %	0.0000 %	22.39 %
2nd order	0.53 %	0.47 %	0.0000 %	21.71 %
3rd order	0.54 %	0.46 %	0.0000 %	20.68 %
4th order	0.56 %	0.44 %	0.0008 %	19.42 %
5th order	0.57 %	0.43 %	0.0008 %	18.13 %
6th order	0.59 %	0.41 %	0.0008 %	16.00 %
7th order	0.61 %	0.39 %	0.0008 %	14.54 %

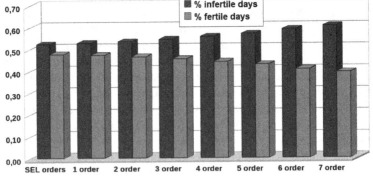

Fig. 14.6 Average percentage of fertile and infertile days during the monthly cycle for each of the compared DBN models.

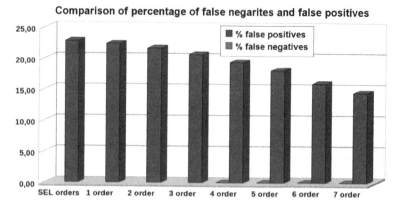

Fig. 14.7   False negatives and false positives during monthly cycle for each of the compared models.

Our results show that higher order models (4th through 7th) show non-zero false negative rate. We investigated this further and found that in each case there was an anomalous cycle, not recognized by the model. It seems that higher order models have the tendency to over-fit the data and be unable to deal with monthly cycles that deviate from typical cycles.

14.8   Conclusion

We have presented the results of an experiment with a series of DBN models monitoring woman's monthly cycle. We have shown that higher order models are more accurate than first order models, as summarized in Fig. 14.6. The lengths of the fertile period for higher order models were shorter, which indicates a better ability of the model to predict ovulation. The percentage of *false negatives* for all models was zero or very close to zero (0.0008 %). Higher order models tend to over-fit the data and have difficulty with anomalous cycles. While we advise to use higher order temporal models for systems with memory, we caution against too high order models when the system exhibit significant noise, as such models may over-fit the data and perform poorly when the course of events departs from typical.

Acknowledgments Our work was supported in part XDATA program of Defense Advanced Research Projects Agency (DARPA), administered through Air Force Research Laboratory contract FA8750-12-C-0332 and the National Institute of Health under grant number U01HL101066-01. We thank Bernardo Colombo, Guido Masarotto, Fausta Ongaro, Petra Frank-Herrmann, and other investigators of the European Study of Daily Fecundability for sharing their data with us. The empirical work described in this chapter was performed using SMILE[©], an inference engine, and GeNIe, a development environment for reasoning in graphical probabilistic models, both developed at the Decision Systems Laboratory, University of Pittsburgh, and available at http://genie.sis.pitt.edu/.

References

1. Barron, M.L., Fehring, R.J.: Basal body temperature assessment: is it useful to couples seeking pregnancy? Am. J. Matern. Child Nurs. **30**(5), 290–296 (2005)
2. Colombo, B., Masarotto, G.: Daily fecundability: first results from a new data base. Demographic Res. **3**(5), (2000)
3. Dean, T., Kanazawa, K.: A model for reasoning about persistence and causation. Comput. Intell. **5**(2), 142–150 (1989)
4. Dunson, D.B., Sinai, I., Colombo, B.: The relationship between cervical secretions and the daily probabilities of pregnancy effectiveness of the TwoDay algorithm. Hum. Reprod. **16**(11), 2278–2282 (2001)
5. Kippley, J., Kippley, S.: The Art of Natural Family Planning, 4th edn. The Couple to Couple League, Cincinnati (1996)
6. World Health Organization: A prospective multicentre trial of the ovulation method of natural family planning. III. Characteristics of the menstrual cycle and of the fertile phase. Fertil. Steril. **40**(6), 773–778 (1983)
7. Pearl, J.: Probabilistic Reasoning in Intelligent Systems: Networks of Plausible Inference. Morgan Kaufmann Publishers Inc., San Mateo (1988)
8. Potter Jr., R.G.: Length of the fertile period. Milbank Q. **39**, 132–162 (1961)
9. Rötzer, J.: Supplemented basal body temperature and regulation of conception. Archiv für Gynäkologie **206**(2), 195–214 (1968)
10. Royston, J.P.: Basal body temperature, ovulation and the risk of conception, with special reference to the lifetimes of sperm and egg. Biometrics **38**(2), 397–406 (1982)
11. Shannon, C.E.: A mathematical theory of communication. Bell Syst. Tech. J. **27**(1), 379–423 (1948)
12. Szymański, Z.: Płodność i Planowanie Rodziny. Wydawnictwo Pomorskiej Akademii Medycznej, Szczecin (2004)
13. Weschler, T.: Taking Charge of Your Fertility: The Definitive Guide to Natural Birth Control, Pregnancy Achievement, and Reproductive Health. Collins (2006)
14. Wilcox, A.J., Weinberg, C.R., Baird, D.D.: Timing of sexual intercourse in relation to ovulation effects on the probability of conception, survival of the pregnancy, and sex of the baby. N. Engl. J. Med. **333**(23), 1517–1521 (1995)

Treatment of Disease

Chapter 15
Treatment of Disease: The Role of Knowledge Representation for Treatment Selection

Jesse Davis, Luis Enrique Sucar and Felipe Orihuela-Espina

15.1 Treatment Selection

Treatment is the care and management of a patient to combat, ameliorate, or prevent a disease, disorder, or injury.[1] It may be *active* if directed to the cure of the disease, *causal* if directed against the cause of the disease, *palliative* if only aimed to relieve pain or distress with no attempt to cure, *preventive* if aimed to prevent the occurrence of a disease, etc. The goal of treatment selection is to help practicing clinicians gain and apply knowledge and standards in order to select the best possible treatment for a patient [3]. Managing a patient's care involves alternating between diagnosis (assessment) and treatment over a period of time [13]. The treatment portion involves a series of decisions, where each one requires selecting among several alternative courses of action [7].

Research on medical judgment has raised deep questions about how clinicians make decisions and plan treatment, particularly when they are faced with uncertainty and information overload. This has lead to the proposal of artificial intelligence methods that support decision making for treatment selection [7]. Knowledge about the effectiveness of treatments must be based on empirical evidence which is, for the most part, produced by scientific research and published in scientific literature. However, extracting this knowledge from research outcomes is not trivial. Indeed, even for someone who is deeply imbued in statistical procedures and nuances, it is very difficult to know what research findings really mean at the level of clinical practice [4]. One of the most significant obstacles in the practice of personalized medicine is the translation of scientific discoveries into better therapeutic outcomes [29].

For most diseases, selecting a treatment is complex because every patient is unique, and many symptoms and diagnoses are imprecise in their definition [30]. For instance, in the case of infectious diseases, the complexity of the problem is so large that it is highly unlikely that clinicians will be capable of delivering optimal treatment to all patients [16]. Therefore, some clinicians believe that providing

---

[1]Mosby's Medical Dictionary, 8th edition in theFreeDictionary.com.

© Springer International Publishing Switzerland 2015
A. Hommersom and P.J.F. Lucas (eds.), *Biomedical Knowledge Representation*, LNAI 9521, DOI 10.1007/978-3-319-28007-3_15

decision support tools may improve the quality of care a patient receives through providing better treatment choices [24].

Helping the clinician select a certain treatment is a multi-objective decision problem that must address different questions [6], such as:

- What would be the most cost-effective treatment?
- How may we plan a treatment regime to cover for possible contingencies?

Knowledge-based systems (KBS) can help practitioners by evaluating the potential outcomes for multiple courses of action. For instance, decision-theoretic KBS can compare alternative treatment policies by combining measures of outcome likelihood with estimates of utility [6].

The next section provides an overview of the main knowledge representation techniques that can be applied for treatment selection. This is followed by a section that presents some representative examples of applications of these techniques. The chapter concludes by introducing the two systems that will described in the following two chapters. The first proposes combining a logical and probabilistic approach for predicting adverse drug reactions from electronic medical records. The second considers a decision-theoretic model for patient-tailored virtual rehabilitation.

15.2 Knowledge Representation Techniques

The following list presents some of the main KR techniques appropriate for treatment selection. The list is not intended to be exhaustive but only to give a broad overview of the possibilities.

- **Rule-based systems**: Rule-based systems are perhaps one the most simple, yet powerful KR methods. Knowledge is encoded in the form of IF-THEN-ELSE rules, and the set of all rules form the *rule base* or *knowledge base*. Finally, the *inference engine* answers questions given to the system by applying the rules to the data in the *working memory*. An example is Lee et al.'s [14] system for monitoring diabetes that combines rule-based knowledge with a k-nearest neighbour classifier to recommend a treatment.
- **Logic of argumentation**: The logic of argumentation is a variant of standard first-order logic where an argument has the form of a proof but does not prove its conclusion [7]. In contrast to classical logic, in argumentation p and $\neg p$ can both be inferred from the same knowledge database. This can occur because the KB is split into subsets, called *theories*, that are internally but not necessarily mutually consistent. The decision making process in argumentation ranks possible solutions in terms of the supporting arguments formed by claims, grounds and confidence. Toxicology and risk assessment in genetics are among the examples where argumentation has been useful [7].
- **Fuzzy set theory and fuzzy logic**: The adjective fuzzy encompasses the notion of a degree of membership. In this sense, a fuzzy set is a set where a bounded function

of membership is defined over its members. Translated to logic, this means that inferences are not restricted to being either true or false, but that they can capture different shades of belief. A number of treatment selection systems use fuzzy set theory and fuzzy logic including the fuzzy-ARDS for the intensive care data of patients with acute respiratory distress syndrome (ARDS) [1] and Ying et al.'s [30] system for determining optimal HIV/AIDS treatment regimens.

- **Bayesian decision-theoretic systems**: In general, Bayesian models are based on probabilities which are updated as new evidence becomes available. Bayes' theorem, which is central to these systems, facilitates inference from existing knowledge. Probabilistic graphical models, which combine an intuitive visual representation with rigourousness of statistics, express (statistical) conditional independencies, which are often admitted as proxies for causality. Perhaps the best known Bayesian decision-theoretic framework is Bayesian networks whose viability for treatment selection is illustrated by a simple pathophysiological model of infection to choose antibiotic treatment [2]. Of course, more advanced models, such as influence diagrams, Markov decision processes (MDPs), and partially observable MDPs (POMDPs) among others, are also appropriate for treatment selection.

In general, a knowledge representation framework optimized for one task, such as diagnosis, might perform poorly in another task, such as treatment selection [20]. Recently, **machine learning** techniques have been incorporated into the library of plausible tools to build or improve recommendation systems based on different representation techniques. This is illustrated in the two examples that are described at the end of this chapter. One uses data from medical records to build a rule-based system for predicting adverse drug reactions. The other uses reinforcement learning to improve a model for adapting a virtual rehabilitation environment to the patient progress.

15.3   Medical Applications

Existing expert and decision support systems tend to focus on diagnosis, and only a few systems deal with treatment selection [23]. Nevertheless, decision-support systems for treatment selection have made an impact in several different medical domains. This section provides some representative examples of treatment selection for a couple of domains.

Treatment selection for infectious diseases is an area that has received attention since the early days of artificial intelligence. The MYCIN system was one of the first rule-based expert systems to attempt to determine anti-infective treatment for septicaemia and meningitis [6]. Since then a number of decision support models focused on treatment selection for infectious diseases have been developed based on different computational techniques including logistic regression, Bayesian approaches, and neural networks [2, 24]. Nosocomial infections are sub-domain of infectious disease that have received particular attention [16, 24], and a canonical system for this task is the Health Evaluation by Logical Processing (HELP) system [17].

The worldwide prevalence of diabetes is overwhelming as currently about 2.2 % of the world population suffers from it. This percentage is estimated to rise to 4.4 % by 2030, which translates to more than 300 million people [28]. Therefore, it is unsurprising that a number of decision-support systems for treatment selection in diabetes have been developed. Some are integrated into the hospital environment, like the DIACONS system [23], while others are developed for ubiquitous healthcare [14].

An exhaustive list of domains is beyond the scope of this section, but it is easy to find examples of knowledge representation-based treatment selection systems in HIV/AIDS [30], breast cancer [13], anemia [22], dyspnoea and bronchospasm [6], glaucoma e.g. CASNET [27], acute respiratory distress syndrome (ARDS) [1], rehabilitation [10] and psychotherapy [3] among others.

Some decision-support systems do not focus on specific diseases but instead intend to be a more comprehensive tool. One example that supports treatment selection is the Oxford System of Medicine [8, 20], which is a project aimed at developing a comprehensive information management and decision support system for general practitioners (GPs).

Next, we briefly introduce the two treatment selection systems presented in the following chapters.

15.4 Personalized Medicine: Predicting Adverse Drug Reactions

One issue that a doctor faces when treating a patient is selecting a medication to prescribe. This task has received increased attention because there have been several dramatic examples of patient variation in response to drugs such as Rofecoxib (Vioxx™) and Coumadin™ [11, 18]. These extreme variations in response are known as Adverse Drug Reactions (ADRs) [9, 12, 19], and they are the fourth-leading cause of death in the United States and represent a major risk to health, quality-of-life and the economy [21]. For example, the pain reliever Vioxx™ alone was earning US$2.5 billion per year before it was found to significantly raise the risk of heart attack and was pulled from the market while other similar drugs remain on the market [11, 18].

These cases have highlighted the need for tools that can help a doctor more accurately determine which drug and dosage to prescribe to a patient. This may be possible now due to the shift in healthcare practice towards the wide spread use of electronic medical records (EMRs), which are databases that store a patient's clinical history. Thus, the relevant data reside on disk as opposed to paper charts. Therefore, machine learning and data mining techniques could be applied to EMR data in order to build decision-support models to help doctors decide which medication to prescribe to which patient.

When EMRs are based on relational databases (a common choice), their relational schemas (i.e., the database contains separate relational tables for diagnoses, prescriptions, labs, etc.) pose challenges from a knowledge representation perspective. When analyzing such data it is important to capture important relationships (e.g., time of diagnosis may be relevant) as well as to model the uncertain, non-deterministic relationships between patients' clinical histories and current and future predictions about their health status. Yet traditional learning and mining paradigms have almost exclusively focused on handling propositional data. That is, data residing in a single table, where each row represents a data point and the rows in the table are assumed to be independent. It is non-trivial to convert an EMR into a single-table because different patients may have dramatically different numbers of entries in any given table, such as diagnoses or vitals. Chapter 16 will discuss three different strategies that address this problem such that statistical models can be learned from relational EMR data. We will present an evaluation of the different methodologies on three real-world ADR tasks.

15.5 Patient-Tailored Rehabilitation: Automatic Adaptation to the Patient

The consequences of strokes worldwide are devastating. They are the first-leading cause of disability, the second-leading cause of dementia, and the third-leading cause of death (more than five million deaths a year). Furthermore, they are a major cause of epilepsy, falls and depression and their prevalence exceeds 30 million people worldwide [5]. In the US alone, the estimated cost of strokes in 2007 surpassed $40 billion USD. Long-term care for stroke rehabilitation will benefit from strengthening health systems, and developing innovative therapies. A rising star among these new generation of therapies is *virtual rehabilitation* [15], which is a therapy paradigm that exploits the power of computers to provide a training environment with unmatched capabilities for tailoring the treatment to a specific patient.

Since the mid nineties, a number of virtual rehabilitation platforms have been developed with different salient features [26]. Gesture Therapy (GT) [25] is an upper limb virtual reality-based motor rehabilitation platform whose major strength is the extensive use of advanced decision theoretic models in order to support adaptation of the therapy to the changing needs of the patient. GT is an example of intelligent rehabilitation, a modality which exploits knowledge representation and reasoning to create assistive technology capable of generating actions, that is, decisions, emulating those of an expert.

Chapter 17 of this book details the probabilistic decision model underlying the critical feature of GT: adaptation. Adaptation is the pillar of intelligent rehabilitation because it is the central feature that allows an otherwise static virtual environment to change its behaviour to fit a patient's overall progress in a manner that imitates the decisions a therapist would make as he observes the advance of the patient.

The decision model of GT is designed to optimize the task challenge expressed by the virtual environment with regards to patient exhibited performance. The knowledge representation formalism is a Markov decision process (MDP) enriched with a reinforcement learning strategy that upgrades the static MDP to a dynamic decision model that keeps the decision policy, i.e., the reasoning, updated throughout the therapy.

Chapter 17 opens with a discussion on the need and importance of adaptation. Then, it proceeds to overview possible alternatives for implementing this feature that capitalize on knowledge representation. Finally, it presents an experimental evaluation of the adaptation model of the GT platform evidencing the general trend of the model decisions to learn and mimic the human therapist's decisions.

References

1. Adlassnig, K.-P.: The section on medical expert and knowledge- based systems at the department of medical computer sciences of the university of vienna medical school. Artif. Intell. Med. **21**, 139–146 (2001)
2. Andreassen, S., et al.: Using probabilistic and decision-theoretic methods in treatment and prognosis modeling. Artif. Intell. Med. **15**, 121–134 (1999)
3. Beutler, L.E., Mark Harwood, T.: Prescriptive Psychotherapy: A Practical Guide to Systematic Treatment Selection, vol. viii, p. 198. Oxford University Press, New York (2000)
4. Beutler, L.E., Moleiro, C., Talebi, H.: How practitioners can systematically use empirical evidence in treatment selection. J. Clin. Psychol. **58**(10), 1199–1212 (2002)
5. Fisher, M., Norrving, B.: The international agenda for stroke. In: First Global Ministerial Conference on Healthy Lifestyles and Noncommunicable Disease Control. World Health Organization, Moscow, Russia (2011)
6. Fox, J.: Formal and knowledge-based methods in decision technology. Acta Psychol. **56**, 303–331 (1984)
7. Fox, J., et al.: Argumentation-based inference and decision making - a medical perspective. IEEE Intell. Syst. **22**(6), 34–41 (2007)
8. Fox, J., et al.: Logic engineering for knowledge engineering: design and implementation of the Oxford System of Medicine. Artif. Intell. Med. **2**, 323–339 (1990)
9. Gurwitz, J.H., et al.: Incidence and preventability of adverse drug events among older persons in the ambulatory setting. JAMA **289**, 1107–1116 (2003)
10. Kan, P., Hoey, J., Mihailidis, A.: Automated upper extremity rehabilitation for stroke patients using a partially observable Markov decision process. In: Association for Advancement of Artificial Intelligence (AAAI) 2008 Fall Symposium on AI in Eldercare (2008)
11. Kearney, P.M., et al.: Do selective cyclo-oxygenase-2 inhibitors and traditional non-steroidal anti-inflammatory drugs increase the risk of atherothrombosis? Meta-analysis of randomised trials. BMJ **332**, 1302–1308 (2006)
12. Lazarou, J., Pomeranz, B.H., Corey, P.N.: Incidence of adverse drug reactions in hospitalized patients. J. Am. Med. Assoc. **279**, 1200–1205 (1998)
13. Leaning, M.S., Ng, K.E.H., Cramp, D.G.: Decision support for patient management in oncology. Med. Inf. **17**(1), 35–46 (1992)
14. Lee, M., Gatton, T.M., Lee, K.-K.: A monitoring and advisory system for diabetes patient management using a rule-based method and KNN. Sensors **10**, 3934–3953 (2010)
15. Levin, M.F.: Can virtual reality offer enriched environments for rehabilitation? Expert Rev. Neurother. **11**(2), 153–155 (2011)

16. Lucas, P.J.F., et al.: A probabilistic and decision-theoretic approach to the management of infectious disease at the ICU. Artif. Intell. Med. **19**, 251–279 (2000)
17. Lumsdon, K.: HELP (health evaluation through logical processing) on the way. Clinical system lays framework for CPR. Hospitals **67**(4), 32 (1993)
18. Mukherjee, D.: Risk of cardiovascular events associated with selective COX-2 inhibitors. J. Am. Med. Assoc. **286**, 954–959 (2001)
19. Naranjo, C.A., et al.: A method for estimating the probability of adverse drug reactions. Clin. Pharmacol. Ther. **30**, 239–245 (1981)
20. O'Neil, M., Glowinski, A.: Evaluating and validating very large knowledge-based systems. Med. Inf. **15**(3), 237–251 (1990)
21. Platt, R., Carnahan, R.: The U.S. food and drug administration's mini- sentinel program. Pharmacoepidem. Drug Safety **21**, 1–303 (2012)
22. Quaglini, S., et al.: A performance evaluation of the expert system ANEMIA. Comput. Biomed. Res. **21**, 307–323 (1988)
23. Schneider, J. et al.: DIACONS - a consultation system to assist in the management of diabetes. In: Rienhoff, O., Piccolo, U., Schneider, B. (eds.) Expert Systems and Decision Support in Medicine. Lecture Notes in Medical Informatics, vol. 36. pp. 44–49. Springer, Heidelberg (1988)
24. Schurink, C.A.M., et al.: Computer-assisted decision support for the diagnosis and treatment of infectious diseases in intensive care units. Lancet Infect. Dis. **5**, 305–312 (2005)
25. Sucar, L.E., et al.: Gesture therapy: A vision-based system for upper extremity stroke rehabilitation. In: 32nd Annual International Conference of the IEEE Engineering in Medicine and Biology Society (EMBS), pp. 3690–3693. IEEE, Buenos Aires (2010)
26. Sucar, L.E., et al.: Gesture Therapy: an upper limb virtual reality-based motor rehabilitation platform. IEEE Trans. on Neural Syst. Rehabil. Eng. **22**(13), 634–643 (2013)
27. Weiss, S.M., et al.: A model-based method for computer aided medical decision-making. Artif. Intell. **1**, 145–172 (1978)
28. Wild, S., et al.: Global prevalence of diabetes: estimates for the year 2000 and projections for 2030. Diabetes Care **27**(5), 1047–1053 (2004)
29. Yan, Q.: Translational bioinformatics and systems biology approaches for personalized medicine. Methods Mol. Biol. **662**, 167–178 (2010)
30. Ying, H., et al.: A fuzzy discrete event system approach to determining optimal HIV/AIDS treatment regimens. IEEE Trans. Inf. Technol. Biomed. **10**(4), 663–676 (2006)

Chapter 16
Predicting Adverse Drug Events from Electronic Medical Records

Jesse Davis, Vítor Santos Costa, Peggy Peissig, Michael Caldwell, and David Page

Abstract Learning from electronic medical records (EMR) poses many challenges from a knowledge representation point of view. This chapter focuses on how to cope with two specific challenges: the relational nature of EMRs and the uncertain dependence between a patient's past and future health status. We discuss three different approaches for allowing standard propositional learners to incorporate relational information. We evaluate these approaches on three real-world tasks where the goal is to use EMRs to predict whether a patient will have an adverse reaction to a medication.

16.1 Introduction

Personalized medicine represents a significant application for the health informatics community [13]. Its objective can be defined as follows:

Given: A patient's clinical history,
Do: Create an *individual* treatment plan.

Personalized medicine is possible due to the fundamental shift in health care practice caused by the advent and widespread use of electronic medical records (EMR). An EMR is a relational database that stores a patient's clinical history: disease diagnoses, procedures, prescriptions, lab results, and more. Figure 16.1 shows one very simplified EMR with two patients that includes phenotypic data, lab tests, diagnoses, and drug prescriptions. With EMR's relevant data residing on disk as opposed to paper charts, it is possible to apply machine learning and data mining techniques to these data to address important medical problems such as predicting which patients are most at risk for having an adverse reaction to a certain drug.

However, working with EMR data is challenging. EMR data violate some of the underlying assumptions made by classical statistical machine learning techniques, such as decision trees [19], support vector machines [22], and Bayesian networks [15]. These techniques are designed to work on propositional (tabulated) data. That is, they operate on data that resides in a single table, where each row represents a data point and the rows in the table are assumed to be independent. Namely, the obstacles of working with EMR data include:

© Springer International Publishing Switzerland 2015
A. Hommersom and P.J.F. Lucas (eds.), *Biomedical Knowledge Representation*, LNAI 9521, DOI 10.1007/978-3-319-28007-3_16

A)

PID	Birth Date	Gender
P1	09/02/50	Female
P2	03/19/75	Male

B)

PID	Date	Lab test	Result
P1	12/23/04	Glucose	43
P1	10/25/04	Glucose	45
P2	04/17/05	Lipid panel	278

C)

PID	Date	Diagnosis
P1	02/01/01	Flu
P1	05/02/03	Bleeding
P2	04/21/05	High Cholestrol

D)

PID	Date	Medication	Dose
P1	05/01/02	Warfarin	10mg
P1	02/02/03	Terconazole	10mg
P2	04/21/05	Zocor	20mg

Fig. 16.1 A simplified electronic health record. Table **A** contains information about each patient. Table **B** contains lab test results. Table **C** lists disease diagnoses. Table **D** has information about prescribed medications.

Multiple relations: Each type of data (e.g., drug prescription information, lab test results) is stored in a different table of a database. Traditionally, machine learning algorithms assume that data are stored in a single table. For example, see the tables in Fig. 16.1.

Uncertainty: The data are inherently noisy. For example, a diagnosis code of 410 for myocardial infarction (heart attack, or MI) may be entered to explain billing for tests to confirm or rule out an MI, rather than to indicate that the patient definitely had an MI on this date. It might even be entered to indicate that an earlier MI is relevant to today's visit.

Non-deterministic relationships: It is important to model the uncertain, non-deterministic relationships between patients' clinical histories and current and future predictions about their health status.

Differing quantities of information: Different patients may have dramatically different numbers of entries in any given EMR table, such as diagnoses or vitals.

Missing and/or incomplete data: Patients switch doctors and clinics over time, so a patient's entire clinical history is unlikely to reside in one database. Furthermore, information, such as the use of over-the-counter drugs, may not appear in the clinical history. In addition, patients rarely return to report when a given condition or symptom ceased, so this information is almost always missing.

Schema not designed to empower learning: Clinical databases are designed to optimize ease of data access and billing rather than learning and modeling.

Large amounts of data: As more clinics switch to electronic medical records, the amount of data available for analysis will exceed the capability of current machine learning techniques.

Longitudinal data: Working with data that contains time dependencies introduces several problems. The central problem we had to address in our work was deciding which data to include in our analysis.

These points raise interesting questions for knowledge representation, especially as they have an effect on the applicability of machine learning and data mining techniques. This chapter will focus on the first two challenges: how to effectively represent uncertainty given the multi-relational nature of the data.

We will discuss three different strategies for learning statistical models from relational data. The first approach, known as *propositionalization*, is to simply handcraft a set of features which are used to represent the multi-relational EMR as a single table. Then it becomes possible to apply traditional techniques from statistical machine learning to the modified data. The second approach builds on the first by employing a *pipeline* that automatically generates a set of features, uses these features to propositionalize the data, and then performs learning on the transformed data. The third approach is more advanced in that it *integrates* feature construction, feature selection and model learning into a single process.

To illustrate and evaluate the different approaches, we focus on the important task of predicting adverse drug reactions (ADRs) from EMR data. ADRs are the fourth-leading cause of death in the United States and represent a major risk to health, quality-of-life and the economy [16]. The pain reliever Vioxx™ alone was earning US$2.5 billion per year before it was found to double the risk of a heart attack and was pulled from the market while other similar drugs remain on the market [7]. Additionally, accurate predictive models for ADRs are actionable. If a model is found to be accurate in a prospective trial, it could be used to avoid giving a drug to those at highest risk of an ADR. Using three real-world ADR tasks, we find that the dynamic approach results in the best performance on two of the three data sets and that the handcrafted approach works reasonably well.

16.2   Background

We briefly review Bayesian networks, which are a well-known technique for representing and reasoning about uncertainty in data. We then discuss Datalog and how it can be used to represent relational data. The rest of the chapter will make use of both of these techniques to tackle the knowledge representation problems posed by EMRs.

16.2.1   Bayesian Networks

Bayesian networks [15] are probabilistic graphical models that encode a joint probability distribution over a set of random variables, where each random variable corresponds to an attribute. A Bayesian network compactly represents the joint probability distribution over a set of random variables by exploiting conditional independencies between random variables. We will use uppercase letters (e.g., X) to refer to a random variable and lower case letters (e.g., x) to refer to a specific value for that random variable. Given a set of random variables $X = \{X_1, \ldots, X_n\}$, a Bayesian network $B = \langle G, \Theta \rangle$ is defined as follows. G is a directed, acyclic graph that contains a node for each variable $X_i \in X$. For each variable (node) in the graph, the Bayesian network has a conditional probability table $\theta_{X_i|Parents(X_i)}$ giving the probability distribution over the values that variable can take for each possible setting of its parents, and $\Theta = \{\theta_{X_1}, \ldots, \theta_{X_n}\}$. A Bayesian network B encodes the following probability distribution:

$$P_B(X_1, \ldots X_n) = \prod_{i=1}^{i=n} P(X_i | Parents(X_i)). \tag{16.1}$$

The Bayesian network learning task can be formalized as follows:

Given: Data set D that contains variables $X_i, \ldots, X_n$.
Learn: Network structure G, that is, which arcs appear in the network, and $\theta_{X_i | Parents}$
(X_i) for each node in the network.

One well-known Bayesian network classification model is called tree-augmented naïve Bayes (TAN) [6]. A TAN model has an outgoing arc from the class variable to each other attribute. It also allows each non-class variable to have at most one other parent in order to capture a limited set of dependencies between attributes. To decide which arcs to include in the augmented network, the algorithm does the following:

1. Construct a complete graph G_A, between all non-class attributes A_i. Weight each edge between i and j with the conditional mutual information, $CI(A_i, A_j | C)$.
2. Find a maximum weight spanning tree T over G_A. Convert T into a directed graph B. This is done by picking a node and making all edges outgoing from it.
3. Add an arc in B connecting C to each attribute A_i.

In step 1, CI represents the conditional mutual information, which is given by the following equation:

$$CI(A_i; A_j | C) = \sum_{a_i}^{A_i} \sum_{a_j}^{A_j} \sum_{c}^{C} P(a_i, a_j, c) log \frac{P(a_i, a_j | c)}{P(a_i | c) P(a_j | c)}. \tag{16.2}$$

This algorithm for constructing a TAN model has two nice theoretical properties [6]. First, it finds the TAN model that maximizes the log likelihood of the network structure given the data. Second, it finds this model in polynomial time.

16.2.2 Datalog

Datalog is a subset of first-order logic whose alphabet consists of three types of symbols: constants, variables, and predicates. *Constants* (e.g., the drug name propranolol), which start with a lowercase letter, denote specific objects in the domain. *Variable* symbols (e.g., Disease), which start with an uppercase letter, range over objects in the domain. *Predicate* symbols P/n, where n refers to the arity of the predicate and $n \geq 0$, represent relations among objects. An *atom* is $P(t_1, \ldots, t_n)$ where each t_i is a constant or variable. A *ground atom* is an atom where each t_i is a constant. A *literal* is an atom or its negation. A *clause* is a disjunction over a finite set of literals. A *definite clause* is a clause that contains exactly one positive literal. Definite clauses are often written as an implication $B \implies H$, where B is a conjunction of literals called the body and H is a single literal called the head. The following is an example of a definite clause:

$$\text{Drug}(\text{Pid}, \text{Date1}, \text{terconazole}) \wedge \text{Weight}(\text{Pid}, \text{Date1}, \text{W})$$
$$\wedge \text{W} < 120 \Rightarrow \text{ADR}(\text{Pid}).$$

All variables in a definite clause are assumed to be universally quantified.

Non-recursive[1] Datalog, in combination with a closed-world assumption, is equivalent to relational algebra/calculus. Therefore, it is natural and easy to represent relational databases, such as EMRs, in Datalog. The most straightforward way to do this is to create one ground atom for each row of each table in the EMR. Consider Tables **C** and **D** in Fig. 16.1, where the data would result in the following ground atoms:

> Diagnosis(p1, 02/01/01, flu)
> Diagnosis(p1, 05/02/03, bleeding)
> Diagnosis(p2, 04/21/05, high cholestrol)
> ...
> Drug(p1, 05/01/02, warfarin, 10mg)
> Drug(p1, 02/02/03, terconazole, 10mg)
> Drug(p2, 04/21/05, zocor, 20mg)
> ...

16.3 Approaches

In this section we describe three different strategies for coping with the multi-relational nature of EMRs.

16.3.1 *Handcrafting Features*

The act of converting a relational database, such as an EMR, into a single table is known as propositionalization [8]. One simple strategy is to handcraft a set of features. While this process usually results in a loss of information, it makes it possible to

---

[1] A Datalog clause is non-recursive by definition if the predicate appearing in its head does not appear in its body. A Datalog program, or theory, is non-recursive if all its clauses are non-recursive.

apply standard machine learning techniques, such as Bayesian network learning, to the transformed data.

The most obvious and straightforward way to do this is to construct a set of binary features for each relevant relation in the domain. For example, consider the diagnosis relation in Fig. 16.1. In this case, one feature for each possible diagnosis code would be constructed that is true of a patient if it appears in the patient's EMR *at any point in the past*. In effect, this conversion makes the assumption that the only thing that matters about a patient's future health status is if they have ever been diagnosed with a specific disease in the past. When in the past the diagnosis was made is irrelevant. The same strategy would then be applied to the other relevant relations in the domain. In the example, this would yield one set of features about lab tests and another set of features about medications.

It is also possible to design more complicated features. One idea would be to incorporate time constraints into the features. For example, one feature could be defined that is true of a patient if he has been diagnosed with a specific disease within the past year. Another idea is to look at pairs of diseases or pairs of medications. One example is a feature that is true of a patient if he was prescribed two specific medicines at any point in the past, regardless of the prescription date (i.e., they do not need to be co-prescribed). Features could be defined that combine both time and diagnoses (or medications) in order to capture co-occurrence. For example, a feature could be proposed that is true of any patient that was prescribed two medications within three months of each other.

While simple, this approach has several potential limitations. Namely, there is a huge space of possible features to consider, and it is challenging to do this in a sensible and systematic way by hand. Furthermore, taking a more directed approach, especially when handcrafting complex features, requires significant domain expertise. Finally, even employing the simplest strategy can result in a very large number of features. For example, creating one binary feature for each diagnosis code that is true of a patient if (s)he has ever been diagnosed with that particular disease would lead to over 5,000 features alone!

16.3.2 *Automatically Generating Features: A Multi-Step Approach*

One way to alleviate the feature construction burden that the previous approach places on a modeler is to use an automated approach to generate the features. Note that it is possible to represent each of the features mentioned in the previous subsection as a query in Datalog. For example, the query Diagnosis(Pid, _, flu) would return the set of all patients that have ever been diagnosed with the flu. Essentially, this corresponds to using the body of a definite clause, whose head is the target concept, to define a feature. This insight suggests that one possibility is to employ techniques from the field of inductive logic programming (ILP) [11]. The goal of ILP is to learn hypotheses expressed as definite clauses in first-order logic. ILP is appropriate for learning in multi-relational domains because the learned rules are not restricted to contain fields or attributes from a single table in a database. Commonly-used ILP systems include FOIL [20], Progol [14] and Aleph [21].

The ILP learning problem can be formulated as follows:

Given: Background knowledge B, a set of positive examples E^+, and a set of negative examples E^- all expressed in first-order definite clause logic.
Learn: A hypothesis H, which consists of definite clauses in first-order logic, such that $B \wedge H \models E^+$ and $B \wedge H \not\models E^-$.

In practice, it is often not possible to find either a pure rule or rule set. Thus, ILP systems relax the conditions that $B \wedge H \models E^+$ and $B \wedge H \not\models E^-$. Typically, this is done by allowing H to cover a small number of negative examples. That is, $B \wedge H \models E'^-$, where $E'^- \subset E^-$ and the goal is to make $|E'^-|$ as small as possible.

ILP systems learn rules for a fixed target concept, such as ADR(Pid), by iteratively learning rules one at a time. Thus, the central procedure is learning a single definite clause. This is usually posed as the problem of searching through the space of possible clause bodies. We briefly describe the general-to-specific, breadth-first search through the space of candidate clauses used by the Progol algorithm [14]. First, a random positive example is selected to serve as the seed example. To guide the search process, it constructs the *bottom clause* by finding all facts that are relevant to the seed example. Second, a rule is constructed that contains just the target attribute, such as ADR(Pid), on the right-hand side of the implication. This means that the feature matches all examples. Third, candidate clause bodies are constructed by adding literals that appear in the bottom clause to the left-hand side of the rule, which makes the feature more specific (i.e., it matches fewer examples). Restricting the candidate literals to those that appear in the bottom clause helps limit the search space while guaranteeing that each generated refinement matches at least one example.

Employing ILP to learn the feature definitions gives rise to the following procedure. In the first step, ILP is employed to learn a large set of rules. In the second step, each learned rule is used to define a binary feature. The feature receives a value of one for an example if the data about the example satisfies (i.e., proves) the clause and it receives a value of zero otherwise. This results in a single table, with one row for each example. In the third step, a classifier is learned from the newly constructed table.

16.3.3 VISTA: An Integrated Approach

Next, we describe VISTA [4], an alternative approach that is based on the idea of constructing the classifier as we learn the rules. VISTA integrates feature construction, feature selection, and model construction into one, dynamic process. Consequently, this approach scores rules by how much they improve the classifier, providing a tight coupling between rule generation and rule usage.

Like the multi-step approach described in the previous subsection, VISTA uses definite clauses to define features for the statistical model. VISTA starts by learning a model M over an empty feature set FS. This corresponds to a model that predicts the prior probability of the target predicate. Then it repeatedly searches for new features for a fixed number of iterations. VISTA employs the Progol algorithm that is described in the previous section to generate candidate features.

VISTA converts each candidate clause into a feature, f, and evaluates f by learning a new model (e.g., the structure of a Bayesian network) that incorporates f. In principle, any structure learner could be used, but VISTA typically uses a tree-augmented naïve Bayes model [6]. VISTA evaluates each f by comparing the generalization ability of the current model FS versus a model learned over a feature set extended with f. VISTA does this by calculating the area under the precision-recall curve (AUC-PR) on a tuning set. AUC-PR is used because relational domains typically have many more negative examples than positive examples, and the AUC-PR ignores the potentially large number of true negative examples.[2] In each iteration, VISTA adds the feature f' to FS that results in the largest improvement in the score of the model. In order to be included in the model, f' must improve the score by a certain percentage-based threshold. This helps control overfitting by pruning relatively weak features that only improve the model score slightly. If no feature improves the model's score, then it simply proceeds to the next iteration. Algorithm 3 provides pseudocode for VISTA.

Algorithm 3. VISTA (Training Set T, Validation Set V, Maximum Iteration $iter$)

$FS = \{\emptyset\}$
$M =$ BuildTANModel(T, FS)
$score =$ AUCPR(M, V)
repeat
  $bestScore = score$
  $f_{best} = \emptyset$
  /*Generate Candidate Features*/
  $Cand =$ GenCandidates()
  for all ($f \in Cand$) **do**
    $M' =$ BuildTANModel($T, FS \cup f$)
    $score' =$ AUCPR(M', V)
    if ($score' > bestScore$) **then**
      $f_{best} = f$
      $bestScore = score'$
    end if
  end for
  if ($f_{best} \neq \emptyset$) **then**
    $FS = FS \cup f_{best}$
    $M =$ BuildTANModel(T, FS)
    $score =$ AUCPR(M, V)
  end if
until Reaching iteration $iter$
return: FS

---

[2] In principle, VISTA can use any evaluation metric to evaluate the quality of the model such as (conditional) likelihood, accuracy, or ROC analysis.

16.4 Empirical Evaluation

In this section, we evaluate the three approaches outlined in Sect. 16.3 on three real-world data sets. In all tasks, we are given patients that take a certain medication, and the goal is to model the patients that have a related ADR. We first describe the data sets we use and our metholodgy. Then we present and discuss our experimental results.

16.4.1 Task Descriptions

Our data comes from a large multi-specialty clinic that has been using electronic medical records since 1985 and has electronic data back to the early 1960s. We have received institutional review board (IRB) approval to undertake these studies. For all tasks, we have access to information about observations (e.g., vital signs, family history, etc.), lab test results, disease diagnoses, and medications. We only use patient data up to one week before that patient's first prescription of the drug under consideration. This ensures that we are building predictive models only from data generated before a patient is prescribed that drug.

The characteristics of the data for each task can be found in Table 16.1. On each task we consider only patients who took a medication, and the goal is to distinguish between patients who went on to experience an adverse event (i.e., positive examples) and those who did not (i.e., negative examples). We now briefly describe each task.

Selective Cox-2 inhibitors (e.g., Vioxx™) are a class of pain relief drugs that were found to increase a patient's risk of having a myocardial infarction (MI) (i.e., a heart attack). For the Cox-2 data set, positive examples consist of patients who had a MI after taking a selective Cox-2 inhibitor. To create a set of negative examples, we took patients that were prescribed a selective Cox-2 inhibitor and did not have an MI. Furthermore, we matched the negative examples to have the same age and gender distribution as the positive examples to control for those risk factors.

Angiotensin-converting enzyme inhibitors (**ACEi**) are a class of drugs commonly prescribed to treat high blood pressure and congestive heart failure. It is known that

Table 16.1 Data set characteristics.

	Selective Cox-2	Warfarin	ACEi
Pos. examples	160	144	102
Neg. examples	2,134	1,440	1,020
Unique drugs	2,590	2,316	2,044
Unique diagnoses	7,912	8,389	7,286
Drug facts	3,518,467	603,503	335,065
Diagnoses facts	3,653,487	691,591	436,934

in some people, ACEi may result in angioedema (a swelling beneath the skin). To create the ACEi data set, we selected all patients with at least one prescription of an ACEi drug in their electronic health record. Within this population, we defined positive examples to be those patients who have a diagnosis of angioedema at any point after their first ACEi prescription.

Warfarin is a commonly prescribed blood thinner that is known to increase the risk of internal bleeding for some individuals. To create the Warfarin data set, we selected all patients who have at least one prescription of Warfarin in their electronic health record. We defined positive examples to be those patients with a bleeding event (any of 219 distinct diagnoses in the ICD9 hierarchy representing bleeding events) at any point after their first Warfarin prescription.

16.4.2 Methodology

We perform stratified, ten-fold cross-validation for each task and compare the following algorithms.

Handcrafted. In this model, we construct a set of handcrafted features to propositionalize the EMR. We create one binary feature for each possible diagnosis code, medication, and lab test. The feature is true of a patient if the appropriate diagnose, medication, or lab test appears in the portion of the patient's EMR used for training. For each test fold, we use information gain on the training set to select the 50 most informative features. A TAN classifier is trained that uses these 50 attributes.

Multi Step. First, we use ILP to learn a set of rules on the training data. We use the Aleph ILP system [21], which is a re-implementation of the Progol algorithm [14], to learn rules. The background knowledge used to construct the rules includes diagnosis codes, medications, and lab tests as before, but also allows temporal relations between events and comparing the results of observations against a learned threshold. We run Aleph under the `induce_max` command in order to fully exploit all the training examples. Second, we create a data set by converting each rule learned by Aleph into a binary attribute, which is true of an example if the rule covers the example. Third, we train a TAN classifier over the newly transformed data set.

VISTA. We follow a greedy algorithm. Starting from a network that contains the class node only, we search for clauses that when added to a classifier will improve its performance. We define a network to be an improvement over a previous classifier if it increases the area under the precision-recall curve (AUC-PR) by at least 2 %. First, we sub-divide the nine folds in the training data into five training and four tuning folds. The training folds are used to generate the candidate classifiers. We first use these folds to discover the clauses and then to train the TAN classifiers. The tuning folds are kept separate. They are used to compute the AUC-PR for the new TAN classifier and decide whether a feature should be included in the model or not. As a stop criteria, we use an arbitrary time limit of three hours for learning each model.

All three approaches make use of a TAN classifier learning algorithm where we compute maximum likelihood parameters of the model and use Laplace smoothing to prevent zero probabilities.

When reporting results, we focus on precision-recall analysis. In precision-recall space, recall is plotted on the x-axis and precision on the y-axis. Recall (also called the true positive rate) is defined as the proportion of positive examples that are correctly classified as positive. Precision reports the fraction of examples classified as positive that are truly positive. Often times, precision-recall analysis is preferred to ROC analysis in domains, such as ours, that have a large class skew [5]. Note that in ROC analysis, a very small false positive rate can correspond to a large number of false positives, if there are a large number of negative examples. In contrast, precision-recall analysis ignores the potentially large number of true negatives. We also report the results for random guessing, which corresponds to an AUC-PR equal to the proportion of positive examples in the test set [2].

16.4.3   Results and Discussion

Table 16.2 shows the average AUC-PR for each of the tasks. First, regardless of the task, each approach also does significantly better than random guessing. Thus, each approach is picking up signal in the data. VISTA results in the best performance on two of the three tasks. This indicates that there is some benefit to using the dynamic, automated approach. The handcrafted approach also exhibits good performance, and has the best performance on the Warfarin task. Interestingly, this approach yields better results than the multi-step approach. One possible explanation is that ILP tends to be biased towards constructing a smaller set of strong, complex features whereas on this task it may be beneficial to have a larger set of weak, simple features. In the future, it is worth exploring a model that uses a combination of simple and complex features. Additionally, ILP systems generate rules that predict the positive examples. In contrast, the other two approaches are able to select features that are predictive of either the positive or negative class, which may yield a benefit.

Figures 16.2, 16.3, and 16.4 show the precision-recall curves for each task. Note that on this task, for drugs on the market it is probably more meaningful to focus on the high precision, low recall (i.e., recall ≤ 0.3) parts of the plots. This is because if we act only based on this portion of the curve then we would only change current clinical practice by denying the drug to patients who will almost all suffer the ADE if

Table 16.2 Average AUC-PR and its standard deviation for each approach. The best result for each task is shown in bold.

	Selective Cox-2	Warfarin	ACEi
VISTA	**0.614 ± 0.11**	0.171 ± 0.06	**0.328 ± 0.06**
Multi Step	0.557 ± 0.14	0.188 ± 0.09	0.261 ± 0.09
Hand Crafted	0.553 ± 0.15	**0.252 ± 0.07**	0.274 ± 0.10
Random Guessing	0.070 ± 0.00	0.091 ± 0.00	0.091 ± 0.00

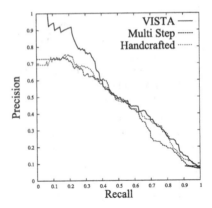

Fig. 16.2 Precision-recall curves for the Selective Cox-2 task.

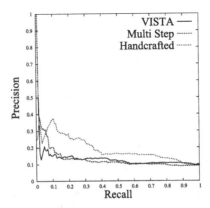

Fig. 16.3 Precision-recall curves for the Warfarin task.

they take the drug, without denying the drug unnecessarily to most individuals who
need it. Exceptions to this preference to operate at the left of the PR curve would be if
(1) the ADR is severe compared with the benefit of the drug, (2) there is an alternative
treatment available, or (3) this is a new drug being added to the market, and we want
to add it as safely as possible. Focusing on this region of PR space shows a similar
picture as looking at average AUC-PR. Again, VISTA has the best performance on
two tasks and the handcrafted approach does the best on the third task.

16.5 Related Work

There has been much previous work on using ILP for feature construction. Such
work treats ILP-constructed rules as Boolean features, re-represents each example
as a feature vector, and then uses a feature-vector learner to produce a final classifier.
The first work on propositionalization is the LINUS system [12]. LINUS transforms
the examples from deductive database format into attribute-value tuples and pairs
these tuples to a propositional learner. LINUS primarily uses propositional algorithms

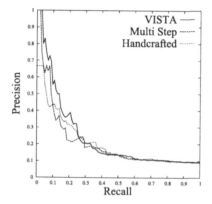

Fig. 16.4 Precision-recall curves for the ACEi task.

that generate `if-then` rules. LINUS then converts the propositional rules back into the deductive database format.

Previous work has also used ILP-learned rules as features in a propositional classifier. For example, [17] do this using a naïve Bayes classifier. Some other work, especially on propositionalization of first-order logic [1], has been developed that converts the training set to propositions and then applies feature vector techniques to the converted data. This is similar to what we do, however we first perform learning in the first-order setting to determine which features to construct. This results in significantly shorter feature vectors than in other work.

The most closely related work to VISTA includes the nFOIL [9] and kFOIL systems [10]. These systems differ in that they use different statistical learners, naïve Bayes for nFOIL and a kernel in kFOIL, and use FOIL instead of the Progol algorithm for proposing the features. Furthermore, VISTA works with AUC-PR which allows it to tackle problems that have significant class skew, which is common in medical domains. The work on structural logistic regression [18] also integrates feature generation and model selection. This work defines features using SQL queries and the statistical learner is logistic regression, but these are not especially important differences. The drawback to this approach is that it is extremely computationally expensive. In fact, they report only searching over queries that contain at most two relations. In ILP, this would be equivalent to only evaluating clauses that contain at most two literals.

In a different context, the issue of converting multiple tables into a single table is also addressed by data warehouses [3]. Typically, data warehouses often use either a star or snowflake schema. These schemas are centered on a single so-called "fact table," which is then connected to several different, multi-dimensional attributes. Each attribute value is often organized according to a hierarchy. For example, a place hierarchy may be city, county, state, and so forth. Traditionally, data warehouses focus on supporting ad-hoc user queries that produce a single table by rolling-up or drilling-down along one of the attribute dimensions. This is in contrast to our focus on building predictive models from data. Additionally, we make no assumption about the schema of data and the work presented in this chapter automatically constructs a single table.

16.6 Conclusions

This chapter addressed the challenges associated with learning statistical models from multi-relational electronic medical record (EMR) data. Specifically, we discussed how to construct features from the multi-relational EMR that can be used by a standard statistical machine learning algorithm such as Bayesian networks. We presented three different approaches: handcrafting a set of features, a multi-step algorithm that automatically learns features, and an integrated algorithm that combines feature construction with model learning. Empirically, we report results on predicting three ADRs from real-world EMR data. We found that the dynamic approach performed the best on two of the three tasks and that handcrafting the features also yielded good results.

Acknowledgements JD is partially supported by the Research Fund K.U.Leuven (CREA/11/015 and OT/11/051), EU FP7 Marie Curie Career Integration Grant (#294068) and FWO-Vlaanderen (G.0356.12). VSC is funded by ERDF through Programme COMPETE and by the Portuguese Government through FCT Foundation for Science and Technology projects LEAP (PTDC/EIA-CCO/112158/2009) and ADE (PTDC/EIA-EIA/121686/2010). MC, PP, EB and DP gratefully acknowledge the support of NIGMS grant R01GM097618-01.

References

1. Alphonse, E., Rouveirol, C.: Lazy propositionalisation for relational learning. In: 14th European Conference on Artificial Intelligence, pp. 256–260. IOS Press (2000)
2. Boyd, K., Davis, J., Page, D., Costa, V.S.: Unachievable region in precision-recall space and its effect on empirical evaluation. In: Proceedings of the 29th International Conference on Machine Learning. Omnipress (2012)
3. Chaudhuri, S., Dayal, U.: An overview of data warehousing and OLAP technology. SIGMOD Rec. **26**(1), 65–74 (1997)
4. Davis, J., Ong, I., Struyf, J., Burnside, E., Page, D., Costa, V.S.: Change of representation for statistical relational learning. In: Proceedings of the 20th International Joint Conference on Artificial Intelligence, pp. 2719–2726 (2007)
5. Davis, J., Goadrich, M.: The relationship between precision-recall and ROC curves. In: Proceedings of the 23rd International Conference on Machine learning, pp. 233–240. ACM Press (2006)
6. Friedman, N., Geiger, D., Goldszmidt, M.: Bayesian networks classifiers. Mach. Learn. **29**, 131–163 (1997)
7. Kearney, P., Baigent, C., Godwin, J., Halls, H., Emberson, J., Patrono, C.: Do selective cyclo-oxygenase-2 inhibitors and traditional non-steroidal anti-inflammatory drugs increase the risk of atherothrombosis? meta-analysis of randomised trials. BMJ **332**, 1302–1308 (2006)
8. Kramer, S., Lavrac, N., Flach, P.: Propositionalization approaches to relational data mining. In: Džeroski, S., Lavrac, N. (eds.) Relational Data Mining Part III, pp. 262–291. Springer, Heidelberg (2001)
9. Landwehr, N., Kersting, K., and Raedt, L. D. nFOIL: Integrating Naive Bayes and FOIL. In: Proceeding of the 20th National Conference on Artificial Intelligence, pp. 795–800 (2005)
10. Landwehr, N., Passerini, A., Raedt, L.D., Frasconi, P.: kFOIL: Learning simple relational kernels. In: Proceedings of the 21st National Conference on Artificial Intelligence (2006)
11. Lavrač, N., Džeroski, S. (eds.): Relational Data Mining. Springer, Heidelberg (2001)

12. Lavrač, N., Džeroski, S.: Inductive learning of relations from noisy examples. In: Muggleton, S. (ed.) Inductive Logic Programming, pp. 495–516. Academic Press, London (1992)
13. McCarty, C., Wilke, R., Giampietro, P., Wesbrook, S., Caldwell, M.: Personalized Medicine Research Project (PMRP): design, methods and recruitment for a large population-based biobank. Personalized Med. **2**, 49–79 (2005)
14. Muggleton, S.: Inverse entailment and Progol. New Gener. Comput. **13**, 245–286 (1995)
15. Pearl, J.: Probabilistic Reasoning in Intelligent Systems: Networks of Plausible Inference. Morgan Kaufmann, San Mateo, California (1988)
16. Platt, R., Carnahan, R.: The US food and drug administration's mini-sentinel program. Pharmacoepidemiol. Drug Saf. **21**, 1–303 (2012)
17. Pompe, U., Kononenko, I.: Naive Bayesian classifier within ILP-R. In: De Raedt, L. (ed.), Proceedings of the 5th International Conference on Inductive Logic Programming, pp. 417–436 (1995)
18. Popescul, A., Ungar, L., Lawrence, S., Pennock, D. Statistical relational learning for document mining. In: Proceeding of the 3rd International Conference on Data Mining, pp. 275–282 (2003)
19. Quinlan, J.R.: Induction of decision trees. Mach. Learn. **1**, 81–106 (1986)
20. Quinlan, J.R.: Learning logical definitions from relations. Mach. Learn. **5**, 239–266 (1990)
21. Srinivasan, A.: The Aleph Manual (2001)
22. Vapnik, V.: The Nature of Statistical Learning Theory. Information Science and Statistics. Springer, Heidelberg (1999)

Chapter 17
User Modelling for Patient Tailored Virtual Rehabilitation

**Luis Enrique Sucar, Shender Maria Ávila-Sansores
and Felipe Orihuela-Espina**

Santiago suffered a stroke 5 years ago, and although he survived, the conse-quences were devastating suffering severe paresis of his left side. However, by looking at him today, you won't notice that for a second; Santiago is playing football with the same skills that he used to before the event. It has taken him long to get here, but his determination and the intelligent rehabilitation *program that he underwent have made the miracle. In the old days, rehabilitation pro-grams were tedious, and most times with limited success; motor recovery was modest, and neurorehabilitation programs were just compensatory in nature. Today, the better understanding of the brain plastic behaviour following stroke, accompanied by the state of the art artificial intelligence incorporated to afford-able robotic devices and virtual training environments have offered Santiago a brand new opportunity to live life to the full.*

Abstract Intelligent rehabilitation is a novel paradigm in motor rehabilitation empowering assistive technology with artificial intelligence (AI). Central to this par-adigm is adaptation, the capacity of the assistive technology to dynamically accom-modate to the therapy evolving demands. This chapter overviews several existing AI solutions to implement a decision making model to provide rehabilitation tools with adaptation capabilities, and provides details of a powerful approach capable of exploiting prior knowledge for a quick start and posterior knowledge to guarantee up-to-dated informed decisions. In this solution, a Markov decision process formu-lates an initial policy optimal within prior knowledge; a policy which is later on allow to evolve on incoming evidence to fit new requirements. This solution ensures short training periods and exhibits convergence with therapists' criteria. In consequence, intelligent adaptation to dynamic circumstances of the patient and therapy plan is demonstrated a feasible endeavour within a real practical timeline. This might endow assistive technology with the necessary competence to be taken home and/or reduce expert surpervision.

© Springer International Publishing Switzerland 2015
A. Hommersom and P.J.F. Lucas (eds.), *Biomedical Knowledge Representation*, LNAI 9521, DOI 10.1007/978-3-319-28007-3_17

259

17.1 Introduction

Of course, the opening futuristic scenario is not yet a reality, and our current rehabilitation technology is merely the one branded above as the "old days". Nevertheless, the progress towards making this a reality that has been in the cook in the last decade has been astonishing. We are still far from a satisfactory recovery of people who have suffered brain lesions, but the foundations of the intelligent rehabilitation are already in the making.

Assistive technology is any product or service designed to enable independence for disabled and older people [19]. Assistive technologies can be realized under many skins; mechanical, robotic, and perhaps ultimately virtual. Regardless of the delivery technology, the core of this intelligent rehabilitation is the extensive use of Artificial Intelligence (AI) providing the assistive technology with human-expert like decision capacities, but enriched with augmented sensing abilities to support neurorehabilitation [55]. This AI capitalizes on *knowledge representation* to encode information about the patient profile, his progress through the therapy and the prognosis, but as well about the medical condition itself. Then, based on this knowledge it *reasons* the optimal decision that can be taken assuming certain therapy goals. Depending on these therapeutic goals, different AI systems will make use of all or only part of this knowledge. The ultimate goal of the AI itself is to *adapt* the behaviour of the assistive technology to the patient progress, yet conciliating the patient necessities with the therapist's long term plan, and achieve this adaptation whilst always acting within the grounds established by neurorehabilitation principles. This chapter overviews some of the technologies underpinning these AI systems and provides examples that have been implemented in the field of virtual rehabilitation.

17.2 Virtual Rehabilitation

Virtual rehabilitation [34] encompasses the use of virtual reality scenarios to afford training environments with an enormous and versatile capacity for feedback and customization. A virtual environment is a simulation of the real world that is generated through computer software and it is experienced by the user through a human-machine interface [22]. The virtual rehabilitation environment can be manipulated at will to offer a more exhaustive and comprehensive learning experience. Within the virtual environment, real world tasks can be replicated with in-depth fidelity to the actual task, or on the contrary, critical elements of the task can be abstracted to eliminate sources of distraction. The virtual environment can offer truly immersive and multisensorial experience, and/or can favour psychological sense of being within the virtual world, a feature known as presence [49, 57].

Several features distinguish virtual environments from other forms of visual imaging such as video and television e.g., different viewpoints, multisensorial input, etc. But arguably the most salient feature is interaction [54]. In virtual rehabilitation, the environments are created to allow the user to interact with the objects represented in the environment and the environment itself. Virtual rehabilitation is mostly administered in the form of serious games [3, 4, 12, 32, 38]; those designed for a serious purpose other than leisure and pure entertainment [38]. A serious game for rehabilitation is presented in a virtual environment and the goal of the game conceals the rehabilitatory task.

The advantages and limitations of virtual rehabilitation in general have been reviewed somewhere else [2, 21, 52, 54], but importantly of course the capacity for adaptation of the virtual environments has not go unnoticed [12, 52].

17.3 Adaptation

As the therapist is helping and guiding the patient over a physical or occupational therapy session, s/he continually monitors with an expert's eye the progress of the patient; demanding more when feeling the patient can do better but also, decelerating the activities program and moderating the requested effort when noticing hints of pain or stress on the patient. The therapist has a long term plan, but continually makes local corrections and adjustments to this plan on the basis of the patient overall progress and dynamic changing necessities. The therapist is adapting the therapy to the patient needs. Adaptation is arguably a central concept in intelligent rehabilitation [52]. It undertakes the responsibility of ensuring that the best possible clinical decision at every moment regarding the therapy delivery and administration. This ultimate goal of adaptation is far from a reality at present, and current solutions, such as the one presented in this chapter, only provide limited decisions commensurate with the knowledge base underpinning the computational model. This decision making process is made autonomously from human experts, but critically learned from prior feedback made by human experts. Adaptation is a necessary element for guaranteeing that the intelligent rehabilitation maximizes fostering of appropriate functional cortical reorganization strategies and stimulates experience dependent plastic changes in the brain motor networks, both critical for the neurorehabilitation process [13, 28, 42].

Adaptation permits controlling the delivery of stimuli in terms of modality (e.g., auditory, haptic, and/or visual), and modulating the parameters of the modality, such as colour, direction, strength/level, speed, duration, and amount of stimulus and, in general, of any property or attribute that may characterise the stimuli. It further can regulate the level and mode of feedback provided to the user. It also has to decide about the chronological succession of rehabilitatory tasks, and the time and intensity with which these should be carried out. It governs the pace of the training.

Adaptation is a more elaborate concept than goal attainment-based challenge adjustment or therapy progress. In the latter, challenge adjustment is unidirectional, it increases as new goals are achieved but it is never revisited downwards. Adaptation, on the other hand, is a patient centered decision making process in which task challenge adjustment and therapy programme scheduling are dynamically fitted to the patient physical and cognitive status. Contrary to systems where game challenge is adapted following a structured approach, e.g., game level increases by achieving a certain goal or target whether explicit or implicit; dynamic adaptation of game difficulty implies monitoring user's in-game performance and ability and using those to maintain an appropriate level of difficulty [12].

Adaptation is also different from customization which is concerned with accommodating the environment to the therapy requirements, for instance, for different pathophysiologies and/or different target groups, perhaps even individuals. Instead, adaptation regulates the dose, frequency, task challenge and variability [52]. Despite both concepts -customization and adaptation- being concerned with tailoring the therapy to the patient, customization is static in nature, whereas adaptation is inherently dynamic and non-linear. Nevertheless, these two concepts are often used interchangeably in the virtual rehabilitation literature.

17.3.1 The Levels of Adaptation

In general, there can be two levels of adaptation in virtual rehabilitation: (i) within-game or game-level adaptation and (ii) inter-game or therapy-level adaptation. The former refers to the level of difficulty in a particular game or task to maintain challenge, whilst the latter refer to therapy task scheduling and is concerned with making the most out of the therapy time. Within-game adaptation can be further performed online as the interaction with the environment occurs, or off-line by which challenge adjustment is guaranteed across tasks performed in sequence. Note a clear difference between ensuring the right level of challenge across subsequent games, i.e., off-line within-game adaptation, and optimizing that sequence of games, i.e., rehabilitatory tasks, as the therapy advances which is controlled by the inter-game adaptation. Both levels can be modelled with decision algorithms and complemented with knowledge-transfer approaches.

17.4 Intelligence and Knowledge Representation Behind the Virtual Environments

The manifestation of the (artificial) intelligence supporting the assistive technology is mainly its adaptation capacity. When the therapist makes a decision over the next action in the therapy, s/he takes into consideration everything that s/he knows about the patient and the medical condition. The therapist exploits his/her *knowledge* by *reasoning* over it to come up with subsequent conduct. Similarly, in developing the AI, these two elements characterise the model underpinning the intelligent rehabilitation technology.

- **Knowledge.** From a rather naive but practical definitions of "useful information" [17] or "understanding of a subject area" (Durkin 1994 in [18]), defining knowledge is a difficult endeavour [5, 29]. Without aiming to settle the argument, knowledge is the repository of information about a certain domain acquired through learning/experience (sensing), discovering (reasoning), or studying (education) and may include facts, concepts, beliefs, skills, as well as relations among these knowledge atoms. Knowledge is more than simply information, it includes context and semantics so that its relevancy to a problem can be determined [5]. To make knowledge available to a certain assistive technology it has to be encoded under certain representation [14]. Familiar basic knowledge representation tools or technologies include logic, rules, frames, semantic nets, graphical models, etc.
- **Reasoning.** Is a process of using known facts and/or assumptions in order to derive a conclusion or make an inference [18]. Reasoning is the engine that allows the AI system to mine the knowledge (i) to make explicit (potentially useful) *new* knowledge that was already implicit in the repository, but more interesting for guiding the intelligent therapy, also (ii) to make an optimal decision about the next action or actions to be carried out in the therapy. There are, of course, pragmatic concerns about the relationship between knowledge and making decisions [16]. Reasoning can be achieved in several fashions; classical logical (inc. inductive, abductive, deductive, syllogistic, modal, etc.), set-based whereby an evidence function maps observed findings to solutions [36, 37], probabilistic whereby new knowledge is derived through probabilistic expressions [33, 43], or semantical where inference rules are specified by means of an ontology language [18].

17.4.1 Knowledge: The State Through Observable and Non-observable Variables

Any intelligent assistive technology possesses some sensing capabilities to experience the environment over which it has to act. Often in artificial intelligence, the actual knowledge about the status of the environment is referred to as *state*. Note that this state can cover self-awareness information as well as information about the target world, and importantly it is not necessarily factual. The state is what ultimately guides the decision making process. The same action might yield very different outcomes when executed under different states.

The sensing abilities will give the system access to some new knowledge about the state which the system will integrate to its knowledge repository. As new knowledge becomes available (feedback to the system), the intelligent system updates its belief over the state of the environment and triggers a new decision making process to confirm or alter accordingly the schedule of actions. Critically, the knowledge of the state by the intelligent system may not necessarily be complete. Thus, a decision evaluated as optimal by the an intelligent system, may actually be suboptimal in real terms. Yet it has to be emphasized that it is still the best decision that can be made with the knowledge at hand.

Regardless of the representation chosen, a factored state can be thought of as variables. In the domain at hand, these variables may encapsulate pieces of information such as the patient performance on a task, the cognitive and psychological state of the patient, the stage on the rehabilitation process, etc. These variables can be directly accessible from the sensing abilities of the intelligent system or on the contrary, have to be inferred from the experienced information. The first type of information is known as *observable variables*, the latter as *non-observable variables*. This distinction should not be overlook when developing decision making processes.

Uncertainty can be present in both, observable and non-observable information, but more often than not, uncertainty in the observable knowledge if considered by the artificial intelligence, it is dealt with *before* its input to the decision making algorithm. At the time the possibility of executing a particular decision is being evaluated by the system, the observable variables are virtually always considered factual.

17.5 State of the Art

In the field of virtual rehabilitation, early systems that appeared back in the 1990s through to the early 2000s lack any form of adaptation e.g., [11, 15, 23, 30, 31, 40, 46, 47]. Even in more recent works, adaptation to the patient is still a luxury feature with many examples still missing it e.g., [4, 6, 24, 48]. Notwithstanding, in the last decade several studies have addressed the task of enriching the system with adaptation, or at least customization capabilities. Representative examples for upper limb virtual rehabilitation platforms are summarized in Table 17.1. They differ both in the chosen knowledge representation as well as in the reasoning modality.

As it emerges from Table 17.1, probabilistic reasoning appears to be the most favoured reasoning modality, perhaps due to the uncertainty inherent to the problem for which probabilistic reasoning excels. Most of these adaptive solutions are based on the observable performance, with only a couple of exceptions [10, 26] attempting to capture the patient's non observable cognitive state.

17.6 Probabilistic Models of Adaptation

A natural and powerful formalism to achieve automatic adaptation are decision-theoretic models, in particular *Markov decision processes* (MDPs) and partially observable MDPs (POMDPs).

A Markov Decision Process [45] models a sequential decision problem, in which a system evolves in time and is controlled by an agent. An MDP is a tuple $\{\mathscr{S}, \mathscr{A}, \mathrm{Pr}, R\}$, where $\mathscr{S}$ is a finite set of states and $\mathscr{A}$ is a finite set of actions. Actions induce stochastic state transitions, with $\mathrm{Pr}(s, a, t)$ denoting the probability with which state t is reached when action a is executed at state s. $R(s, a)$ is a real-valued reward function, associating with each state s and action a its immediate

Table 17.1 Summary of virtual reality based rehabilitation solutions for the upper limb including some form of customization or adaptation sorted by year of publication. dof: degrees of freedom; VR: Virtual Reality; RL: Reinforcement Learning.

Given Name, References (Year)	Brief Description	Virtual Environments	Adaptability / Customizability	Artificial Intelligence
Virtual Environment Training System [22] (2002)	A desktop display and electromagnetic motion-tracking devices	Putting envelope in mailbox. Reaching exercises.	Allow to tailor feedback to each patient's need	Not described
Gentle/s [35] (2003)	Large computer screen with a 3 dof haptic interface. Requires elbow orthosis.	Empty room, real room and detail room.	Different levels of guidance and correction can be programmed.	Predefined polynomial models
TheraGame [27] (2006)	Video capture (Webcam) VR system	Games inc. Tetris, frog, colorSok and motion music	Level of difficulty of games may be graded to patient's level	Not described
Universities of Derby and Ulster's serious games for movement therapy [12, 38] (2008)	Immersive head mounted display (HMD) and gloves	Games inc. Rabbit chase, arrow attack, orange catching, and whack-a-mouse	Difficulty increases or decreases based on patient's performance.	Preset conditions dynamically checked.
Toronto Rehabilitation Institute (TRI) device [26] (2008)	1 dof robot + virtual environment interface	Reaching task	Probabilistic decision theoretic models adjust within-game challenge	POMDP
Virtual Piano Trainer [1] (2009)	Cyberglove + Cybergrasp + two arm tracking sensors combined with a virtual piano	Virtual piano	Haptic assistance regulated in proportion to subject performance	Two adaptive differential algorithms
Gesture Therapy [10, 50, 51] (2009-11)	A game console enhanced with a gripper with pressure sensor	3 games based on classical concepts and physical rehabilitation movements	Probabilistic models adjust within-game challenge	POMDP
iStretch [19, 20] (2010)	1 dof robotic system for the early stages of physiotherapy. The evolution of [26].	Reaching task	Probabilistic decision theoretic models adjust within-game challenge	POMDP
None given [3] (2010)	Wii based + vision system	A set of 8 games inc. baseball catch, helicopter flying, frog Simon and under-the-sea	Detects and filters motion compensation. Calibrates through example motions.	Preset conditions dynamically checked.
Gesture Therapy II [7, 52] (2013)	A game console enhanced with a gripper with pressure sensor	5 games based on classical concepts and physical rehabilitation movements	Probabilistic models adjust within-game challenge	MDP + RL

utility $R(s, a)$. A policy for an MDP is a mapping $\pi : S \rightarrow A$ that selects an action for each state. A solution to an MDP is a policy that maximizes its expected value. The expected value is a certain value function; this could be the average reward over certain time horizon, or the expected accumulated reward in the future. Two popular methods for finding an optimal policy for an MDP are the value iteration and the policy iteration algorithms [45].

MDPs assume that the state of the system is known with certainty, that is that the state is observable. In many domains such as virtual rehabilitation, it is not always possible to observe the complete state, e.g., the cognitive and psychological state of the patient is not directly observable. In this case, an extension of the MDP model, known as partially observable Markov decision processes (POMDPs) becomes handy. In addition to the elements of an MDP, a POMDP has the following elements: a set of observations O, the conditional probability of observing o while in state s, denoted by $\Omega(s, o)$, and finally, the initial state probability distribution $\Pi(s)$. A solution for a POMDP is a mapping from belief states to actions, which is a more complex problem than the MDP counterpart as in principle the number of belief states is infinite. POMDPs have been so far a popular solution to support adaptation in virtual rehabilitation systems [10, 20, 26]. However, exact solutions are feasible only for very small problems, and in general approximate solution techniques are used [44]. Moreover, using a POMDP to model the adaptation process of a virtual rehabilitation system in isolation assumes that the same policy that was learn over *a priori* static knowledge would remain valid longitudinally across the therapy and cross-sectionally for different patients. None of these premises hold in a real therapy and consequently a smarter artificial intelligence must be sought.

Ideally, the adaptation model of the virtual rehabilitation system must be able to deliver actions based on a policy that remains optimal regardless of the dynamically changing knowledge. Recently, we have proposed an intelligent adaptation system [9] for our virtual rehabilitation platform, Gesture Therapy [52] (see Sect. 17.6.4), that aims to address this necessity. This adaptation model is based on MDPs, ergo assuming, for now, that we can observe the patient's state. However, the initial policy rather than being left immutable is allowed to accommodate new knowledge as it becomes available. This up-to-date knowledge comes from sensing the performance of the user but also from educative rewards from the therapist. From the seed policy returned by the MDP over *a priori* knowledge, the new dynamic policy thus built by means of reinforcement learning may vary from patient to patient, as well as for the same patient as the therapy progresses. In other words, an initial, general model to the patient is iteratively refined ensuring the policy remains optimal to fit the actual circumstances, and in turn the actions chosen by the dynamic policy permit adaptation of the virtual environment. In the following sections we describe this model and its adaptation using reinforcement learning algorithms.

17.6.1   A Model for Adaptive Rehabilitation

In a nutshell, the model deals with within-game adaptation; after each game is played for a certain amount of time, the speed and control exhibited by the patient during the game are evaluated. Depending on the evaluation the decision-theoretical adaptation system proposes a new level of challenge for the next game to match the patient's progress thorough the therapy. Although different strategies can be designed regarding performance response, we have chosen one that favours levelled improvement in speed and control.

More formally, the model has two major elements. First, an MDP, defined based on expert knowledge, is solved to obtain an initial, general policy. This is in a sense a general model not specific to any patient. As we have shown in [9], this *a priori* optimized seeding reduces the time needed to dynamically evolve an adapted patient-specific model with respect to random or null initialization. Second, a reinforcement learning algorithm progressively tailors this initial model to keep the policy optimal to the patient's needs throughout the therapy.

17.6.2   The General Default Policy

The initial general model is an MDP in which the system set of states, S, is described by a discretized bivariate performance space relying on the subject *speed* and *control*. Speed is measured from task onset until task completion. It is calculated as the on-screen avatar trace pathlength over the time needed to fulfill the task, and expressed relatively against empirically found values normal for a healthy subject, with three possible intervals: *low*, *medium* and *high*; determined by preset hard thresholds. Control is calculated as the deviation in pixels from a straight path in the screen going from the user avatar location at task onset to the location of the task target. Control is also expressed relatively against empirically found ranges considered normal for a healthy subject, with three possible intervals: *poor*, *fair* and *good*; again separated by hard thresholds. Although this adaptation model is grounded on an MDP since the performance metrics monitored in this case are observable, it is possible to extend the present solution to a POMDP for a more educated model that perhaps incorporates psychological and cognitive variables.

The actions considered by the MDP are either to *increase*, *maintain* or *decrease* the challenge level of the task. The practical realization of this in the virtual rehabilitation platform Gesture Therapy (see Sect. 17.6.4) enforces lower and upper boundary limits to the challenge levels, in other words, increments or decrements of challenge are limited by each game capacity. As aforementioned, the transition and reward functions implemented have been designed to favour a match between speed and control encouraging a balanced progression in both performance metrics. The full details can be found in [8].

The optimal policy of the MDP is found with a value iteration algorithm [44]. The policy is the result of optimizing the expected accumulated rewards. This initial policy provides a reasonable default response, and it is optimal for the given *a priori* knowledge. However, it is not optimal for all patients and all conditions. Thus, in a second stage, this inceptive policy is allowed to evolve using reinforcement learning techniques to meet arriving evidence, whether sensed e.g., patient's performance, or taught e.g., therapist's feedback.

17.6.3 Improving the Policy by Reinforcement Learning

Reinforcement learning [25] is a machine learning paradigm inspired by how a human learns. A child attempts some act and his progenitor either praises (positive reward) or disapproves (negative reward) his actions. With time, as the child seeks to maximize praise and minimize disapproval, he learns the behaviour that his progenitor is predicating. Analogously, an agent or process evolves to maximize expected rewards as it receives feedback from the environment [53]. Different reinforcement learning algorithms are available in literature but they can coarsely be classified as off-policy or on-policy. In off-policy algorithms, the policy is learned greedily ignoring of the actions that the agent performs. The policy value is updated using hypothetical actions separating exploration from control. Consequently, the optimal policy is learnt even when a non-optimal policy is being followed. In contrast, on-policy algorithms are unable to distinguish exploration from control and the policy value is updated implying the results of the executed actions. In other words, the optimal policy is learnt only by using the systematic departures from the true optimal. Archetypical examples of off-policy and on-policy algorithms are Q-*Learning* [56] and Sarsa [53], respectively.

Q-*Learning*, stated in Algorithm 1, is an off-policy learning algorithm because the policy being learned may be different from the policy being executed. The quality function $Q(s; a)$ specifies the value (expected accumulated reward) of

---

Algorithm 1. Q-*Learning*
___
Input: $< S, A, R >$
Output: The table Q

1 Initialize the table entry $Q(s_t, a_t)$ arbitrarily
2 **for** *(each episode)* **do**
3   Initialize s_t
4   **repeat**
5   Choose a_t and s_t using the policy derived from $Q(e.g., \varepsilon - greedy)$
6   Take action a_t, observe the reward r_{t+1} and the next state s_{t+1}
7   Update the table entry for $Q(s_t, a_t)$ as follows:
8       $Q(s_t, a_t) \leftarrow Q(s_t, a_t) + \alpha[r_{t+1} + \gamma max_{a_{t+1}} Q(s_{t+1}, a_{t+1}) - Q(s_t, a_t)]$
9       $s_t \leftarrow s_{t+1}$
10   **until** *(s_t is a terminal state)*
11 **end**

executing action a whilst in state s. Often, the states and actions are discrete, and thus $Q(s; a)$ can be specified by a matrix. This quality function $Q(s_t, a_t)$ evaluates the rewards obtained through the course of actions. In Q-*Learning*, the value of the quality function $Q(s_t, a_t)$ (line 8) is updated considering the action that maximizes the expected utility i.e. $max_{a_{t+1}}(Q(s_{t+1}, a_{t+1}))$. The goal of the learning agent is consequently to maximize its accumulated reward and it does so by learning which action is optimal for each state. Often, the initial policy quality table $Q_{S \times A}$ is initialized to some random value e.g. zero, minimal rewards, etc., and the value of Q is updated as the learning progresses.

In contrast, the Sarsa (state-action-reward-state-action) algorithm stated in Algorithm 2 behaves on-policy. Line 9 is the on-policy equivalent for updating the quality function $Q(s_t, a_t)$. However, in contrast to Q-*Learning*, in this case it strictly updates the value on the basis of the experience gained through the implementation of the policy. The substantial difference between the two algorithms is the fact that Q-*Learning* is a greedy agent that always takes the action with the best Q-values and then backs up the best Q-value from the state reached; while Sarsa waits until an action is taken and then backs up the Q-value from that action.

Algorithm 2. Sarsa

Input: $< S, A, R >$
Output: The table Q

12 Initialize the table entry $Q(s_t, a_t)$ arbitrarily **for** *(each episode)* **do**
13 | Initialize s_t Choose a_t and s_t using the policy derived from $Q(e.g., \varepsilon - greedy)$ **repeat**
14 | | Take action a_t and observe r_{t+1}, s_{t+1} Choose a_{t+1} from s_{t+1} using the policy derived
 | | from $Q(e.g., \varepsilon - greedy)$ Update the $Q(s_t, a_t)$ as follows: $Q(s_t, a_t) \leftarrow Q(s_t, a_t) +$
 | | $\alpha[r_{t+1} + Q(s_{t+1}, a_{t+1}) - Q(s_t, a_t)]$ $s_t \leftarrow s_{t+1}$ $a_t \leftarrow a_{t+1}$
15 | **until** *(s_t is a terminal state)*
16 **end**

In both cases, the learning rate α determines to what extent the newly acquired information will override the old information. A factor of 0 will make the agent not learn anything, while a factor of 1 would make the agent consider only the most recent information. A second parameter, the discount factor γ regulates the relevance given to short or long term rewards. A value $\gamma = 0$ considers only the most immediate future reward, whereas as γ approximates 1, progressively more weight is given to long-term rewards. The policy derived from Q was considered $\varepsilon - greedy$, that is, this strategy assumes the probability $(1-\varepsilon)$ to choose the action with the highest value and probability estimate of ε to choose randomly among all actions. The value of ε emphasizes the balance (or unbalance) between exploration and exploitation.

The original versions of the Q-*Learning* and Sarsa algorithms were formulated to consider only a single source of rewards i.e. those given by the environment. In virtual rehabilitation this is clearly insufficient as the adaptation must abide both patient's status and therapist's dictations, in other words, we have two sources of incoming educational knowledge. In addition, the domain at hand, i.e., virtual rehabilitation

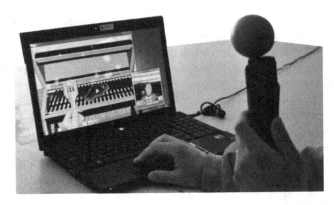

Fig. 17.1 Gesture Therapy, a virtual rehabilitation platform for the upper limb. The picture presents one of the serious games of the platform to camouflage the abduction/adduction movement. On the right of the photograph, the user is holding the gripper for controlling the games.

demands that actions issued have to be acceptable from onset, forbidding any chances to thoroughly explore the policy space before a confident action can be issued. To overcome these two issues, we capitalize on *reward shaping* [41].

Given any definition of optimality, there are infinitely many reward functions that are consistent with it [39]. The choice of the reward function has a strong effect on how long it takes to learn an optimal policy. Reward shaping [41] can accelerate learning by providing localized useful advice. The heuristic supporting reward shaping is to focus learning on the most promising areas of the search space whereby a second shaping reward funds efforts towards the goal.

In order to incorporate reward shaping ideas into the Q-*Learning* and Sarsa's algorithms, these have to be modified to accept this additional shaping reward f which further complements the regular reward r received by the original algorithms. To distinguish these reward shaping-based versions from the original algorithms we refer to them as Q+ and S+, respectively. The full description of these versions of the algorithms can be found in [8]. The Q+ algorithm is essentially the same as Q learning, except for the reward considered when the Q values are updated, that in the Q+ version is the sum of the environment reward, r, and the shaping reward, f. S+ is derived analogously from Sarsa. Although shaping can be accomplished under many forms here we opted for a sum, likely the most popular implementation. In the case of virtual rehabilitation, the shaping reward is provided by the therapist. The reward shaping alteration is (i) convenient to accommodate more than one reward source, and (ii) critical to achieve good adjustment of the dynamic policy within the timeframe imposed by the rehabilitation schedule.

17.6.4   Gesture Therapy: A Virtual Rehabilitation Platform

In order to test the proposed adaptation algorithm it has been implemented in an existing virtual rehabilitation platform. Gesture Therapy [50–52], developed at our laboratory, is a virtual platform for the rehabilitation of the upper limb, from shoulder to hand. Figure 17.1 shows the external appearance of the platform and Fig. 17.2 illustrates the internal architecture of the platform. Central to this work, is the adaptation module which communicates with the game set, overseeing user's performance and adjusting the challenge in return. Prior to this work, the Gesture Therapy platform had an adaptation module based on POMDP [10] which for the reasons explained above was upgraded to this new model of adaptation.

17.6.5   Integration of the Dynamic Adaptation Model to Gesture Therapy

The adaptation model based on MDPs and reinforcement learning has been integrated to the Gesture Therapy rehabilitation system to govern the setting of the task

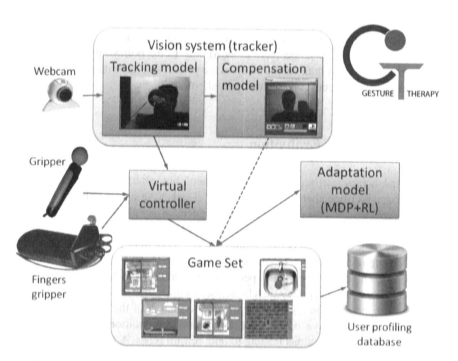

Fig. 17.2 Schematic representation of the Gesture Therapy architecture. The adaptation module interacts with the game set to regulate the challenge.

challenge level within games based on both the patient's performance and the therapist's didactics.

As aforementioned, the system state is characterized by the patient's observable performance in terms of the exhibited control and speed. The user proceeds with the task for a given time (usually 3 to 5 min), and after this period, the system evaluates the demonstrated performance. Based on its current policy, the adaptation model issues an action, i.e., a decision setting the difficulty level of the task for the next game. The reward function yields an environmental reward r_{t+1} appraising the patient's interaction with the system in terms of the current state. In addition, the shaping reward is obtained from the therapist by informing the expert about the decision taken and the conditions leading to that decision, and asking whether s/he agrees with that decision. The clinician binary response (agree or disagree with the decision) is mapped to the shaping reward f_{t+1}. This reward feeds from the clinician experience and the *in-situ* assessment that the clinician makes of the patient's status. The decision made by the current policy will be carried out whether right or wrong in the eyes of the therapist, but the reward associated to the clinician's statement is not ignored and will still shape future decisions. In other words, it is used to update the policy.

This policy dynamic optimization process continues iteratively until the decision policy is tuned to the therapy contemporary needs. For convenience, learning can be switched on or off. While off is chosen, the ongoing policy continues to rule the challenge adaptation decisions and remains unchanged until a new adjustment is required when the learning process is switched back on. The requirement for the presence of the clinician is therefore reduced only to the policy updating periods. This permits that the system can be taken to the patient's home with guarantees that the system carries the most up-to-date optimal policy.

17.7 Preliminary Evaluation

If the virtual therapy is to be deployed to the patient's home without continuous expert supervision, it is critical that the adaptation model makes the system to behave intelligently to replicate what the expert would recommend at any given time. Thus, a high level of congruence between the model and expert recommended actions is desirable. Ideally, any policy updating period should not last more than 2–3 therapeutics sessions. Considering a common rehabilitation session of about 45 min, and assuming that during each session the patient performs in average 10 to 15 tasks (games) of about 3 min per game; the policy shall be adjusted within 30 to 45 feedback iterations.

We have conducted an initial experimental evaluation of the adaptation system through a small feasibility study in laboratory controlled conditions. This experiment considered human interactions leading to both reward types. A few subjects played the role of patients and two experts, representing therapists, assessed the model decisions. For this study, since interaction with the virtual platform and underlying decision taking mechanisms are independent of the user's level of impairment, yet healthy users facilitate reproducible and controlled conditions, healthy subjects were preferred over real patients. The tests were carried out using Gesture Therapy [51, 52] as the virtual rehabilitation platform.

Importantly, the experiment although carried out in controlled laboratory conditions, it was still susceptible to noise in data acquisition, thus permitting assessing the learning performance under realistic conditions. Moreover, it allows us to elaborate on the congruency between the decisions taken by the adaptation model and the corresponding dis/agreement statement made by the expert. This is critical if the system is to be taken home with limited clinical supervision for certain therapy periods.

17.7.1   Experimental Set-up

The experiment has been described elsewhere [8, 9] and it is briefly summarized here. Four subjects participated in the study (age mean 28; range 23–30). All the participants had previous experience in using computers. No training or familiarization with the platform or the games were allowed, however, one participant being internal to the developing team had gaming experience with Gesture Therapy. A physician and an experienced researcher played the roles of the therapists. The experiment was carried out in a single session, where all participants were in the laboratory concurrently. Each expert was in charge of monitoring two of the participants.

Each participant played 25 blocks of 2 tasks (50 learning policy updates episodes) selected among a set of the five rehabilitation games available. Each block lasted for two minutes in average. At each feedback episode, the adaptation model took a decision about next game challenge level, and subsequently gathered appropriate double rewards.

The adaptation model used the MDP solution as the initial policy and the Q+ was used as the reward shaping mechanism. Model parameterization was as follows: $\alpha = 0.5$, $\varepsilon = 0.2$ and $\gamma = 0.95$. The learning algorithm and parameters used during the experiment were chosen based upon previous simulations carried out on synthetic data [8]. These previous simulations permitted studying model theoretical response and convergence under different (i) reward shaping algorithm, (ii) compromises between exploration and exploitation, (iii) user behaviours and (iv) policy initialization.

17.7.2   Results

Table 17.2 summarizes the congruence between the model and the expert expressed as a percentage of agreements over the total decisions. Congruence levels surpassed 90% for 3 of the subjects. Congruence in the remaining subject was lower following some initial disagreements at the beginning of the session, strongly influencing subsequent decisions as further discussed below.

Table 17.2 Agreement of the expert with the decisions taken by the adaptation model (in percentage over the total feedback episodes) per participant.

Subject	1	2	3	4
Congruence	56%	92%	96%	100%

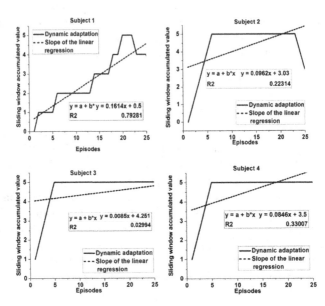

Fig. 17.3 A graph per subject is depicted showing temporal evolution of the congruence between the expert and the recommendations of the adaptation module (solid line) during the experiment. The overall learning progress can be characterized by the slope of the linear regression (dashed line). Positive slopes indicate a growing congruence between model and expert as times progress. Negative slopes (none occurred) indicate a departure in congruence.

The overall agreement is a good indicator of the model performance but is insufficient to show that the learning process has occurred. For this, the temporal evolution of the congruence was analyzed, affording further insight about the dynamics of how the congruence with the therapist was achieved.

The most recent dis/agreement statements were aggregated along a 5 episodes wide a sliding window. A value 0 represents total "recent" disagreement between the model recommended actions and the expert feedback, whereas a value 5 represent full "recent" agreement of the expert with the actions recommended by the system. Figure 17.3 shows the progress of the congruence over the experiment. The positive slopes suggest that the agreement between the model decisions and the expert increases over time. Figure 17.3 suggests that the bad decisions taken by the model at the beginning clearly hindered the progress for the subject 1. Notwithstanding, the model eventually managed to recover from this initial missteps and succeeded to learn the therapist's doctrine. This highlights two important issues. First, the early decisions have an important weight over the learning curve, which further stresses the importance of a good initialization, i.e., the MDP seeding. Second, the MDP solution built over *a priori* solution, despite being optimal for that knowledge is insufficient to characterize all participants, thus critically confirming our driving motivation that the decision making policy has to be adjusted and not left immutable.

17.8   Conclusions

It will still be a few years before our knowledge of neuro-rehabilitation is solid enough as to permit a motor recovery as the one envisaged in the futuristic scenario opening the chapter. It is likely that when the time comes, assistive technologies will be part of the rehabilitation therapy, and with them their companion artificial intelligence granting these technologies the capacity to optimally adapt the administration of the therapy. Adaptation is a central issue in this intelligent decision processes and can be achieved by a number of techniques. Probabilistic reasoning is emerging as the most favoured approach to support the modelling of adaptation according to the current trend in literature, perhaps because of its inherent capacity to deal with uncertainty.

Taking virtual rehabilitation as the paradigm of intelligent rehabilitation, this chapter has discussed different possible probabilistic solutions to model adaptation and has highlighted the need to accommodate new knowledge as it becomes available and further permitting this new knowledge to influence the future decision making events. A solution addressing this necessity that is further capable of affording decisions with high agreement with human experts within a feasible timeframe has been discussed in deeper detail.

Adequate exploitation of neuro-rehabilitation knowledge, and reasoning over this knowledge, are the fundamental elements over which newborn intelligent rehabilitation shall be grounded.

References

1. Adamovich, S.V., et al.: Design of a complex virtual reality simulation to train finger motion for persons with hemiparesis: a proof of concept study. J. NeuroEng. Rehabil. **6**, 28 (10 p.) (2009)
2. Adamovich, S.V., et al.: Sensorimotor training in virtual reality: a review. NeuroRehabilitation **25**(1), 29 (2009)
3. Alankus, G., et al.: Towards customizable games for stroke rehabilitation. In: Mynatt, E., et al. (eds.) ACM Conference on Human Factors in Computing Systems (CHI) Therapy and Rehabilitation, pp. 2113–2122. ACM, Atlanta, Georgia, USA (2010)
4. Taylor, A.-S.A., et al.: Gamers against All Odds. In: Chang, M., et al. (eds.) Learning by Playing. Game-Based Education System Design and Development. LNCS, vol. 5670, pp. 1–12. Springer, Heidelberg (2009)
5. Alterovitz, G., Ramoni, M. (eds.): Knowledge-Based Bioinformatics: From Analysis to Interpretation, 1st edn. Wiley, New York (2010)

6. August, K., Bleichenbacher, D., Adamovich, S.: Virtual reality physical therapy: a telerehabilitation tool for hand and finger movement exercise monitoring and motor skills analysis. In: Proceedings of the IEEE 31st Annual Northeast Bioengineering Conference, pp. 73–74. IEEE, New Jersey, USA, April 2005

7. Shender, Á.-S., Felipe, O.-E., Luis, E.S.: Patient tailored virtual rehabilitation. In: International Conference on NeuroRehabilitation (ICNR 2012), Toledo, Spain, pp. 879–883, November 2012

8. Shender Maríya Á.-S.: Adaptación en línea de una política de decisión utilizando aprendizaje por refuerzo y su aplicación en rehabilitación virtual. M.Sc thesis, Division of Computational Sciences, National Institute for Astrophysics, Optics and Electronics (INAOE), Puebla, Mexico, February 2013

9. Shender Maríya Á.-S., et al.: Adaptive decision models for virtual rehabilitation environments. In: International Conference on Machine Learning (ICML 2013) Workshop on Role of Machine Learning in Transforming Healthcare (WHEALTH), Atlanta, USA, June 2013

10. Avilés, H., et al.: Gesture Therapy 2.0: adapting the rehabilitation therapy to the patient progress. In: Hommerson, A., Lucas, P. (eds.) Workshop on Probabilistic Problem Solving in Biomedicine in 13th Conference on Artificial Intelligence in Medicine (AIME 2011), Bled, Slovenia, pp. 3–14, July 2011

11. Burdea, G., et al.: Virtual reality-based orthopedic telerehabilitation. IEEE Trans. Rehabil. Eng. **8**(3), 430–432 (2000)

12. Burke, J.W., et al.: Serious games for upper-limb rehabilitationfollowing stroke. In: Rebolledo-Mendez, G., Liarokapis, F., de Freitas, S. (eds.) 2009 Conference in Games and Virtual Worldsfor Serious Applications. Coventry, UK, pp.103–110, March 2009

13. Carey, L.M., et al.: Motor impairment and recoveryin the upper limb after stroke: behavioral and neuroanatomicalcorrelates. Stroke **36**, 625–629 (2005)

14. Davis, R., Shrobe, H., Szolovits, P.: What is a knowledge representation? AI Mag. **14**(1), 17–33 (1993)

15. Ellsworth, C., Winters, J.: An innovative system to enhance upper-extremity stroke rehabilitation. In: Clark, J.W., et al. (eds.) 2nd Joint Engineering in Medicine and Biology Society and Biomedical Engineering Society (EMBS/BMES) Conference, vol. 3, pp. 2367–2368. IEEE, Houston, Texas, USA, October 2002

16. Fagin, R., et al.: Reasoning About Knowledge. MIT Press, London (1995)

17. Fayyad, U., Piatetsky-Shapiro, G., Smyth, P.: From data mining to knowledge discovery in databases. Artif. Intell. Mag. **17**(3), 37–54 (1996)

18. Gašević, D., Djurić, D., Devedžić, V.: Model Driven Engineering and Ontology Development, 2nd edn. Springer, Heidelberg (2009)

19. Department of Health (UK): Research and development work relating to assisstive technology 2009–2010. Presented to Parliament Pursuant to Section 22 of the Chronically Sick and Disabled Persons Act 1970, November 2010

20. Hoey, J., Monk, A., Mihailidis, A.: People, sensors, decisions: customizable and adaptive technologies for assistance in healthcare. In: POMDP Practitioners Workshop: Solving Real-World POMDP Problems at 20th International Conference on Automated Planning and Scheduling (ICAPS 2010), Toronto, Canada, p. 9, May 2010

21. Holden, M.K.: Virtual environments formotor rehabilitation: review. Cyberpsychol. Behav. **8**(3), 187–211 (2005)

22. Holden, M.K., Dyar, T.: Virtual environment training: a new tool for neurorehabilitation. Neurobiol. Rep. **26**(2), 62–71 (2002)

23. Johnson, M.J., et al.: Driver's SEAT: Simulation Environment for Arm Therapy. In: van der Loos, M. (ed.) 6th International Conference on Rehabilitation Robotics (ICORR 1999), Stanford, California, USA, pp. 227–234, July 1999

24. Johnson, M.J., et al.: TheraDrive: a new stroke therapy concept for homebased, computer-assissted motivating rehabilitation. In: Donna, H., Zhi-Pei, L. (eds.) 26th Annual International Conference of the IEEE Engineering in Medicine & Biology Society (EMBS), pp. 4844–4847. San Francisco, CA, USA, September 2004

25. Kaelbling, L.P., Littman, M.L., Moore, A.W.: Reinforcement learning: a survey. J. Artif. Intell. Res. **4**, 237–285 (1996)
26. Kan, P., Hoey, J., Mihailidis, A., Automated upper extremity rehabilitation for stroke patients using a partially observable Markov decision process. In: Association for Advancement of Artificial Intelligence (AAAI) 2008 Fall Symposium on AI in Eldercare (2008)
27. Kizony, R., et al.: TheraGame - a home basedvirtual reality rehabililtation system. In: Brooks, T., Cobb, S. (eds.) 6th InternationalConference on Disability, Virtual Reality and Associated Technologies (ICDVRAT 2006), Esbjerg, Denmark, pp. 209–214, September 2006
28. Kleim, J.A., Jones, T.A.: Principles of experience-dependent neural plasticity: implications for rehabilitation after brain damage. J. Speech Lang. Hear. Res. **51**, S225–S239 (2008)
29. Klein, P.D.: A proposed definition of propositional knowledge. J. Philos. **68**(16), 471–482 (1971)
30. Krebs, H.I., et al.: Robot-aided functional imaging: application to a motor learning study. Hum. Brain Mapp. **6**, 59–72 (1998)
31. Kuhlen, T., Dohle, C.: Virtual reality for physically disable people. Comput. Biol. Med. **25**(2), 205–211 (1995)
32. Lange, B., et al.: Development and evaluation of low cost game-based balance rehabilitation tool using the microsoft kinect sensor. In: Bonato, P. (ed.) 33rd Annual International Conference of the IEEE Engineering in Medicine and Biology Society (EMBS 2011), pp. 1831–1834. IEEE, Boston, Massachussets, USA (2011)
33. Lassiter, D., Goodman, N.D.: How many kinds of reasoning? Inference, probability, and natural language semantics. In: 34th Annual Conference of the Cognitive Science Society (2012)
34. Levin, M.F.: Can virtual reality offer enriched environments for rehabilitation? Expert Rev. Neurother. **11**(2), 153–155 (2011)
35. Loureiro, R., et al.: Upper limb robot mediated stroke therapy - GENTLE/s approach. Auton. Robots **15**, 35–51 (2003)
36. Lucas, P.: Modelling interactions for diagnosis. In: CESA 1996 IMACS Multiconference, Symposium on Modelling, Analysis and Simulation, p. 6 (1996)
37. Lucas, P.J.F.: Analysis of notions of diagnosis. Artif. Intell. **105**, 295–343 (1998)
38. Ma, M., Bechkoum, K.: Serious games for movement therapy after stroke. In: IEEE International Conference on Systems, Man and Cybernetics, 2008 (SMC 2008), Singapore, pp. 1872–1877, October 2008
39. Marthi, B.: Automatic shaping and decomposition of reward functions. In: Sammut, C., Ghahramani, Z. (eds.) 24th International Conference on Machine Learning (ICML 2007), Oregon, USA, pp. 601–608, June 2007
40. Merians, A.S., et al.: Virtual reality-augmented rehabilitation for patients following stroke. Phys. Ther. **82**(9), 898–915 (2002)
41. Ng, A.Y., Harada, D., Russell, S.J.: Policy invariance under reward transformations: theory and application to reward shaping. In: 16th International Conference on Machine Learning (ICML 1999), pp. 278–287. Morgan Kaufmann Publishers Inc., San Francisco, CA, USA (1999)
42. Orihuela-Espina, F., et al.: Neural reorganization accompanying upper limb motor rehabilitation from stroke with virtual reality-based Gesture Therapy. Top. Stroke Rehabil. **20**(3), 197–209 (2012)
43. Pearl, J.: Probabilistic reasoning in intelligent systems: networks of plausible inference. Representation and Reasoning, 2nd edn, p. 552. Morgan Kaufmann, Burlington (1988)
44. Poupart, P.: An introduction to fully and partially observable Markov decision processes (Ch. 3). In: Sucar, L.E., Morales, E.F., Hoey, J. (eds.) Decision Theory Models for Applications in Artificial Intelligence: Concepts and Solutions, pp. 33–62. IGI Global, Pennsylvania (2011)
45. Puterman, M.L.: Markov Decision Process-Discrete Stochastic Dynamic Programing, 1st edn. Wiley, New York (1994)
46. Reinkensmeyer, D.J., et al.: Java Therapy: Web-Based Robotic Rehabilitation (2001)
47. Reinkensmeyer, D.J., et al.: Understanding and treating arm movement impairment after chronic brain injury: progress with the ARM guide. J. Rehabil. Res. Dev. **37**(6), 653–662 (2000)

48. Sanchez, R.J., et al.: Automating arm movement training following severe stroke: functional exercises with quantitative feedback in gravityreduced environment. IEEE Trans. Neural Syst. Rehabil. Eng. **14**(3), 378–389 (2006)
49. Slater, M., et al.: Immersion, presence, and performance in virtual environments: an experiment with tri-dimensional chess. In: ACM Virtual Reality Software and Technology (VRST), Hong Kong, China, pp. 163–172, July 1996
50. Sucar, L.E., et al.: Clinical evaluation of a low-cost alternative for stroke rehabilitation. In: IEEE International Conference on Rehabilitation Robotics (ICORR 2009), pp. 863–866. IEEE, Kyoto International Conference Center, Japan, June 2009
51. Sucar, L.E., et al.: Gesture Therapy: a vision-based system for upper extremity stroke rehabilitation. In: 32nd Annual International Conference of the IEEE Engineering in Medicine and Biology Society (EMBS), pp. 3690–3693. IEEE, Buenos Aires, Argentina (2010)
52. Sucar, L.E., et al.: Gesture Therapy: an upper limb virtual realitybased motor rehabilitation platform. IEEE Trans. Neural Syst. Rehabil. Eng. **22**(13), 634–643 (2013)
53. Sutton, R.S., Barto, A.G.: Reinforcement Learning: An Introduction, 1st edn. MIT Press, Cambridge (1998)
54. Sveistrup, H.: Motor rehabilitation using virtual reality. J. NeuroEng. Rehabil. **1**(10), 8 (2004)
55. Rosalie H. Wang, Jennifer Boger, and Babak Taati. Creating intelligent rehabilitation technology: an interdisciplinary effort. In: Pons, J.L., Torricelli, D., Pajaro, M. (eds.) International Conference on NeuroRehabilitation (ICNR 2012), Converging Clinical and Engineering Research on Neurorehabilitation, vol. Part I, Springer, Heidelberg, pp. 1199–1202, November 2012
56. Watkins, C., Dayan, P.: Learning from delayed rewards. Ph.D thesis, King's College, Cambridge University (1989)
57. Weiss, P.L., et al.: Virtual reality in neurorehabilitation (Ch. 13). In: Selzer, M.E., et al. (eds.) Textbook of Neural Repair and Neurorehabilitation: Volume II Medical Neurorehabilitation, pp. 182–197. Cambridge University Press, Cambridge (2006)

Recommendation

Chapter 18
Supporting Physicians and Patients Through Recommendation: Guidelines and Beyond

Luca Anselma, Alessio Bottrighi, Arjen Hommersom, Paolo Terenziani and Anthony Hunter

18.1 Clinical Practice Guidelines

The recommendation task, intended as the task of supporting physicians in their activity (and, in particular, in decision making) by providing them indications of the most appropriate way of treating patients, has a long story in Medical Informatics that dates back, for instance, to the first medical expert systems (MYCIN [19]). Many different tools and techniques have been devised, within the Medical Informatics area, in order to provide physicians with recommendations about the most appropriate treatment of patients. Recently, Clinical Practice Guidelines (CPG) have gained a major role in this context. CPGs are, in the definition of the USA Institute of Medicine, 'systematically developed statements to assist practitioner and patient decisions about appropriate health care in specific clinical circumstances' (Institute of Medicine, 2001, p. 151). They are conceived as a way of putting Evidence-Based Medicine into practice, as well as a mean to grant both the quality and the standardization of healthcare services, and the minimization of costs. Thousands of CPGs have been devised in the last years. For instance, the Guideline International Network (http://www.g-i-n.net) groups 77 organizations of 4 continents, and provides a library of more than 5000 CPGs. CPGs aim to reduce errors, unjustified practice variation and wasteful commitment of resources, and encourage best practices and accountability in medicine. Clinical guidelines are typically created by medical experts or panels convened by specialty organizations, who review the relevant studies, perform meta-analysis by contrasting and combining results from different studies and, using a consensus-based process, compile a set of evidence-based recommendations. Their focus may be on screening, diagnosis, management, treatment, or referral of patients with specific clinical conditions. The recommendations are typically written as narrative text and tables, which point back to background material and evidence, ranking the strength of clinical validity, and the strength with which recommendations should be followed according to the guideline authors.

The adoption of computerized approaches to acquire, represent, execute and reason with CPGs can further increase the advantages of CPGs, providing crucial advantages to:

© Springer International Publishing Switzerland 2015
A. Hommersom and P.J.F. Lucas (eds.), *Biomedical Knowledge Representation*, LNAI 9521, DOI 10.1007/978-3-319-28007-3_18

281

- patients, granting them that they will receive the best quality medical treatments (since CPGs are actually a way of putting EBM into practice);
- physicians, providing them with a standard reference which they may consult, with a way of certifying the quality of their activity (e.g., for insurance or legal purposes), as well as with advanced support to their decision-making activity;
- hospitals and healthcare centers, providing them with tools to grant the quality and the standardization of their services, as well as with a means to evaluate quality, and to optimize costs and resources.

However, the main purpose of CPGs is to support physicians in their everyday knowledge-based decision making when treating patients, providing them evidence-based recommendations at the point of care.

Unfortunately, there are several obstacles for a full exploitation of CPGs in the clinical practice. For instance, since CPGs are usually written as standard text in natural language, they tend to be quite long, so that it is difficult for the physician at the point of care to find out the specific part of the guideline that is relevant for the specific patient at hand. Additionally, natural language is inherently ambiguous, so that textually written CPGs are usually not "rigorous" and "formal" enough, possibly leading to incorrect interpretations of physicians using them. Last, but not least, one of the main goals of CPGs is to capture medical evidence. However, from one side, evidence is essentially a form of statistical knowledge, capturing the generalities of classes of patients, rather than the peculiarities of a specific patient. From the other side, demanding to expert committees to characterize all possible executions of a CPG on any possible specific patient in any possible clinical condition is an unfeasible task. Thus, CPGs assume to deal with ideal patients, i.e., patients that have just the single disease considered in the CPG (thus excluding the concurrent application of more than one CPG), and are "statistically relevant" (they model the typical patient affected by the given disease), not presenting rare peculiarities/side-effects. Also, CPGs assume to operate in ideal context of execution, so that all necessary resources are available. Unfortunately, however, not all patients and execution contexts are "ideal" (in the above sense). As a consequence, there is always a gap between the generality of CPGs and the specificities of their execution on a specific patient in a specific context. Fulfilling such a gap is a difficult and challenging task, which is usually completely demanded to user physicians.

18.2 Computer Interpretable Guidelines

In the last two decades, Computer Interpretable Guidelines (CIGs) have been introduced in order to overcome some the above problems, and different formalisms and software systems have been developed to support them. CIG formalisms are usually based on a Task-Network Model (TNM): a (hierarchical) model of the guideline control flow as a network of specific tasks. Such formalisms are "formal" and allow one to unambiguously represent guideline procedures and recommendations. Besides supporting formal languages to acquire and represent CPGs, CIG systems usually also provide execution engines that allow user physicians to "instantiate" general guidelines on specific patients: by accessing the patient clinical data, the execution engine shows to the user physicians only those paths of actions that are applicable to the patient at hand. In such a way, they provide patient-oriented recommendations to physicians, allowing them to fulfill the gap between the generality of the CPG and the specificity of the patient at hand. Given such advantages, many CIG formalisms and systems have been designed/built in the last two decades. Some of them (the list is in alphabetic order, and is far from being exhaustive) are: Asbru [15], EON [9], GEM [18], GLARE [22], GLIF [12], GUIDE [13], PRODIGY [6], PROforma [2], SAGE [23].

A survey and/or a comparative analysis of these systems is outside the goals of this chapter. A comparison of Asbru, EON, GLIF, Guide, PROforma, PRODIGY can be found in [10]. The recent book by Ten Teije et al. [21] represents a consensus of a large part of the computer-oriented CPG community. It presents an assessment of the state of the art, as well as a collection of several recent approaches. Comprehensive surveys of the state of the art in CIGs have been already published [1, 3–5, 7, 24].

These surveys show that a relative consensus has been achieved concerning the representation formalisms. Although there are notable differences among the various approaches, partly due to the different goals they pursue, some important commonalities have been reached. For example, most approaches model guidelines in terms of a Task-Network Model (TNM): a (hierarchical) model of the guideline control flow as a network of specific tasks. Although the terminology may differ, all approaches support a basic set of core guideline tasks, such as decisions, actions and entry criteria. Decisions for example are represented by means of *logic* slots in the Arden Syntax, *Decision steps* in GLIF, *Decision tasks* in PRO*forma* and GLARE, *conditions* in Asbru, and *Decisions* in EON. The TNMs of most approaches define a fixed set of guideline tasks (one remarkable exception is EON, in which new types of tasks may be introduced). Most approaches also provide explicit support for controlled nesting of guidelines in order to model complex guidelines in terms of subguidelines (e.g., GLIF and EON) or subplans (e.g., PRO*forma*, Asbru, GLARE). GLIF also supports the representation of common guideline structures through Macros, which facilitates the reuse of guidelines that are employed often (e.g., 'if-then' rules). EON, PRO*forma* and Asbru also support the use of goals and intentions to formally specify a guideline on a higher level of abstraction.

From the architectural point of view, most CIG approaches provide specific support for at least two subtasks: (i) CPG acquisition and representation and (ii) CPG execution. Concerning acquisition, different issues have been addressed, ranging from the definition of suitable graphical interfaces to enhance the physician-system interaction, to the definition of set of tools supporting the progressive transformation from a textual CPG to its formal representation [8, 11, 14, 16, 17, 20].

With respect to execution, most approaches have developed execution engines that support the execution of an acquired CPG on a specific patient. Execution engines access the patient clinical data and use them to discriminate between alternative diagnostic/therapeutic paths, providing user physicians with recommendations about the next actions to be executed on the specific patient at hand.

18.3 Verification of Computer Interpretable Guidelines

While the representation and the execution of CIGs seem nowadays to be at least partly consolidated, a very important open issue regards reasoning on CPGs. Indeed, CPGs are, first of all, knowledge sources and, as such, the Artificial Intelligence tradition demonstrates that they may be object of different forms of reasoning. Indeed, Artificial Intelligence widely demonstrates that representation and reasoning are strictly related tasks complementing each other. In many Artificial Intelligence contexts, knowledge representation is useless without proper reasoning mechanisms operating on it. Indeed, reasoning mechanisms are the tool to "qualify" the represented knowledge, determining its implicit implications and, at the very end, showing its intrinsic underlying semantics.

In the last years, some reasoning tasks concerning CIGs have started to attract increasing attention. CIG *verification* and *conformance* are two of them. Roughly speaking, conformance analysis concerns the execution of a CIG on a specific patient, and is used in order to check whether the CIG recommendations have been followed in the treatment of the patient. A technical description and an advanced investigation of conformance are proposed in Chap. 5 of this book. On the other hand, in Chap. 19 we focus on CIG verification.

As regards verification, it is worth remembering that, in general, CPGs are a very extensive body of knowledge, which, as long as no formal language is used to represent it, is expressed in an "imprecise" (or partially ambiguous) way. The acquisition and formal representation of a CPG is thus a complex process, so that there is no guarantee that the final formal representation exactly achieves all the desired objectives in terms of correctness and completeness of the specified therapeutic and/or diagnostic treatments. Indeed, there are at least two potential sources of errors. On the one hand, given the large amount of knowledge it contains, there is no guarantee that even the original (textual) guideline correctly covers all the desired cases. On the other hand, the formalization of original (textual) guidelines into some CIG formalism is a complex process that may introduce errors. As a consequence of these problems (and, in general, of the complexity of CPGs), automatic or semi-automatic supports to verification are important to check, e.g., whether an acquired CIG allows to cope in the desired way with its eligible patients. Only after the check that a CIG verifies the desired properties, physicians can fully trust it and the recommendation it provides. However, CIG verification is a complex task, also in consideration of the fact that CPGs contain heterogeneous forms of knowledge. As a consequence, the adoption of different methodologies (each one appropriate for a specific type of knowledge/verification) seems to be the best option. In particular, the GLARE system emerges in the literature for the attention devoted to different forms of verification, through the adoption of different Artificial Intelligence formal techniques. In particular, Chap. 19 considers three different forms of verification:

1. verification that the temporal constraints in a CIG are consistent, through constraint-based temporal reasoning techniques;

2. verification of different medical properties of a CIG (e.g., its capability of coping with a given type of patients, or to support specific types of treatments), through model checking;
3. verification of probabilistic properties of a CIG in the context of a probabilistic knowledge base, through probabilistic modelling.

18.4 Aggregation of Evidence Using Argumentation

Whilst guidelines are important vehicles for the systematic use of evidence in healthcare, and thereby support evidence-based decision making, they do have some shortcomings. Producing a guideline requires substantial resources and time to acquire and process the evidence in order to produce robust recommendations, and yet they can rapidly become out-of-date when new evidence is published. They are written for general populations and so do not consider specific circumstances of individual patients, and they often do not consider co-morbidities. Also they do not take into account the preferences of the individual patient or clinician with regard to possible options. Finally, it is important to note that aggregations of evidence such as in systematic reviews and guidelines can interpret and aggregate the evidence in a particular way, but often there are multiple ways that the evidence can interpreted and aggregated leading to alternative recommendations being derived from the evidence.

Recent research in knowledge representation and reasoning is offering a new method to derive recommendations from evidence. This addresses the above shortcomings by automatically generating recommendations from a database of evidence taking into account the quality of the evidence according to specified criteria as well as contextual information concerning the patient. This allows for different evidence quality criteria and different patient criteria to be considered so that their effect on the recommendations can be explored. Furthermore, the criteria considered for the recommendations can be published with the recommendations to make the process systematic, transparent, and reproducible. In Chap. 20, this knowledge representation methodology based on argumentation is presented as a tutorial.

References

1. de Clercq, P.A., et al.: Approaches for creating computer-interpretable guidelines that facilitate decision support. Artif. Intell. Med. **31**(1), 1–27 (2004)
2. Fox, J., Johns, N., Rahmanzadeh, A.: Disseminating medical knowledge: the PROforma approach. Artif. Intell. Med. **14**(1), 157–182 (1998)
3. Grando, M.A., Glasspool, D., Fox, J.: A formal approach to the analysis of clinical computer-interpretable guideline modeling languages. Artif. Intell. Med. **54**(1), 1–13 (2012)
4. Heller, B., et al. (eds.): Computer-Based Support for Clinical Guidelines and Protocols. Studies in health technology and informatics, vol. 83. IOS Press, Amsterdam (2001)
5. Isern, D., Moreno, A.: A computer based execution of clinical guidelines: a review. Int. J. Med. Inform. **77**(12), 787–808 (2008)

6. Johnso, P. D., et al.: Using scenarios in chronic disease management guidelines for primary care. In: Proceedings of the AMIA Symposium, pp. 389–393. American Medical Informatics Association (2000)
7. Kaiser, K., Miksch, S., Tu, S.W. (eds.): Computer-Based Support for Clinical Guidelines and Protocols. Studies in Health Technology and Informatics, vol. 101. IOS Press, Amsterdam (2004)
8. Kaiser, K., Miksch, S.: Versioning computer-interpretable guidelines: semi-automatic modeling of living guidelines using an information extraction method. Artif. Intell. Med. 46(1), 55–66 (2009)
9. Musen, M.A.: EON: a component-based approach to automation of protocol-directed therapy. J. Am. Med. Inform. Assoc. 3(6), 367–388 (1996)
10. Peleg, M., et al.: Comparing computer-interpretable guideline models: a casestudy approach. J. Am. Med. Inform. Assoc. 10(1), 52–68 (2003)
11. Peleg, M., Tu, S.W.: Design patterns for clinical guidelines. Artif. Intell. Med. 47(1), 1–24 (2009)
12. Peleg, M., et al.: GLIF3: the evolution of a guideline representation format. In: Proceedings of the AMIA Symposium, p. 645. American Medical Informatics Association (2000)
13. Quaglini, S., et al.: Guideline-based careflow systems. Artif. Intell. Med. 20(1), 5–22 (2000)
14. Serban, R., Ten Teije, A.: Exploiting thesauri knowledge in medical guideline formalization. Methods Inf. Med. 48(5), 468–474 (2009)
15. Shahar, Y., Miksch, S., Johnson, P.: The Asgaard project: a task-specific framework for the application and critiquing of time-oriented clinical guidelines. Artif. Intell. Med. 14(1–2), 29–51 (1998)
16. Shalom, E., et al.: A quantitative assessment of a methodology for collaborative specification and evaluation of clinical guidelines. J. Biomed. Inform. 41(6), 889–903 (2008)
17. Shiffman, R.N., et al.: Building better guidelines with BRIDGE-Wiz: development and evaluation of a software assistant to promote clarity, transparency, and implementability. J. Am. Med. Inform. Assoc. 19(1), 94–101 (2012)
18. Shiffman, R.N., et al.: GEM: a proposal for a more comprehensive guideline document model using XML. J. Am. Med. Inform. Assoc. 7(5), 488–498 (2000)
19. Shortliffe, E.: Computer-Based Medical Consultations: MYCIN. Elsevier, NewYork (1976)
20. Svatek, V., Ruzicka, M.: Step-by-step mark-up of medical guideline documents. Int. J. Med. Inform. 70(23), 329–335 (2003)
21. Ten Teije, A., Miksch, S., Lucas, P. (eds.): Computer-Based Medical Guidelines and Protocols: A Primer and Current Trends. Studies in Health Technology and Informatics, vol. 139. IOS Press, Amsterdam (2008)
22. Terenziani, P., Molino, G., Torchio, M.: A modular approach for representing and executing clinical guidelines. Artif. Intell. Med. 23(3), 249–276 (2001)
23. Tu, S.W.: The SAGE guideline model: achievements and overview. J. Am. Med. Inform. Assoc. 14(5), 589–598 (2007)
24. Wang, D.: Representation primitives, process models and patient data in computer-interpretable clinical practice guidelines: a literature review of guideline representation models. Int. J. Med. Inform. 68(13), 59–70 (2002)

Chapter 19
A Hybrid Approach to the Verification of Computer Interpretable Guidelines

Luca Anselma, Alessio Bottrighi, Laura Giordano, Arjen Hommersom, Gianpaolo Molino, Stefania Montani, Paolo Terenziani and Mauro Torchio

Abstract Computer Interpretable Guidelines (CIGs) are assuming a major role in the medical area, in order to enhance the quality of medical assistance by providing physicians with evidence-based recommendations. However, the complexity of CIGs (which may contain hundreds of related clinical activities) demands for a verification process, aimed at assuring that a CIG satisfies several different types of properties (e.g., verification of the CIG correctness with respect to several criteria). Verification is a demanding task, which may be enhanced through the adoption of advanced Artificial Intelligence techniques. In this paper, we propose a general and hybrid approach to address such a task, suggesting that, given the heterogeneous character of the knowledge in CIGs, different forms of verification should be supported, through the adoption of proper (and different) methodologies.

19.1 Introduction

Clinical Practice Guidelines (CPGs) can be defined as a means for specifying the "best" clinical procedures and for standardizing them. The adoption of CPGs, by supporting physicians in their decision making and diagnosing activities, may provide crucial advantages, both in individualized health care, and in the overall service offered by a health care organization. In particular, it has been shown [35] that CPGs can improve the quality of patient care, reduce variations in quality of care, and reduce costs. These observations justify the increasing number of CPGs which have been defined in the last decade, covering a large spectrum of diseases and medical procedures. Given the relevance of this phenomenon, in the last two decades a lot of efforts has been devoted in order to provided formal representations of guidelines, that can be treated by computer systems (usually called Computer Interpretable Guidelines CIGs for short). Many approaches have focused on the development of guideline representation formalisms, and/or systems to acquire, store and execute CIGs. However, the effort in defining and disseminating CIGs has not always been coupled by a parallel effort in guaranteeing their "quality" [45]: despite the fact that

© Springer International Publishing Switzerland 2015
A. Hommersom and P.J.F. Lucas (eds.), *Biomedical Knowledge Representation*, LNAI 9521, DOI 10.1007/978-3-319-28007-3_19

CPGs and/or CIGs are issued by recognized experts' committees, they might be ambiguous or incomplete [32], or even inconsistent. The need for guideline quality verification is thus clearly emerging. As we will show in this paper, computer-based approaches can provide crucial advantages in this context.

In particular, in this paper we suggest that, given the heterogeneous character of the knowledge contained in CIGs, different forms of verifications should be supported, demanding for an hybrid approach in which different representation formalisms are used (to properly capture different types of knowledge) and different methodologies are devised (to properly reason with the different formalisms). In particular, in this paper, we focus on three different forms of verification:

1. verification that the temporal constraints in a CIG are consistent, through constraint-based temporal reasoning techniques;
2. verification of different medical properties of a CIG (e.g., its capability of coping with a given type of patients, or to support specific types of treatments), through model checking;
3. verification of probabilistic properties of a CIG in the context of a probabilistic knowledge base, through probabilistic modelling.

19.2 Representing and Reasoning with Temporal Constraints

Representing and reasoning with temporal constraints is an essential feature for computer-based approaches to clinical guidelines. In particular, a temporal manager coping with time-related issues can be exploited in different ways in the management of clinical guidelines. For instance, during the acquisition of a new guideline, the consistency of the temporal constraints it contains can be automatically checked; during the execution of a guideline on a specific patient, the temporal manager can be used to check whether the specific actions have been executed in such a way that the constraints in the guideline have been respected, or to determine the times when the next actions need to be executed. However, although many domain-independent temporal managers have been devised within the Artificial Intelligence (AI) literature, and several approaches to time-related issues have been faced within the clinical guideline literature, several new challenges have to be addressed when dealing with temporal representation and temporal reasoning about clinical guidelines.

19.2.1 Desiderata for a CIG Temporal Reasoner

As in most AI approaches to the treatment of time, also in the context of CIGs we must take into account the fundamental trade-off between the expressiveness of temporal formalisms and the computational complexity of the correct and complete temporal reasoning algorithms operating on them.

While expressiveness is an obvious desideratum, we will now briefly motivate the second term of the above trade-off: correctness, completeness, and tractability. First, it is important to stress that a formalism for temporal constraints is not very useful if it is not paired with algorithms for temporal reasoning, performing temporal inferences on a set of constraints (expressed in the given formalism) and/or checking their consistency. Consider, for instance, a Knowledge Base KB containing the temporal constraints (i) and (ii) among three events A, B and C.

$$KB = \{(i)\ A\ before\ B; (ii)\ B\ before\ C\}$$

The constraint *(iii) A before C* can be inferred because it is logically implied by *(i)* and *(ii)*, so that, given KB, one can correctly assert *(iii)*, but not *(iv) A after C*, which is actually inconsistent with KB. In other words, the set of constraints $KB' = \{(i), (ii), (iv)\}$ cannot be satisfied. Temporal reasoning is necessary in order to support such an intended semantics. With no temporal reasoning, a CIG may contain the above set of temporal constraints, and thus be not executable (since there is no way of satisfying the constraints).

Of course, temporal reasoning algorithms are computationally expensive. An important desideratum is tractability, i.e., the fact that the running time of the algorithms grows as a fixed power of the number of the actions and/or constraints in the knowledge base (i.e., in polynomial time).

However, temporal reasoning algorithms should also be correct, i.e., such that they only infer constraints that are logically implied by the initial set of constraints (in fact, correctness grants that no wrong inference is made). Completeness (i.e., the fact that all logically implied constraints are actually inferred) is a fundamental desideratum as well, since it is essential in order to grant that the system's answers are fully reliable (e.g., if (iii) is not inferred from $\{(i), (ii)\}$, the answer to the question "Is (iv) consistent with $\{(i), (ii)\}$?" may be yes).

In particular, as in most AI approaches, the main task of our temporal reasoning algorithms is that of checking the consistency of temporal constraints in a guideline. In fact, real-world guidelines usually consist of hundreds of actions, often related by temporal constraints. This means that: (i) the fact that hundreds of constraints are mutually consistent cannot be taken for granted and (ii) consistency checking cannot be directly performed by physicians (and/or by a knowledge engineer), since making explicit all the possible implications of such a large number of constraints is an overwhelming and too complex task.

19.2.1.1   Dealing with Temporal Constraints in Clinical Guidelines: New Challenges and Open Problems

Despite the large amount of valuable works, there still seems to be a gap between the range of phenomena covered by current AI constraint-based approaches and the needs arising from clinical guidelines management. In essence, while many AI approaches to temporal constraints are focused on the treatment of a specific type of constraints only (e.g., qualitative temporal constraints), in the CIG context several different issues and types of constraints need to be taken into account:

(i) qualitative (e.g., 'at the same time') and quantitative (e.g., at least ten days after) constraints between actions;
(ii) repeated/periodic events (and constraints between them);
(iii) all the above types of constraints may be imprecise and/or partially defined;
(iv) temporal constraints involved by part-of relations between actions in the CIGs
(v) the distinction between (temporal constraints between) classes of actions (e.g., an action in a general guideline) and instances of such actions.

As regards issue (iv), notice that most CIG formalisms support multiple levels of abstraction, through the definition of composite actions, and the specification of their components. However, part-of decomposition involves temporal constraints, since each composite action temporally contains its components. Finally, issue (v) points out that actions in CIGs can be conceived as classes of actions, which admit multiple instantiations, whereas CIGs are applied to specific patients. This involves the treatment of some form of temporal constraint inheritance from classes to instances. As a real example of the temporal complexity of the CIG domain, consider Example 19.1 (which is a simplified part of a guideline about multiple myeloma).

Example 19.1. The therapy for multiple myeloma is made by six cycles of 5-day treatment, each one followed by a delay of 23 days (for a total time of 24 weeks). Within each cycle of 5 days, 2 inner cycles can be distinguished: the melphalan treatment, to be provided twice a day, for each of the 5 days, and the prednisone treatment, to be provided once a day, for each of the 5 days. These two treatments must be performed in parallel.

Temporal constraints such as the ones in Example 19.1 are challenging for the constraint-based formalisms developed within the AI literature.

Obviously, the interplay between issues (i)–(v) needs to be dealt with, too. For example, the interaction between composite and periodic events might be complex to represent and manage. In fact, in the case of a composite periodic event, the temporal pattern regards the components, which may, recursively, be composite and/or periodic events. For instance, consider Example 19.1. The instances of the melphalan treatment must respect the temporal pattern "twice a day, for 5 days", but such a pattern must be repeated for six cycles, each one followed by a delay of 23 days, since the melphalan treatment is part of the general therapy for multiple myeloma.

While some of the above issues have been treated in an ad-hoc way in the literature, in our approach we aim at devising a general module coping in an integrated way with all of them. The temporal knowledge server will act as an independent module and the temporal problems in different clinical guidelines will be delegated to such a server. The strategy we chose to adopt in order to achieve our goal is that of devising a two-layer approach:

1. the high-level layer provides a high-level language to represent the above-mentioned temporal phenomena and to offer several temporal reasoning facilities;

2. the low-level layer consists of an internal representation of the temporal constraints, on which temporal constraint propagation algorithms operate.

We designed our high-level language with specific attention to modelling repeated
actions, and in such a way that tractable temporal reasoning can be supported. At
the low-level layer, we chose to exploit as much as possible STP (Simple Temporal
Problem), a standard AI temporal reasoning framework [9]. In a certain sense, our
approach uses STP as an "assembly language" and builds an expressive "high-level
temporal reasoning framework" on top of it. Obviously, the gap between our high-
level language and STP is very large. Filling such a gap is the main contribution of
our approach, and has involved the design of suitable temporal reasoning algorithms
to cope with issues (i)-(v) above, as well as an extension of the STP framework itself
(to consider labelled trees of STPs).

19.2.2   High-Level Formalism for CIG Temporal Constraints

Our high-level language allows one to express temporal constraints of the different
types discussed above.

   Dates can be expressed by the predicate **date(A, L1, U1, L2, U2)**, stating that
the action A must start between dates L1 and U1 and end between dates L2 and U2.
Precise dates can be expressed imposing L1 = U1 or L2 = U2. Please note that also
unknown dates are allowed by imposing that the extremes assume value $-\infty$ or $+\infty$.
Other constructs include the predicate **duration(A, L, U)**, stating that the duration
of action A must be included between L and U, **delay(P1, P2, L, U)**, stating that the
delay between P1 and P2 must be between L and U, where P1 and P2 are time points
(i.e., starting or ending points of actions). Also qualitative temporal constraints such
as **"before"**, **"after"**, **"during"** are supported by our language: in fact all and only
the qualitative constraints that can be mapped to conjunctions of STP constraints are
supported.

   For representing composite actions we support the predicate **partOf(A', A)**, stating that the action A' is part of the composite action A. Please note that the partOf
relation induces a temporal constraint between the actions: i.e., action A' must be
during action A. The predicates described above can be also used for representing
temporal constraints between instances of actions.

   In order to describe the relation between instances and classes, we need to introduce a further predicate, **instanceOf(I, A, p)** to represent the fact that the instance
of action I is an instance of the class of actions A. If A is a repeated action, then p
represents the fact that I is an instance of the pth repetition of A (if A is not a repeated
action, $p = 0$).

   Regarding repetition of actions, we provide the predicate **repetition(A, RSpec)**,
to state that the (possibly composite) class of action A is repeated according to the
specification RSpec. $RSpec$ is a recursive structure of arbitrary depth of the form

$$RSpec = \langle R_1, \ldots, R_n \rangle,$$

where each level R_i states that the actions described in the next level (i.e., R_{i+1}, or by convention the action A, if $i = n$) must be repeated a certain number of times in a certain time span. To be more specific, any basic element R_i consists of a quadruple

$$R_i = \langle nRepetitions_i, I\text{-}Time_i, repConstraints_i, conditions_i \rangle,$$

where the first term represents the number of times that R_{i+1} must be repeated, the second one represents the time span in which the repetitions must be included, the third one may impose a pattern that the repetitions must follow, and the last one allows to express conditions that must hold so that the repetition can take place. Informally, we can roughly describe the semantics of a quadruple R_i as the natural language sentence repeat R_{i+1} $nRepetitions_i$ times in exactly $I\text{-}Time_i$, if $conditions_i$ hold.

A detailed treatment of such a specification is outside the goals of the current paper. Indeed, in [4] the expressiveness of the language for repetitions has been studied, on the basis of both the classification criteria provided by Egidi and Terenziani [11, 12] and by Bettini [6].

Additionally, in [4] the semantics of such specifications has been formally studied.

For example, the melphalan treatment in Example 19.1 can be represented as $Repetition(melphalan, \langle R_0 = \langle 5, 5d, , \rangle, R_1 = \langle 2, 1d, , \rangle \rangle)$, meaning that the treatment is composed by two levels: R_0 states that R_1 must be repeated five times in five days and R_1 states that melphalan must be administered twice a day.

19.2.3 Reasoning with Temporal Constraints in CIGs

Regarding the instances of actions, we designed the high-level language in such a way that all constraints can be mapped onto bounds on differences and, thus, internally represented as a "standard" STP framework [9].

However, regarding the classes of events, while dates, delays, durations and qualitative temporal constraints might be represented with an STP about classes, it is not possible to represent in such a basic way also the temporal constraints about repeated/periodic and/or composite actions. We thus introduce STP-trees, as a suitable low-level representation of temporal constraints, on which temporal reasoning algorithms can operate.

19.2.3.1 STP-Tree

In our approach, the overall set of constraints between actions in the CIG is represented by a tree of STPs (STP-tree henceforth). The root of the tree is the STP which represents the constraints between all the actions in the guideline, except the components of repeated actions.

The STP-tree corresponding to a guideline can be automatically constructed on the basis of the temporal constraints in the guideline (expressed using the high-level

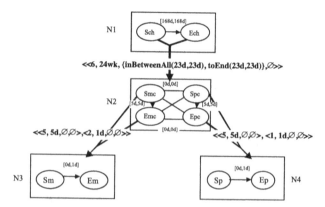

Fig. 19.1 STP-tree for the multiple mieloma chemotherapy guideline in Example 19.1. Thin lines and arcs between nodes in a STP represent bound on differences constraints. Arcs from a pair of nodes to a child STP represent repetitions. Arcs between any two nodes X and Y in a STP of the STP-tree are labeled by a pair [n,m] representing the minimum and maximum distance between X and Y. Sch, Ech, Smc, Emc, Spc, Epc, Sm, Em, Sp and Ep stand for the starting (S) and ending (E) points of chemotherapy, melphalan cycle, prednisone cycle, melphalan treatment and prednisone treatment, respectively.

language in Subsect. 19.2.2) by executing an algorithm which operates recursively, from the root to the leaves, by putting in each STP-node all the actions except the components of repeated actions, which are represented in separate STP-nodes. On the other hand, the partOf relations not involving repeated actions are represented in the same STP as the composite action by adding to such an STP-node the constraints that all the components are contained into the corresponding composite action.

To summarize, in the STP-tree there are as many STP-nodes as the number of repeated actions, and in each STP-node there are as many actions as the number of actions in the guideline that are parts of the repeated action that the STP-node represents. Specifically, each action is represented in the STP-node as a pair of time points, while constraints between (not repeated) actions are represented by arcs connecting them.

For instance, in Fig. 19.1, we show the STP-tree representing (at the low-level) the temporal constraints in Example 19.1.

Additionally, an independent STP must be used in order to represent the temporal constraints about the specific instances of the actions of the guidelines, as emerging from executions of the guidelines on specific patients.

19.2.3.2   Checking the Consistency of a Guideline

Given an STP-tree, it is possible to check its consistency in an intensional way, i.e., without generating every repetition of repeated actions. However, it is not sufficient to check the consistency of each STP contained in the STP-nodes separately. In such a case, in fact, we would neglect the repetition/periodicity information. Temporal consistency checking, thus, proceeds in a top-down fashion, starting from the root of the STP-tree towards its leaves. Basically, the root contains a "standard" STP, so that the Floyd-Warshall's algorithm can be applied to check its consistency. Thereafter, for each node X in the STP-tree (except the root), we proceed as shown in the algorithm STP_tree_consistency (see Algorithm 5).

Algorithm 5. Algorithm for checking the consistency of a guideline (represented as an STP-tree).

---

function $STP\_tree\_consistency(X : STPNode,$
$RSpec = (R_1 = \langle nRepetitions_1, I\text{-}Time_1, repConstraints_1, conditions_1 \rangle, \ldots,$
$R_n = \langle nRepetitions_n, I\text{-}Time_n, repConstraints_n, conditions_n \rangle)) : STP$

1: check that the repetition/periodicity constraint is well-formed (i.e., that repetitions nest properly)
2: compute Max, i.e. the maximum duration of a single repetition of X according to $RSpec$
3: impose in X that the maximum distance between each pair of points is less or equals Max
4: $X \leftarrow FloydWarshall(X)$
5: if X = INCONSISTENT return INCONSISTENT else return X

STP_tree_consistency takes in input the STP-node that must be checked (i.e. X) and the repetition/periodicity constraint (i.e., the repetition specification in the arc of the STP-tree entering node X), and gives as an output an inconsistency or, in the case of consistency, the local minimal network of the constraints in X considering also the repetition/periodicity constraints. In step 1 it checks whether the repetition/periodicity constraint is well-formed, i.e. if it is consistent when it is taken in isolation (e.g., $I\text{-}Time_2$ must be contained into $I\text{-}Time_1$). In step 2 it computes the maximum duration of a single repetition. This is obtained by considering the time that allows to perform a repetition assuming that all the other repetitions have the minimum possible duration. In step 3 it adds to the STP X the constraints stating that the maximum duration of X must be the computed maximum duration of a single repetition of X. Finally, in step 5 it checks the consistency of the augmented STP X via the Floyd-Warshall's algorithm.

Property. STP_tree_consistency is correct and complete (see [4]). Considering that the number of nesting levels, in the worst case, is less than the number of classes, the algorithm is dominated by step 4, that is $O(C^3)$, where C is the number of actions in the guideline.

19.2.3.3   Reasoning with the Executions of the Guideline

We have also devised an algorithm for checking the consistency of the execution of a guideline instance with respect to its related guideline. In our work, as in most approaches to clinical guidelines, we suppose that one has full observability of instances (i.e., all the instances of actions which have been executed have been observed and inserted into the knowledge base), and that, for each instance, one knows the corresponding class of actions and/or repetition in the guidelines. The procedure integratedConsistency accepts three parameters: T (the STP-tree that describes the constraints about classes of actions in the guideline), E (the STP that describes the temporal constraints between the instances of actions – i.e., the actions that have been executed on specific patients), and NOW, that corresponds to the time of the present. The basic idea is to:

(a) check that in the executionSTP there are all and only the instances that the STP-tree predicts to be. Possible missing instances are hypothesized because they may happen in the future;
(b) inherit the repetition/periodicity constraints and the temporal (non-periodic) constraints from the classes to the instances;
(c) propagate the temporal constraints on the executionSTP, thus obtaining the minimal network [9];
(d) check whether the hypothesized instances expected in the future may actually start in the future (i.e., after NOW).

Property. Let us denote with C the number of classes in the STP-tree, with I the number of instances. We have that the complexity of the procedure is $O(max\{I^3, C^3\})$. Also, integratedConsistency is correct and complete as regards consistency checking of the constraints among the instances and among the classes in the STP-tree [4].

19.3 Clinical Guideline Verification

The verification capabilities concerning the general properties of CIGs and their execution available in the conventional CIG management systems in the literature are usually rather limited. In many cases, such systems do associate only very specific and ad-hoc inferential mechanisms to the knowledge represented in the guideline. To overcome such limitations, the adoption of theorem proving techniques has been proposed within the Protocure European project starting in 2003 [30, 45]. As an alternative of the theorem-proving methodology, the adoption of model-checking techniques has been independently proposed a few years later in the Protocure project [5] and in our project GLARE [17, 18, 47], mainly motivated by the simplicity and efficiency of model-checking techniques with respect to the theorem proving approach [20].

Specifically, in our approach we propose a modular solution in which a CIG management system is loosely coupled with a model checker via a translator, which maps any guideline expressed in the formalism of the CIG management system into the formalism of the model-checker. In such a way, the advantages of adopting a CPG management system from one side, and a general-purpose model-checker on the other side are retained and combined. In particular, once the mapping has been defined, any class of properties that can be formalized in the logic of the model checker can be easily verified, without requiring the definition of a new verification software module from scratch. This obviously facilitates a real interaction between the physician examining the CIG and the system itself. Thanks to its modularity, such an approach can be easily implemented, since it does not require any modification to either the CIG management system or the model-checker.

Although our proposal is mostly application-independent, as a proof of concept, we have integrated within the system GLARE [46] a verification tool which models a CIG in Promela, the specification language of the model checker SPIN [21], and verifies the CIG properties to be checked by formalizing them as Linear time Temporal Logic (LTL) formulas.

19.3.1   Integrating GLARE with SPIN

We have applied the general methodology introduced above in order to couple GLARE with the model checker SPIN. We have implemented a translator which takes in input a GLARE CIG, expressed in the XML format, and transforms it into the corresponding CIG in the Promela language. Analogously, the patient data (in XML) are also translated into the Promela language.

Promela allows a high level model of a distributed system to be defined by modeling each process in an extended pseudo C code, including synchronization primitives and message exchange primitives. Promela provides the usual *if-then-else* and iteration constructs of imperative languages, but it also allows for goto statement (allowing jumps to labels), for the non-deterministic choice construct, as well as for the parallel execution of processes. Processes may share global variables and they also may exchange messages through asynchronous communication channels.

In the following, we briefly describe the general principles we adopt to convert a GLARE CIG into the corresponding agent-based program in the Promela language. First, we describe how a CIG is mapped to a set of interacting processes (called agents henceforth), i.e. to a set of Promela processes and to a set of proper synchronization primitives and message exchange primitives. Then, we shortly describe our translator module.

19.3.1.1   Guidelines as Agents

Obviously, the basic object we need to represent in Promela for the purpose of verification is the CIG itself. A CIG can be seen as a set of actions, to be executed in the order specified by a set of control flow primitives. We have mapped each construct (action or control flow primitive) in the CIG to a Promela statement or to a Promela piece of code.

However, CIG execution is a complex phenomenon that cannot be modeled just by representing the CIG per se.

In the following, we propose a possible, more realistic way of capturing the dynamics of the CIG and of its execution environment, based on the idea of modeling a set of processes, whose interaction models the CIG execution itself.

One of the required processes, which we will call agents, is of course the CIG itself. The other agents represent the (human or not) components interacting with the CIG at execution time.

In particular, the Database agent has to be represented. Actually, patient's characteristics need to be specified, and, rather naturally, we characterize a patient by relying on her data, which are typically maintained in the clinical database. The Database agent thus provides data on demand, and is able to store new data values.

Updated data values are sometimes obtained from additional sources (e.g. from the hospital laboratory service). We have generically modeled such sources and services by means of a further agent, called Outside world.

Last but not least, CIG execution is performed by a physician; therefore, the physician's behavior needs to be modeled as an agent as well. In particular, we have identified two main tasks that the Physician agent is expected to cover when applying a CIG to a specific patient. Obviously, it is required to make decisions, i.e. it has to select exactly one diagnosis or therapy, among a set of alternative ones. Moreover, it has to evaluate data recency and reliability: if a data value, extracted from the database, is judged as unreliable or not up-to-date (i.e. too old), the Physician agent has to rise the problem, thus triggering the generation of a newer data value from the outside world.

In summary, the model of the distributed system we propose to simulate CIG execution can be described by the interaction among the following agents, interpreted as Promela processes:

1. the Guideline agent, which models the overall behavior of the CIG;
2. the Database agent, which models the behavior of the patient database, allowing for data insertion and retrieval;
3. the Outside agent, which represents the outside world and provides up to date values for patient data (together with the time of their measurement) when they are not already available in the database or are evaluated as being not reliable by the physician. It also stores data in the database, and simulates the execution of actions by reporting their success or failure;
4. the Physician agent, which interacts with the CIG by evaluating the patient data, choosing among the different alternative feasible paths as a physician would do, and judging data reliability. Observe that we model the Physician agent as a non-deterministic process, since it is not possible to know a-priori all the possible choices of physicians in all the possible situations. We therefore model the uncertainty about the choice of physicians using non-determinism: from the point of view of the simulation, choices are taken randomly by the Physician agent.

19.3.1.2   The Translator

As explained above, we have defined a translator which takes a set of XML documents representing any GLARE CIG and automatically transforms them into the corresponding CIG in the language Promela.

A CIG in GLARE is a hierarchical graph, in which it is possible to have composite actions (i.e. plans), which can be defined in terms of their components via the has-part relation. In the XML document such a structure is maintained. Thus, the translator works as a top-down parser.

In particular, the translator takes in input a graph defined as a couple $\langle N, E \rangle$ (where N is the set of nodes and E is the set of edges), which is the XML document representing the CIG, and a vocabulary V, which contains the medical data information. To make the translation, the parser visits the graph twice. The first time it makes a preprocessing in order to obtain the data concerning the requests of information.

In the second step, the parser visits the graph for the second time, in order to build the agents which model the CIG behavior.

19.3.2 CIG Verification in SPIN

After the translation, SPIN can be used in order to "reason" about the guidelines. In particular, verification can be managed by expressing properties in LTL, and giving them in input to SPIN, together with the representation of a guideline obtained through the translation process. SPIN translates each Promela process into a finite automaton, and the global behaviour of the system is obtained by computing an asynchronous interleaving product of automata. The resulting automaton represents the global state space of the system (the model containing all the possible executions - runs - of the CIG) and can be built on-the-fly during the verification process. The correctness claims, that have to be checked on the model of the system, are then specified as temporal logic formulas in LTL. Given a property (specification) as an LTL formula, SPIN verifies if the property is true on all the executions of the system. Namely, each run of the system is regarded as a linear temporal model, on which the truth of the property is verified from the initial state.

As a matter of fact, temporal logics such as LTL allow one to express a wide range of formulas. Such an expressiveness and generality motivates a deeper analysis of what kinds of properties, expressible in LTL, are useful in the CIG context. We show some examples, dividing the properties on the basis of the CIG life-cycle phases. Specifically, we single out three main phases (namely, (1) design and acquisition, (2) contextualization, and (3) execution), and we highlight how verification can be fruitfully exploited in each phase.

For the sake of exposition, we describe the properties to be verified by distinguishing two components: (1) a quantifier on "runs": ∀, stating that we verify if the property holds on all the runs, and ∃, stating that we look for one run satisfying the property; (2) an LTL formula. In the following we assume that the variable "done" in each state is set to the action performed in that state.

19.3.2.1 Design and Acquisition

CIGs are usually defined by a national or international committee of specialists, and can be acquired into a computer-based system, usually through a cooperation between some specialists and some knowledge engineers. In such a phase, verification through model checking is useful in order to take into account at least two different classes of properties, namely structural properties and medical validity properties. In particular:

(i) **Structural properties** concern the existence of the appropriate clinical requirements. These properties regard the actions, conditions and paths of actions in the CIG considered "per se", without any reference to the specific context of execution and to the specific patients on which the CIG will be applied, and are relevant in order to ensure the appropriate management of any patients.

Example: verify that any run contains antibiotic treatment (community acquired pneumonia guideline)

$$< \forall run, \Diamond(done = antibiotic\_treatment) >$$

Comment: The property evaluates to true if all possible runs contain a state in which an antibiotic treatment is administered.
Relevance: The antibiotic treatment is mandatory in the case of community acquired pneumonia.

(ii) **Medical validity properties** concern both the exclusion of dangerous treatments and the inclusion of the most appropriate treatments for the considered class of patients. These properties are relevant in order to ensure best practice.

Example: verify that whenever hepatic encephalopathy is present, diuretics are not administered (ascites guideline)

$$< \forall run, liver\_state = encephalopathy \rightarrow \Box(done \neq diuretics\_administration) >$$

Comment: Diuretics are contraindicated in hepatic encephalopathy.
Relevance: Diuretics can worsen the liver perfusion and precipitate the encephalopathy or worsen its severity.

Both structural and medical validity properties are verified during the acquisition phase, in which both medical experts and knowledge engineers are usually involved. Specifically, medical experts can identify the structural and validity properties that are relevant for the CIG under consideration, and knowledge engineers can formulate and run the corresponding verifications, reporting the results to the experts. In case the checks show that a desired property does not hold, the domain experts should identify the appropriate corrections to the CIG, which will be modified accordingly, in cooperation with the knowledge engineers.

19.3.2.2 Contextualization

Once a CIG has been defined and acquired (e.g., by a national or international committee), it has to be applied to several different local structures (e.g., hospitals). Unfortunately, in several cases, the original CIG is too "general" to be applied on any specific environment. For instance, depending on the local availability of resources, certain actions of a general CIG cannot be executed in specific contexts (e.g., small hospitals). A phase of contextualization is thus usually needed: when a new CIG is introduced in a hospital, the medical personnel can use verification (possibly in cooperation with knowledge engineers) in order to identify which resources the CIG (or specific paths of the CIG itself) requires. Specifically:

(iii) **Contextualization properties** concern the resources needed for the CIG execution and can be checked to adapt the CIG to locally available resources.

Example: verify that there is a run in which the CT scanner is not used (ischemic stroke guideline)

$$< \exists run, \Box done \neq TC >$$

Comment: If this condition holds, the GL (or, at least a part of it) can be applied also in hospitals where the case the CT scanner is not available.

Relevance: The CT scanner is very important in some cases, but not always accessible.

The results of such verifications can be used for modifying the original CIG, or for improving the hospital resources, in order to conform the hospital to the CIG requirements (to grant the best practice). In the last case, the intervention of administrator personnel is also necessary.

19.3.2.3   Execution

Finally, the acquired and contextualised CIGs are used in clinical practice. In such a case, a specific user-physician selects and applies a specific CIG to a specific patient. Verification is a crucial support also in such a phase:

(iv) **Properties concerning the application of a CIG to a specific patient** allow to check which are the best actions (as indicated in the CIG) to be executed on the patient at hand, on the basis of the patient's status and symptoms; they also allow to check whether the CIG (or some specific path of it) contains the specific actions which the user-physician expects to be necessary for the patient at hand.

Example: verify that there is a treatment in which growth factors are administered, when leukopenia appears (lymphoma treatment guideline)

$$< \exists run, \Box (leukopenia\_value = present \rightarrow$$
$$\Diamond (done = growth\_factors\_administration)) >$$

Comment: The growth factors administration can positively reduce the duration of the leukopenia and the risk of infections.

Relevance: If leukopenia is not severe, there are also alternative treatments to the administration of growth factors (e.g., expectant treatment and monitoring). That is why we check the existence of one run in which (in a given status) growth factors are administered, without forcing that they are administered in all runs (in contrast with the verification above).

19.4 Probabilistic Verification

While many of the logical verification methods that have been proposed can be used to verify existing guidelines, a possible shortcoming of the logical methods is that they cannot deal with uncertainty stemming from the use of scientific evidence. On the other hand, many probabilistic methods do not have the representational benefits of logic for modelling temporal constraints between tasks.

In the last few years, there has been a surge of interest in the field of statistical relational learning [16]. In this endeavour, many probabilistic logics have been developed. We believe that these kind advances provide the right ingredients to represent and reason with such heterogeneous medical knowledge.

We think this type of probabilistic verification could particularly be important during the development of a CIG. In this section, we will first introduce a language that can be used to represent guidelines and a probabilistic knowledge base. After this, we show that such a language may be used to represent a guideline. Finally, we illustrate the approach by means of an example in the development of a hypothetical guideline for diabetes mellitus type 2.

19.4.1 Causal Probabilistic Decision Logic

We use CP-logic as a starting point, which we will briefly introduce. CP-logic theories consist of a multi-set of causal probabilistic laws (CP-laws), which are statements of the form:

$$\forall x : (h_1 : \alpha_1) \vee \cdots \vee (h_n : \alpha_n) \leftarrow b_1, \ldots, b_m \qquad (19.1)$$

where the $\alpha_1 : [0, 1]$ are probabilities with $\sum \alpha_i \leq 1$, $n \geq 1$, and $m \geq 0$. In this formula, h_i and b_j are atoms, that is, expressions of the form $p(t_1, \ldots, t_m)$ in which p/m is the name of a predicate of arity m and t_i are terms, i.e., constants or variables. We call the set of all $(h_i : \alpha_i)$ the head of the law, and the conjunction of literals b_i the body of the law. We also refer to all h_i as consequences, and to b_i as conditions. If the head contains only one atom $h : 1$, we may write it as h. Informally, the law states that in case the body is true, then at most one of the consequents becomes true, i.e., a consequent is caused by the body. The probabilities in the consequents reflect the probability that the body causes the consequent to become true.

The semantics of CP-logic relies on the notion of a Herbrand interpretation. This is essentially a set of ground atoms that can be constructed using the constant and predicate symbols occurring in the theory. We shall denote Herbrand interpretations by M and we shall write $M \models \varphi$ if the logical formula φ satisfies the interpretation M. Moreover, for simplicity of presentation, we assume a finite set of constants and also that all laws are grounded, i.e., each law is replaced by the set of laws where the variables are replaced by constants. For more details on notions of first-order logic and logic programming, we refer to [28].

CP-logic was designed as a probabilistic logic for modelling causal processes. Actions, too, can be incorporated into these processes, in which case CP-logic requires that the actions that agents take when the body holds is modelled using probabilities. In some cases, one wants to abstract from such actions, for example, to abstract from scheduling decisions when reasoning about concurrent systems. In other situations, there is no probabilistic information about the behaviour of agents, e.g., the course of action of physicians. To be able to model this, we introduce non-determinism into the CP-logic models by adding causal decision laws (CD-laws) to CP-logic. The resulting language is called Causal Probabilistic Decision Logic (CPDL).

Causal decision laws (CD-laws) are of the form:

$$\forall x : h_1 \vee \cdots \vee h_n \leftarrow b_1, \ldots, b_m \tag{19.2}$$

with $n \geq 1$ and $m \geq 0$, which can be seen as CP-laws without any probabilities attached to the elements in the head of the clause. The intuitive reading is also similar to CP-laws, i.e., $b_1, \ldots, b_m$ causes one of the heads, but in this case non-deterministically. That is, again exactly one of the heads is caused by the body, but we do not know which one and also do not know the probabilities.

To obtain a probability distribution for CPDL, the nondeterminism has to be resolved. For this we introduce a policy, which is a function π which maps each ground CD-law to one of its heads. For this function it holds that if $\pi(R) = h_i$, then R is a CD-law of the form:

$$h_1 \vee \cdots \vee h_n \leftarrow b_1, \ldots, b_m.$$

and $1 \leq i \leq n$. The intended semantics is that if $(b_1, \ldots, b_n)$ holds, and $\pi(R) = h_i$, then h_i becomes true. Therefore different groundings will produce different choices (as in CP-logic).

In [50], the semantics of this CP-logic is presented by relating the set of laws to a possible probabilistic causal process. We briefly introduce the semantics of CPDL in the spirit of CP-logic. Consider a CPDL theory T, a policy π, a Herbrand interpretation M, and a grounded law R_k where $R_k = head \leftarrow body$. If R_k is a CP-law and $M \models body$, then the law can be applied for $h_i : \alpha_i \in head$, which we denote by $M \longrightarrow_{\alpha_i} M \cup \{h_i\}$. A CD-law can be applied if also $\pi(R_k) = h_i$ holds, which is denoted by $M \longrightarrow M \cup \{h_i\}$. We then write $M \longrightarrow_p^* M'$ if there exists a chain of applications of laws from M to M' such that each ground law has been applied at most once, no other laws can be applied, and $p = \prod_i \alpha_i$ where α_i are all the probabilities of the applied CP-laws. CPDL defines a joint probability distribution over Herbrand interpretations given a interpretation M by $P_\pi(M') = \sum_{M \longrightarrow_p^* M'} p$. Note that a uniform probability distribution over heads in a CP-law is quite different from a CD-law. If a theory consists of CP-laws, then this models a unique probability distribution. For theories that contain CD-laws, each policy defines a possibly different probability distribution over the Herbrand interpretations.

As a first-order language, CPDL is of course sufficiently rich to model discrete-time models. For representation, we propose a small syntactical extension to the language, which we call CPDTL (Causal Probabilistic Decision Time Logic). We introduce a predicate $\overrightarrow{\cdot}$ which denotes a transition, i.e., $\overrightarrow{a(v)}$ denotes that $a(v)$ holds after a transition. A CPDTL theory contains a set of CPDL laws which may contain $\overrightarrow{\cdot}$, and also a set of *initial laws* of the following form:

$$(a_i(v_{i1})) : \alpha_{i1} \vee \cdots \vee (a_i(v_{in})) : \alpha_{in} \leftarrow \mathbf{M}$$

where $\mathbf{M}$ is called the *starting state*. A CPDTL theory can be mapped to CPDL by replacing all predicates a/m by $a/m + 1$ and indexing the predicates by time. Predicates in the initial law get indexed by time 0, i.e., $a_i(v_i)$ becomes $a_i(v_i, 0)$; the atoms $\overrightarrow{a(v)}$ are replaced by $a(v, t + 1)$; all other atoms $a(v)$ are replaced by $a(v, t)$. Consider the following example to illustrate this language.

Example 19.2. Each year, you can decide whether or not to get a flu shot, which affects the chance of becoming infected with influenza (with probability 0.01 when vaccinated, 0.1 when not vaccinated). Influenza might cause other disorders, such as angina (with probability 0.2) and pneumonia (with probability 0.1). Angina causes pneumonia (with probability 0.1), and vice versa (with probability 0.8). Pneumonia might be lethal (with probability 0.01), although there is also a chance of dying of other causes (with probability 0.001). This medical knowledge of influenza can be represented in CPDTL as follows.

> state(alive) ← **M**
> vaccine(true) ∨ vaccine(false) ← state(alive)
> disorder(influenza) : 0.1 ← vaccine(false)
> disorder(influenza) : 0.01 ← vaccine(true)
> disorder(angina) : 0.2 ∨ disorder(pneumonia) : 0.1
>   ← disorder(influenza)
> disorder(pneumonia) : 0.1 ← disorder(angina)
> disorder(angina) : 0.8 ← disorder(pneumonia)
>
> $\overrightarrow{\text{state(dead)}}$: 0.01 ∨ $\overrightarrow{\text{state(alive)}}$: 0.99
>   ← disorder(pneumonia)
> $\overrightarrow{\text{state(dead)}}$: 0.001 ∨ $\overrightarrow{\text{state(alive)}}$: 0.999
>   ← state(alive)

Note that the choice for vaccination has been represented by a CD-law, whereas the rest of the knowledge is represented by a set of CP-laws.

While it is already obvious in this specification that vaccination increases chances of survival, medical researchers are often more interested in relative measures such as the relative risks and the number needed to treat (NNT), i.e., the number of patients who need to be treated to prevent one additional bad outcome. For example, if vaccination decreases the chance on flu from 0.1 to 0.01, then the NNT is $1/(p_{max} - p_{min}) = 1/(0.1 - 0.01) \approx 11$, which means that if 11 people are vaccinated, 10 people are not expected to benefit. The NNT for preventing death, however, is not so clear given the interactions between variables. If, however, we would have the minimal and maximal probability of death, then such measure can be easily computed (similar for other relevant measures). If there is one binary decision variable, then this can be solved by computing the outcome of both decisions, but more generally this approach is not feasible.

19.4.2 Application to Guideline Verification

The idea of probabilistic verification is now as follows. CPDTL is expressive enough to formalize a non-deterministic automaton using CD-laws. Hence, in principle, a SPIN model derived from a GLARE CIG as described in Sect. 4.2 can be represented in CPDTL. Furthermore, probabilistic information may be combined with this model. The resulting model can be mapped to a probabilistic automaton that can be used to reason with.

19.4.2.1 Probabilistic Automata

Probabilistic automata model discrete-time stochastic systems consisting of a (finite) set of states S, an initial state $s_0 \in S$, a (finite) set of actions A and transition probabilities $\mathbf{P}: A \times S \times S \to [0, 1]$ such that for all a and s, $\mathbf{P}(a, s, s')$ is a probability distribution over s'. Furthermore, we assume a labelling function $L: S \to 2^{AP}$ that labels each state with a set of atomic propositions that are true in that state.

A policy $\hat{\pi}: S \to A$ is used to decide which action is taken in a state. Given this, a PA can be interpreted as a joint probability distribution over states and actions indexed by time. It is clear that $P(S_0 = s_0) = 1$. Furthermore, the transition probabilities define the conditional probability $P(S_{t+1} = s' \mid S_t = s, A_t = a) = \mathbf{P}(a, s, s')$. Finally, we can interpret policies as a deterministic probability distribution $P(A_t = a \mid S_t = s) = 1$ if $\hat{\pi}(s) = a$.

Given the assumptions above in addition to a Markov assumption, the joint probability of a path, given a policy $\hat{\pi}$, is the product of all transitions that occur in the path, i.e., $P(\mathbf{M}, s_0, \ldots, s_n) = \prod_{t=1}^{n} \mathbf{P}(\hat{\pi}(s_{t-1}), s_{t-1}, s_t)$. In the formal methods community, standard solvers exist to compute lower and upper bounds on probabilities. For this paper, we use the most well-known probabilistic model checker PRISM [27].

19.4.2.2 Translation

To model a CPDTL theory as a PA, we require that we have a set of attributes *Attr*, with a known domain $dom(a)$ for $a \in Attr$, corresponding to a set of predicates in the theory for modelling a state. It should hold that these attributes in the theory are both mutually exclusive and complete. States can be defined as the set of attributes with particular values. As in many other probabilistic logics, this property is not being checked by the system, but should be ensured by the modeller. However, if this holds, then consider a CPDTL theory T with dynamic attributes *Attr* for which we define a PA $M = \langle S, s_0, A, L, P \rangle$ such that:

- $s \in S$ iff $s = \mathbf{M}$ or for all $a \in Attr$ there exists a unique $v \in dom(a)$ such that $a(v) \in s$
- $A = \{\pi \mid \pi$ a CPDL policy for $T\}$
- $s_0 = \mathbf{M}$
- $L(s) = s$
- For all states $s_i, s_k \in S$ and policies $\pi \in A$:

$$\mathbf{P}(\pi, s_i, s_k) = \begin{cases} P_\pi(\overrightarrow{s_k} \mid s_i) & \text{if } s_i \neq s_k \\ 1 - \sum_{j \neq i} P_\pi(\overrightarrow{s_j} \mid s_i) & \text{if } s_i = s_k \end{cases}$$

Note that in this definition, the probability of not transitioning to a new state means that you will end up in the same state, which can be seen as a frame axiom. This is a small semantic difference with the original semantics. However, when the transitions are fully specified, i.e., for all π and s_i holds $\sum_k P_\pi(\overrightarrow{s_k} \mid s_i) = 1$, such as in Example 19.2, then the models will be equivalent in the following sense.

Proposition 19.1 (Fundamental Connection PA and CPDTL). *Given a CPDTL theory with state variable s made from the dynamic attributes such that the transitions are fully specified. Let P_{CPDTL} be the corresponding probability distribution and P_{PA} the probability distribution of the corresponding PA. Then*

$$P_{PA}(M, S_0 = s_0, \dots, S_t = s) = P_{CPDTL}(s(t))$$

Note that for representation, it can be quite useful to have the frame axiom.

Example 19.3. The knowledge base presented in Example 19.2 can be graphically represented as a probabilistic automaton as follows:

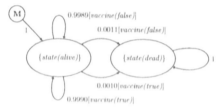

The state of the PA is defined by the predicate '*state*' and knowledge that models transitions have been abstracted into a single number for each possible policy choice.

19.4.3 Case Study

Using the machinery that has been introduced so far, we investigate a problem of deciding an appropriate treatment for diabetes mellitus type 2. This model is significantly more complex than the influenza example as diabetes is a complicated disease: various metabolic control mechanisms are deranged and many different organ systems may be affected by the disorder. For the individual patient, there is a lot of uncertainty to which extent physiological phenomena occur, which has an impact on the effectiveness of a treatment. We will focus here on a well-known drug called metformin, which is commonly prescribed as the primary oral anti-diabetic, of which the efficacy is known [15]. Moreover, we consider a genetic variation in the encoding of a protein called organic cation transporter 1 (OCT1) which affects the response to metformin [44]. Such knowledge was used to build a set of logical sentences that can be used to explore a simple model of a guideline that recommends treating diabetes with metformin. We answer a number of relevant questions that may come up during the design of such a diabetes guideline. In total, the knowledge base consists of about 50 rules and 10 facts, of which most rules are CD-laws (describing the guideline) and about 10 rules describing background knowledge based on medical literature. For example, it is stated as two CP-laws that there is a 20% chance of carrying the genetic OCT1 variation:

$$\frac{oct\_variant(true) : 0.2 \vee oct\_variant(false) : 0.8 \leftarrow \mathbf{M}}{oct\_variant(\overrightarrow{X}) \leftarrow oct\_variant(X)}$$

From a practical modelling point of view, variables are not restricted to a finite domain using this logic. For example, in this application, it is convenient to count the number of days that metformin has been given to a patient. This is easily modelled using a counting variables *applied* defined by:

$$\overrightarrow{applied(T+1)} \leftarrow state(activated), applied(T)$$

which says that, whenever metformin is given to the patient (*state(activated)*), then the counter *applied* is incremented. While this results in an infinite number of states, queries are always related to a time-point. Hence, we can dynamically restrict the domain of T to an appropriate upperbound.

Given such a model, we show a number of queries that explores relevant questions for the practical treatment of diabetes mellitus type 2 patients with metformin.

Question 1: How long should metformin be applied before it can be decided to stop the treatment?

There is a trade-off for deciding to stop a treatment: if the treatment with oral anti-diabetics is stopped too early then patients may be injecting themselves with insulin for no good reason; if the treatment is stopped too late, then patients who need treatment with insulin are not treated appropriately. In Fig. 19.2, we plot minimal

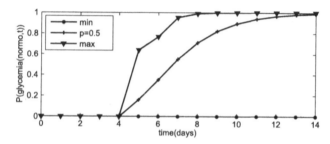

Fig. 19.2 Probabilistic simulation of metformin application with minimal (min) and maximal (max) probabilities. Furthermore, we consider a model where the physician acts with a probability $p = 0.5$.

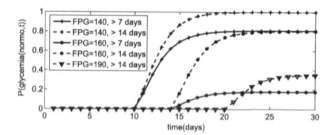

Fig. 19.3 Probabilistic simulation of metformin application to patients with different fasting blood glucose (FPG) at baseline. Time of metformin application is varied as well.

and maximal probabilities over time. In this case, minimal probabilities are zero, because the guideline did not force the physician to start treatment within a certain time bound, which can be considered a shortcoming of the guideline. We therefore consider another choice where physicians start treatment every day with a certain probability, which in this case is set to a probability 0.5. Furthermore, in Fig. 19.3, we plot a number of dose-response curves for different patients (also with a physician that acts with probability 0.5). For people with an initial low fasting plasma glucose (FPG), the effect of treatment is relatively quick, whereas people with an initial high fasting plasma glucose, the effect is much slower and might not be effective at all even after prolonged treatment. Hence, a recommendation of metformin should take the differences with respect to the baseline fasting plasma glucose into account.

Question 2: What improvement could we gain using genetic information?

As the OCT1 protein affects the efficacy of metformin, it might be useful to test whether a patient has a variation in this gene before treatment. In Fig. 19.4, patients are plotted with the same FPG at baseline, but given different evidence with respect to having a variation in the OCT1 protein. On average, patients in this population have a good chance that metformin is effective. However, for the patients with the OCT1-variant, the chance that metformin is effective is rather small and it might be better

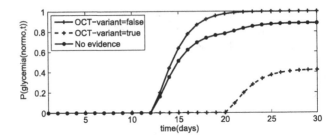

Fig. 19.4 Probabilistic simulation of metformin application to patients with or without a variation in the OCT1 protein.

to prescribe an alternative drug, whereas for patients with a normal OCT1 protein, metformin seems like a good choice. This illustrates that such pharmacogenetics could thus be used for the personalisation of treatments if tests for variations in the OCT1 protein become available.

19.5   Related Works

19.5.1   Reasoning About Temporal Constraints

Many AI approaches focused their attention to the definition of suitable formalisms to represent time-related phenomena and to reason with them. Besides "logical" approaches (e.g., temporal or non-monotonic logics), starting from the early 80's, many constraint-based approaches have been developed in AI [22]. Such approaches are mostly concerned to define domain-independent knowledge servers which temporal reasoning, in the form of propagation of temporal constraints, can be delegated to, and which can be coupled with other modules (e.g., a planner, or a system which manages guidelines) to solve complex problems.

The aim towards specialization led these approaches to focus on specific classes of constraints (e.g., qualitative constraints such as "A before B", quantitative constraints such as dates, delays and durations) [22], or to devote great attention to granularities and/or periodic/repeated constraints [23–25]) or to the integration of different sorts of constraints (e.g., qualitative and quantitative constraints [26]).

In the area of clinical guidelines several interesting approaches have been devised to represent temporal constraints. For instance, GLIF [37] deals both with temporal constraints on patient data elements and with duration constraints on actions and decisions. In PRO*forma* [14], guidelines are modelled as plans, and each plan may define constraints on the accomplishment of tasks, as well as task duration and delays between tasks. Moreover, temporal constructs can also be used in order to specify the preconditions of actions. DILEMMA and PRESTIGE [32] model temporal constraints within conditions. EON [33] uses temporal expressions to allow the scheduling of guideline steps, and deals with duration constraints about activities. Moreover, by incorporating the RESUME system, it provides a powerful approach to cope with temporal abstraction. In EON, the Arden Syntax allows the representation of delays between the triggering event and the activation of a Medical Logic Module (MDL), and between MDLs [43].

A rich ontology to deal with temporal information in clinical trial protocols has been proposed in [53], considering also relative and indeterminate temporal information and cyclical event patterns.

Despite the large amount of work devoted to the representation of temporal constraints, and the very rich and expressive formalisms being identified, little attention has been paid to temporal reasoning. Notable exceptions are represented by the approaches by Shahar [42] and by Duftschmid et al. [10].

In Shahar's approach, the goal of temporal reasoning is not to deal with temporal constraints (e.g., to check their consistency), but to find out proper temporal abstractions to data and properties. Therefore, temporal reasoning is not based on constraint propagation techniques, in fact, e.g., interpolation-based techniques and knowledge-based reasoning are used.

Miksch et al. have proposed a comprehensive approach based on the notion of temporal constraint propagation [10, 42]. In particular, in Miksch et al.'s approach, different types of temporal constraints deriving from the scheduling constraints in the guideline, from the hierarchical decomposition of actions into their components and from the control-flow of actions in the guideline are mapped onto an STP framework [9]. Temporal constraint propagation is used in order to (1) detect inconsistencies, and to (2) provide the minimal constraints between actions. In [10], there is also the claim that (3) such a method can be used by the guideline interpreter in order to assemble feasible time intervals for the execution of each guideline activity. Moreover, advanced visualization techniques are used in order to show users the results of temporal reasoning [26].

19.5.2 Verification

Our work about model-checking verification has started in the context of the Italian (two-years) project MIUR-PRIN 2003 "Logic-based development and verification of multi-agent systems" whose main objective was the development of logical and computational formalisms for the specification and verification of agents and their interactions. Our approach to LTL verification of clinical guidelines in SPIN has been described in detail in [7].

Automatic verification of clinical guidelines has first been explored in [30], where a theorem proving approach is proposed to deal with the problem of protocol verification. This activity has been developed within the European projects Protocure and Protocure II. Here, a medical protocol is modelled in the Asbru language as a hierarchical plan and then it is mapped to a specification in KIV, an interactive theorem prover for higher order logic. Properties are expressed in a variant of Interval

Temporal Logic. [45] has provided an evaluation of the feasibility of this approach based on the formalization and verification of the "jaundice" protocol and the "diabetes mellitus" protocol.

In the Protocure II project, model checking techniques for the verification of clinical guidelines have also been explored [5]. In contrast to interactive verification, model checking is fully automatic. In particular, Protocure II exploits CTL model checking and the tool SMV [31]. The Asbru model is translated into the input language of SMV model checker by making use of a suitable abstraction which eliminates time. The compiler takes the algebraic specification of Asbru models in KIV as input and generates an SMV document. CTL model checking is used in the verification of a wide range of properties of guidelines modelled in Asbru, namely structural and medical properties. In particular, in [5] properties of the jaundice protocol are formalized as ACTL formulas (that is, CTL formulas only allowing universal path quantifiers) [8].

The main difference between our approach and Protocure's one is that our approach is based on LTL temporal logic while Protocure's one is based on CTL temporal logic. The adoption of CTL (and ACTL) or LTL model checking allows for the verification of different temporal properties, as CTL and LTL are expressively incomparable (as well as ACTL and LTL). A further difference between our approach and Protocure one is due to the availability in SPIN of a higher-level input language, as compared with the input language of SMV. The fact that Promela is well suited for modelling guidelines as processes interacting with their environment by exchanging messages over channels, substantially simplifies the task of providing a translation of guidelines into Promela code (which does not require intermediate levels of representation), as well as that of interpreting the results of Concerning the type of the properties to be verified, as observed in [5] the model checking approach is well suited for the verification of structural and simple medical properties of the guideline, that normally do not require an incremental verification strategy.

19.5.3 Probabilistic Verification

Since the last two decades, probabilistic graphical models, PGMs for short, have become the state of the art for knowledge representation involving uncertainty. PGMs, and in particular Bayesian and Markov networks, have been successfully applied to various problem areas, including medicine. There is a considerable body of work (e.g. [3, 29, 36, 49, 54]) indicating that Bayesian networks offer a natural and intuitive formalism for constructing clinically relevant models. Unfortunately, PGMs are unsuitable for capturing knowledge that goes beyond statistical dependence and independence information, like clinical guidelines. In contrast, it has been shown that CP-logic that the probabilistic verification introduced in this chapter is based upon, can also represent various PGMs [22, 50].

With the recent introduction of probabilistic logics more powerful, relational languages for the representation of uncertain knowledge have become available, which are more suitable for dealing with combinations of logical and probabilistic knowledge. For example, there now exist logical versions of Markov networks, called *Markov logic networks* [40], and of Bayesian networks, called *Bayesian logic programs* [24]. Influential is also Poole's independent choice logic [38, 39], in addition to ProbLog [25] and CP-Logic [50]. These probabilistic logics offer a very natural and flexible choice for modelling complex domains involving uncertainty. On the other, all these languages are general probabilistic logics and do not deal with the particular requirements for representing CIGs, in particular temporal information. A notable exception is CPT-L [48], where CP-logic is used for modelling Markov models. The difference to our approach in the fact that in CPT-L each rule determines a transition. In the logic proposed in this chapter, each derivation determines a transition, which allows for richer modelling of the transitions.

The CPDTL logic proposed here can also been as a hierarchical models, with on the top-level a Markov model and in each state transition a CP-logic program. In this sense, logical hierarchical HMM (LoHiHMM) [34] can be seen as a related approach. The difference with this approach is two-fold. In the probabilistic sense, the LoHiHMM is more expressive, as it is a hidden Markov model rather than a Markov chain. On the other hand, the logical representation is weaker. LoHiHMMs are called logical, because each state is abstracted using predicate logic, rather than a propositional state. However, logic is not used to model the transitions, which makes it unsuitable to model the dynamic behaviour using a symbolic language.

19.6 Conclusions

CIGs are assuming an important role in the standardization and optimization of healthcare. In particular, CIG systems can be used by physicians as recommendation tools, to provide high-quality medical treatments to patients, on the basis of evidence-based medicine.

However, given the dimensions of CIGs (which may consist of hundreds of inter-related actions), and the large amount of knowledge they contain, verification is important to guarantee the quality of the provided recommendations. As described in this chapter, verification is important at different stages in the CIG life-cycle: during design and acquisition, to check structural and medical validity properties, during contextualization, to support the adoption of general CIGs in specific application contexts, and during execution, to look for the most appropriate treatments of specific patients, possibly considering probabilistic information on treatments outcomes and patient evolutions.

In this chapter, we investigate such issues, proposing a range of methodologies covering the different aspects of verification. The core idea of this chapter is that, given the heterogeneous character of the knowledge contained in CIGs, different forms of verifications should be supported, demanding for an hybrid approach in which different representation formalisms are used (to properly capture different types of knowledge) and different methodologies are devised (to properly reason with the different formalisms). In particular, we focused on three different issues, and methodologies.

Considering the temporal constraints in CIGs, we propose to adopt the 'classical' AI approach to devise a specialized constraint-propagation-based temporal reasoner [2, 51]. Such approaches focus on temporal constraints only, so that specific representation formalisms can be devised, in such a way that correct and complete temporal reasoning can be performed efficiently (in cubic time, in our approach). While such approaches are advantageous when considering temporal constraints only, they are not general enough to deal with more general forms of knowledge, and of verification.

We then considered the verification of various medical properties of CIGs, with an emphasis on the temporal evolution of CIGs actions. In that case, we considered two kinds of properties: logical properties, which can be used to investigate whether the guideline adheres to *hard outcomes*, e.g., whether an action will be done or not, and probabilistic properties, which considers *soft outcomes*, for example, the effect of particular actions on the survival rate. During design time, probabilistic verification could be used to analyse the available evidence, and to potentially derive appropriate treatment. Given this knowledge, whether derived by probabilistic methods or traditional analysis techniques in evidence-based medicine, logical verification can be used to check whether or not the CIG adheres to such a medical validity properties. At this stage, it is sensible to verify hard outcomes only, as clinical guidelines should codify the most appropriate for a given disease [13].

A more direct application of probabilistic verification is in the execution of a CIG when treating a particular patient. Again, in some cases, we may have hard constraints, as illustrated in the example in Sect. 19.3.2. However, deviation of a guideline does not imply by itself malpractice. For example, the guideline may prescribe penicillin as the drug of choice for certain infections, but may allow other antibiotics for patients who are allergic to penicillin. Another example are patients with comorbidities, which is very common in the elderly (e.g. [1] for the Dutch population), to which standard treatments in the guideline very often do not apply [19, 23]. Yet another example is the growing trend to involve the patient in the decision making process [41, 52], where preferences about treatment alternatives could be taken into account to select the most appropriate treatment for that particular patient. In such cases, a probabilistic approach may be appropriate.

In summary, we have proposed a mixture of verifying both logical and probabilistic outcomes. To enable logical verification, we have proposed the adoption of constraint-propagation based verification and model-based verification techniques based on temporal logics (LTL), which proved to be well-suited for many medical verification tasks. Similarly, to enable probabilistic verification, we have proposed to adopt a probabilistic logic, which can be mapped to probabilistic automata. Using probabilistic model checking, properties can be checked using probabilistic temporal logics (see e.g. [27]). While logical approaches already had significant success for the verification of CIGs, further experimentation with probabilistic verification is necessary. It is expected that this approach is especially when considering the application of CIGs to specific patients, to identify those treatment which, probabilistically speaking, are the best option for them.

References

1. van den Akker, M., et al.: Multimorbidity in general practice: prevalence, incidence, and determinants of co-occurring chronic and recurrent diseases. J. Clin. Epidemiol. **51**(5), 367–375 (1998)
2. Allen, J.F.: Maintaining knowledge about temporal intervals. Commun. ACM **26**(11), 832–843 (1983)
3. Andreassen, S., et al.: Using probabilistic and decision-theoretic methods in treatment and prognosis modeling. Artif. Intell. Med. **15**(2), 121–134 (1999)
4. Anselma, L., et al.: Towards a comprehensive treatment of repetitions, periodicity and temporal constraints in clinical guidelines. Artif. Intell. Med. **38**(2), 171–195 (2006)
5. Bäumler, S., Balser, M., Dunets, A., Reif, W., Schmitt, J.: Verification of medical guidelines by model checking – a case study. In: Valmari, A. (ed.) SPIN 2006. LNCS, vol. 3925, pp. 219–233. Springer, Heidelberg (2006)
6. Bettini, C., De Sibi, R.: Symbolic representation of user-defined time granularities. In: Proceedings of the Sixth International Workshop on Temporal Representation and Reasoning, TIME 1999, pp. 17–28 (1999)
7. Bottrighi, A., et al.: Adopting model checking techniques for clinical guidelines verification. Artif. Intell. Med. **48**(1), 1–19 (2010)
8. Clarke, E.M., Grumberg, O., Peled, D.A.: Model Checking. MIT Press, Cambridge (1999)
9. Dechter, R., Meiri, I., Pearl, J.: Temporal constraint networks. Artif. Intell. **49**(1), 61–95 (1991)
10. Duftschmid, G., Miksch, S., Gall, W.: Verification of temporal scheduling constraints in clinical practice guidelines. Artif. Intell. Med. **25**(2), 93–121 (2002)
11. Egidi, L., Terenziani, P.: A lattice of classes of user-defined symbolic periodicities. In: Proceedings of the 11th International Symposium on Temporal Representation and Reasoning, TIME 2004, pp. 13–20 (2004)
12. Egidi, L., Terenziani, P.: A mathematical framework for the semantics of symbolic languages representing periodic time. In: Proceedings of the 11th International Symposium on Temporal Representation and Reasoning, TIME 2004, pp. 21–27 (2004)
13. Field, M.J., Lohr, K.N.: Guidelines for Clinical Practice: From Development to Use. National Academies Press, Washington, DC (1992)
14. Fox, J., Johns, N., Rahmanzadeh, A.: Disseminating medical knowledge: the PRO*forma* approach. Artif. Intell. Med. **14**(1), 157–182 (1998)
15. Garber, A.J., et al.: Efficacy of metformin in type II diabetes: results of a double-blind, placebo-controlled, dose-response trial. Am. J. Med. **103**(6), 491–507 (1997)
16. Getoor, L., Taskar, B. (eds.): Introduction to Statistical Relational Learning. Adaptive Computation and Machine Learning. MIT Press, Cambridge (2007)
17. Giordano, L., et al.: Model checking for clinical guidelines: an agent-based approach. In: AMIA Annual Symposium Proceedings, vol. 2006, p. 289. American Medical Informatics Association (2006)
18. Giordano, L., et al.: A temporal approach to the specification and verification of interaction protocols. In: WOA, pp. 171–176 (2005)
19. Guthrie, B., et al.: Adapting clinical guidelines to take account of multimorbidity. BMJ **345**, e6341 (2012)
20. Halpern, J.Y., Vardi, M.Y.: Model checking vs. theorem proving: a manifesto. In: Artificial Intelligence and Mathematical Theory of Computation, vol. 212, pp. 151–176. Academic Press, Inc. (1991)
21. Holzmann, G.J.: The model checker spin. IEEE Trans. Softw. Eng. **23**(5), 279–295 (1997)

22. Hommersom, A., Ferreira, N., Lucas, P.J.F.: Integrating logical reasoning and probabilistic chain graphs. In: Buntine, W., Grobelnik, M., Mladenić, D., Shawe-Taylor, J. (eds.) ECML PKDD 2009, Part I. LNCS (LNAI), vol. 5781, pp. 548–563. Springer, Heidelberg (2009)

23. Huges, L.D., McMurdo, M.E.T., Guthrie, B.: Guidelines for people not for diseases: the challenges of applying UK clinical guidelines to people with multimorbidity. Age Ageing **42**(1), 62–69 (2013)

24. Kersting, K., De Raedt, L.: Towards combining inductive logic programming with Bayesian networks. In: Rouveirol, C., Sebag, M. (eds.) ILP 2001. LNCS (LNAI), vol. 2157, pp. 118–131. Springer, Heidelberg (2001)

25. Kimmig, A., et al.: On the implementation of the probabilistic logic programming language problog. Theory Pract. Logic Program. (2010)

26. Kosara, R., Miksch, S.: Visualization methods for data analysis and planning in medical applications. Int. J. Med. Inform. **68**(1), 141–153 (2002)

27. Kwiatkowska, M., Norman, G., Parker, D.: PRISM: probabilistic symbolic model checker. In: Field, T., Harrison, P.G., Bradley, J., Harder, U. (eds.) TOOLS 2002. LNCS, vol. 2324, pp. 200–204. Springer, Heidelberg (2002)

28. Lloyd, J.W.: Foundations of Logic Programming, 2nd edn. Springer, Heidelberg (1987)

29. Lucas, P.J.F., et al.: A probabilistic and decision-theoretic approach to the management of infectious disease at the ICU. Artif. Intell. Med. **19**(3), 251–279 (2000)

30. Marcos, M., Balser, M., ten Teije, A., van Harmelen, F., Duelli, C.: Experiences in the formalisation and verification of medical protocols. In: Dojat, M., Keravnou, E.T., Barahona, P. (eds.) AIME 2003. LNCS (LNAI), vol. 2780, pp. 132–141. Springer, Heidelberg (2003)

31. McMillan, K.L.: Symbolic Model Checking. Springer, Heidelberg (1993)

32. Musen, M.A., et al.: Knowledge engineering for a clinical trial advice system: uncovering errors in protocol specification. Bull. du Cancer **74**(291), 296 (1987)

33. Musen, M.A., et al.: EON: a component-based approach to automation of protocol-directed therapy. J. Am. Med. Inform. Assoc. **3**(6), 367–388 (1996)

34. Natarajan, S., Bui, H.H., Tadepalli, P., Kersting, K., Wong, W.-K.: Logical hierarchical hidden markov models for modeling user activities. In: Železný, F., Lavrač, N. (eds.) ILP 2008. LNCS (LNAI), vol. 5194, pp. 192–209. Springer, Heidelberg (2008)

35. Overhage, J.M., et al.: A randomized trial of corollary orders to prevent errors of omission. J. Am. Med. Inform. Assoc. **4**(5), 364–375 (1997)

36. Paul, M., et al.: Improving empirical antibiotic treatment using treat, a computerized decision support system: cluster randomized trial. J. Antimicrob. Chemother. **58**, 1238–1245 (2006)

37. Peleg, M., et al.: GLIF3: the evolution of a guideline representation format. In: Proceedings of the AMIA Symposium, p. 645. American Medical Informatics Association (2000)

38. Poole, D.: The independent choice logic and beyond. In: de Raedt, L., Frasconi, P., Kersting, K., Muggleton, S.H. (eds.) Probabilistic ILP 2007. LNCS (LNAI), vol. 4911, pp. 222–243. Springer, Heidelberg (2008)

39. Poole, D.: The independent choice logic for modelling multiple agents under uncertainty. Artif. Intell. **94**(1–2), 7–56 (1997)

40. Richardson, M., Domingos, P.: Markov logic networks. Mach. Learn. **62**(1–2), 107–136 (2006)

41. Sacchi, L., Rognoni, C., Rubrichi, S., Panzarasa, S., Quaglini, S.: From decision to shared-decision: introducing patients' preferences in clinical decision analysis - a case study in thromboembolic risk prevention. In: Peek, N., Marín Morales, R., Peleg, M. (eds.) AIME 2013. LNCS (LNAI), vol. 7885, pp. 1–10. Springer, Heidelberg (2013)

42. Shahar, Y.: A framework for knowledge-based temporal abstraction. Artif. Intell. **90**(1), 79–133 (1997)

43. Sherman, E.H., et al.: Using intermediate states to improve the ability of the arden syntax to implement care plans and reuse knowledge. In: Proceedings of the Annual Symposium on Computer Application in Medical Care, p. 238. American Medical Informatics Association (1995)

44. Shu, Y., et al.: Effect of genetic variation in the organic cation transporter 1 (OCT1) on metformin action. J. Clin. Invest. **117**, 1422–1431 (2007)

45. Ten Teije, A., et al.: Improving medical protocols by formal methods. Artif. Intell. Med. **36**(3), 193–209 (2006)
46. Terenziani, P., Molino, G., Torchio, M.: A modular approach for representing and executing clinical guidelines. Artif. Intell. Med. **23**(3), 249–276 (2001)
47. Terenziani, P., et al.: Spin model checking for the verification of clinical guidelines. In: ECAI 2006 Workshop on AI Techniques in Healthcare: Evidence-Based Guidelines and Protocols (2006)
48. Thon, I., Landwehr, N., De Raedt, L.: A simple model for sequences of relational state descriptions. In: Daelemans, W., Goethals, B., Morik, K. (eds.) ECML PKDD 2008, Part II. LNCS (LNAI), vol. 5212, pp. 506–521. Springer, Heidelberg (2008)
49. Velikova, M., et al.: Improved mammographic cad performance using multi-view information: a Bayesian network framework. Phys. Med. Biol. **54**, 1131–1147 (2009)
50. Vennekens, J., Denecker, M., Bruynooghe, M.: CP-logic: a language of causal probabilistic events and its relation to logic programming. Theory Pract. Logic Program. **9**, 245–308 (2009)
51. Vila, L.: A survey on temporal reasoning in artificial intelligence. AI Commun. **7**(1), 4–28 (1994)
52. van der Weijden, T., et al.: Clinical Practice Guidelines And Patient Decision Aids. An Inevitable Relationship. J. Clin. Epidemiol. **65**(6), 584–589 (2012)
53. Weng, C., Kahn, M., Gennari, J.: Temporal knowledge representation for scheduling tasks in clinical trial protocols. In: Proceedings of the AMIA Symposium, p. 879. American Medical Informatics Association (2002)
54. Zalounina, A., et al.: A stochastic model of susceptibility to antibiotic therapy-the effects of cross-resistance and treatment history. Artif. Intell. Med. **40**(1), 57–63 (2007)

Chapter 20
Aggregation of Clinical Evidence Using Argumentation: A Tutorial Introduction

Anthony Hunter and Matthew Williams

Abstract In this tutorial, we describe a new framework for representing and synthesizing knowledge from clinical trials involving multiple outcome indicators. The framework offers a formal approach to aggregating clinical evidence. Based on the available evidence, arguments are generated for claiming that one treatment is superior, or equivalent, to another. Evidence comes from randomized clinical trials, systematic reviews, meta-analyses, network analyses, etc. Preference criteria over arguments are used that are based on the outcome indicators, and the magnitude of those outcome indicators, in the evidence. Meta-arguments attack (i.e. they are counterarguments to) arguments that are based on weaker evidence. An evaluation criterion is used to determine which are the winning arguments, and thereby the recommendations for which treatments are superior. Our approach has an advantage over meta analyses and network analyses in that they aggregate evidence according to a single outcome indicator, whereas our approach combines evidence according to multiple outcome indicators.

20.1 Introduction

Evidence-based decision making is well established in medicine. However, the scale and pace of new evidence makes it difficult for clinicians and researchers to acquire and assimilate that evidence. As a consequence, understanding and reviewing the literature is difficult and time-consuming. This problem is exacerbated by the fact that the evidence is uncertain, incomplete and inconsistent. In this tutorial, we describe a new framework for aggregating evidence from clinical trials. This provides a systematic, transparent, and robust process that operates over multiple outcome indicators. The formal presentation of our framework has been presented in [8], but given the novelty of our approach can seem forbidding for a non-technical audience. So with this tutorial, we provide a more accessible introduction for clinical and scientific readers interested in reasoning with clinical evidence. We assume the reader has some basic familiarity with clinical trials, in particular randomised clinical trials.

© Springer International Publishing Switzerland 2015
A. Hommersom and P.J.F. Lucas (eds.), *Biomedical Knowledge Representation*, LNAI 9521, DOI 10.1007/978-3-319-28007-3_20

20.2 Motivation

To cope with the problems of volume, complexity, inconsistency and incompleteness of evidence, organizations supporting decision makers, such as the UK National
Institute for Clinical Excellence, (NICE, www.nice.org.uk), compile and aggregate
evidence into evidence-based guidelines for decision makers. Such guidelines systematically appraise available evidence so as to encode best-practice *recommendations*. These typically specify what tests should be done, and what treatments should
be considered, for particular classes of patient. The advice is supported by reference
to the primary literature (such as published randomized clinical trials, cohort studies,
etc.), together with available systematic reviews of evidence, such as by the Cochrane
Collaboration (www.cochranecollaboration.org).

As valuable as guidelines are for drawing the best available evidence into decision
making in healthcare, there are also some important limitations.

1. Constructing guidelines can involve **assimilating massive amounts of evidence**.
   For instance, medical guidelines are based on a rapidly growing body of biomedical evidence, such as clinical trials and other scientific studies (for example,
   PubMed, the online repository of biomedical abstracts run by the US National
   Institute of Health has over 20 million articles). Production of evidence-based
   guidelines therefore requires **considerable human effort and expenditure** since
   the evidence needs to be systematically reviewed and aggregated.
2. Guidelines can become **out-of-date** quite quickly. For example, in medicine,
   even when major trials are published on topics, it may take years before the
   guidelines are rewritten to take account of the large amounts of newly available
   evidence (for example, PubMed is growing at the rate of 2 articles per minute).
   Decision makers are thus faced with the problem of assimilating and processing
   guidelines in combination with large amounts of newly available evidence which
   may warrant recommendations that conflict with, and so suggest revisions to,
   those recommendations provided by the guidelines.
3. Often there are **overlapping guidelines** to consider (from different agencies or
   bodies, and international, national, and local sources), and when there are multiple
   problems to be resolved (e.g. a patient with both cancer and liver problems). Thus,
   different guidelines may offer conflicting guidance.
4. Guideline recommendations are often written keeping in mind a **general population** so they need to be interpreted for individual cases with specific features.
   For example, given a patient with some particular symptoms and test results, the
   clinician needs to decide if the patient falls into any of the classes of patients for
   which the guideline offers guidance (e.g. if the patient is from a particular ethnic
   group, or if they are very young, or if their symptoms do not exactly correspond).
   If the clinician has doubts, then turning to the primary literature for fuller descriptions of the relevant clinical trials may be useful. However, the clinician may then
   need to assimilate and aggregate the results from a number of articles which can
   be challenging. So after what may be an incomplete study of the evidence, the

clinician decides whether or not to accept the recommendation from the guideline for the specific case.

5. Guidelines are **not sensitive to local needs** or circumstances. This may also result in non-compliance by the decision maker in using a guideline. For example, an international guideline may recommend a particular kind of scan for patients with a particular combination of symptoms, but a particular hospital using the guideline might not be able to provide such a scan, and would deviate from the recommendations by the guideline.

6. Use of guidelines can **decouple a decision maker from the evidence** which can be problematical since the decision maker may have valuable knowledge and experience for use in interpreting the evidence.

These shortcomings suggest that there is a need for knowledge aggregation technologies for making evidence-based recommendations based on large repositories of complex, rapidly expanding, incomplete and inconsistent evidence. These technologies should aim to overcome the limitations of guidelines listed above, and offer tools for users who need to make evidence-based decisions, as well as users who need to draft systematic reviews and guidelines, and users who need to undertake research in order to fill gaps or resolve conflicts in the available evidence.

20.3 Argument-Based Evidence Aggregation

In this section, we provide some background to our approach. We consider the kind of input we assume, and we briefly discuss what we mean by argumentation.

20.3.1 Input to Our Aggregation Process

We concentrate on clinical trials that compare two different treatments (i.e. "two-armed" trials"), but where different trials may measure and report different outcome indicators.

Consider two treatments τ_1 and τ_2 for some heart condition. These may be compared on their efficacy in treating the condition, and on their side-effects. For example, we may have evidence from a trial that compares treatment τ_1 with τ_2 on the relative risk of mortality within 5 years is 0.95 (i.e. the risk of mortality with τ_1 is 0.95 of that with τ_2), and we may have evidence from a trial that compares treatment τ_2 with τ_1 on the relative risk of causing drowsiness is 0.5 (i.e. the risk of drowsiness with τ_2 is 0.5 of that with τ_1). Our framework takes this evidence as input, and determines which treatment is superior. In order to do this, we need to also take into account preferences (of clinicians or patients) over the outcome indicators and their magnitude.

- (Option 1) The relative risk of mortality within 5 years is 0.95 (if taking τ_1 instead of τ_2)
- (Option 2) The relative risk of causing drowsiness is 0.5 (if taking τ_2 instead of τ_1)

These preferences may vary from person to person. For some people, even a modest reduction in the risk of mortality is preferred to a reduced risk of drowsiness, and therefore they would prefer option 1, whereas for other people (e.g. HGV drivers), the risk of drowsiness would be problematical, and they would therefore prefer option 2. Whilst such preferences are subjective, once we have captured them we can use them systematically when aggregating evidence with multiple outcome indicators.

So to summarize, the input to our aggregation process is the evidence concerning pairwise comparisons of treatments, and the preferences over outcome indicators (and their magnitude) that appear in the evidence. Note, in Sect. 20.4, we consider how to consider different choices of preference when we do not have a specific preference.

20.3.2 Our Aggregation Process Is Based on Argumentation

Argumentation is an important cognitive activity for handling incomplete and inconsistent information. It involves identifying individual arguments and counterarguments, and it may involve identifying winning arguments. For example, diagnosis involves argumentation. There may be competing diagnoses for a patient. For each diagnosis, there may be one or more arguments that support it. Furthermore, there may counterarguments to some of these arguments (perhaps based on conflicting results from tests, or other reasons to doubt individual diagnoses). Deciding on which is the diagnosis for the patient can be regarded as a process of deciding on which arguments win.

In recent years, there has been substantial interest in developing theoretical and computational models of argument that can be used in diverse applications (for a review, see [3]). In theoretical models of argument, each argument has a formally specified claim, and some specified premises from which the claim can be derived using some formal reasoning process. For example, consider the following premises

```
The shape is square
If the shape is square, then the shape has four sides
```

From these premises, we have the claim "The shape has four sides" by logical reasoning (syllogism). Hence, we can construct an argument with these premises and claim.

A counterargument is an argument that contradicts the premises or claim of an argument. So a counterargument is an argument that "attacks" another argument. For example, from the premise that "The shape is triangular", we could construct a counterargument to the above argument.

```
The shape is triangular
If the shape is triangular, then the shape
does not have four sides
```

So that claim of the second argument contradicts the claim of the first argument, and so the second argument is a counterargument to the first argument. Furthermore, the claim of the first argument contradicts the claim of the second argument, and so the first argument is a counterargument to the second argument. So each argument attacks the other in this example.

Argumentation is useful when there is uncertainty in the information available. Here for instance, it may be that there is uncertainty about the shape of the observed object. One source believes it is square and the other source believes it is triangular.

Different formalisms for argumentation provide different ways of formalizing arguments and counterarguments, and for deciding on which arguments win. We do not provide a review of the field in this tutorial. Rather, we just outline (in the next section) the notions we require for our framework. However, what is common amongst these formalisms is that they provide an explicit representation of the conflicts arising in the available information, and that they provide principled ways of deciding what are winning arguments.

20.4 Step-by-Step Tutorial on Our Approach

In this section, we provide an introduction to our process for aggregating evidence. We do this in seven steps starting with the representation of the set of evidence as input (at Step 1) and a decision on which treatment is superior as output at (Step 7).

20.4.1 Tabulating the Evidence (Step 1)

We start with a set of 2-arm superiority trials, i.e., clinical trials whose purpose is to determine whether, given two treatments, one is superior to the other. Each trial will typically report more than one outcome (perhaps a measure of effectiveness, and a measure of a side-effect). We collect these as an evidence table. Each row represents data about the trial and a single outcome; thus each trial may generate more than one row. The columns of the table depend on the particular trial, but we assume the following columns as a minimum for an evidence table. We give an example of an evidence table in Example 20.1.

- The **left** and **right** attributes signify the treatments compared in each item of evidence (i.e. the left and right arms of the trial for each item of evidence).

- The **outcome indicator** attribute is the specification of the particular outcome that is being considered when comparing the two treatments. For example, it could be the relative risk of mortality.
- The **outcome value** attribute is the value obtained for the outcome indicator for the left arm compared to the right arm. For example, if the outcome indicator is relative risk of mortality, then it would be the value obtained for the left arm compared to the right arm.
- The **net outcome** attribute is a binary relation over the two treatments that is determined from the value of the outcome and an evaluation of whether the outcome indicator is desirable or undesirable for the patient class. In this tutorial, we consider outcome indicators that are evaluated in terms of relative risk. In this case, there are four possibilities for this.

1. If the outcome indicator is something that we want to decrease, and the outcome value is less than 1, then the left arm is superior is to the right arm, and so the net outcome is "superior".
2. If the outcome indicator is something that we want to decrease, and the outcome value is greater than 1, then the left arm is inferior is to the right arm, and so the net outcome is "inferior".
3. If the outcome indicator is something that we want to increase, and the outcome value is less than 1, then the left arm is inferior is to the right arm, and so the net outcome is "inferior".
4. If the outcome indicator is something that we want to increase, and the outcome value is greater than 1, then the left arm is superior is to the right arm, and so the net outcome is "superior".

For example, if the outcome indicator is relative risk of mortality, and the value is below 1, then the net outcome is desirable, and so the left arm is superior to the right arm. Whereas, if the outcome indicator is relative risk of mortality, and the value is above 1, then the net outcome is undesirable, and so the left arm is inferior to the right arm.

The set of attributes we have discussed here is the minimum that we require. There are numerous other optional attributes that are useful for assessing and aggregating evidence, such as the following, and so each such attribute could be captured as a further column in the evidence table (depending on the kind of evidence available and how it might be regarded).

- the p-value for the study
- the number of patients involved in each trial
- the geographical location for each trial
- the drop-out rate for the trial
- the methods of randomization
- the evidence type (meta-analysis, cohort study, network analysis, etc.)

For a general introduction to the nature of clinical trials, and a discussion of a wider range of attributes, see [7].

Example 20.1. For our running example, we will use the following evidence table. There are four items of evidence e_1 to e_4. For each item of evidence, the left arm is CP (standing for contraceptive pill) and the right arm is NT (standing for no treatment). For e_1, the outcome indicator is relative risk of pregnancy, for e_2, the outcome indicator is relative risk of ovarian cancer, for e_3, the outcome indicator is relative risk of breast cancer, and for e_4, the outcome indicator is relative risk of deep vein thrombosis (DVT). There is one optional column in this evidence table which is the p value for the RCT in each item of evidence.

ID	Left	Right	Outcome indicator	Outcome value	Net outcome	p
e1	CP	NT	pregnancy	0.05	superior	0.01
e2	CP	NT	ovarian cancer	0.99	superior	0.07
e3	CP	NT	breast cancer	1.04	inferior	0.01
e4	CP	NT	DVT	1.02	inferior	0.05

20.4.2 Generation of Structured Arguments (Step 2)

From the input evidence, a particular kind of argument that we call an structured argument is generated. Each structured argument is a pair $\langle X, \varepsilon \rangle$ where X is a subset of the evidence concerning two treatments τ_1 and τ_2. If all the evidence in X indicates that τ_1 is better in some respects than τ_2 (i.e. for the evidence in X, the net outcome is superior), then the claim ε is that τ_1 is superior to τ_2. Whereas if all the evidence in X indicates that τ_2 better in some respects to τ_1, then the claim ε is that τ_1 is inferior to τ_2 (i.e. for the evidence in X, the net outcome is inferior). And if all the evidence in X indicates that τ_2 equal in some respects to τ_1, then the claim ε is that τ_1 is equal to τ_2 (i.e. for the evidence in X, the net outcome is equal). Note, we assume the evidence in an argument is homogeneous in the sense that X only contains evidence that indicates τ_1 better in some respects to τ_2, or X only contains evidence that indicates τ_1 equal in some respects to τ_2, or X only contains evidence that indicates τ_2 better in some respects to τ_1

Example 20.2. Continuing Example 20.1, we have six structured arguments. Given two items of evidence that support the claim $CP > NT$, we get three arguments with the claim $CP > NT$. Similarly given two items of evidence that support the claim $CP < NT$, we get three arguments with the claim $CP < NT$

$$\langle \{e_1\}, CP > NT \rangle \quad \langle \{e_3\}, CP < NT \rangle$$
$$\langle \{e_2\}, CP > NT \rangle \quad \langle \{e_4\}, CP < NT \rangle$$
$$\langle \{e_1, e_2\}, CP > NT \rangle \quad \langle \{e_3, e_4\}, CP < NT \rangle$$

Each of the arguments on the left provides the case for the claim that τ_1 is superior to τ_2, and each of the arguments on the right provides the case for the claim that τ_2 is superior to τ_1 (or equivalently $.\tau_1$ is inferior to τ_2). Informally, we want to have each of the possible subsets of the evidence that supports a claim as an argument because we want to consider all possible ways that the evidence could be used as a winning argument. We will explain this in the rest of this section.

Looking at Example 20.2, we see intuitively that the arguments with differing claims conflict. Obviously it cannot be the case that both of the claims are true. So in this sense these arguments attack, or rebut, each other. We can represent the arguments and the attacks between them by a network (technically, a directed graph): Each node is an argument, and each arc (i.e. arrow) denotes one argument attacking another.

Example 20.3. Continuing Example 20.2, we can see that each argument with claim $CP > NT$ attacks each argument with claim $CP < NT$ and vice versa. In other words, each argument with claim $CP > NT$ is a counterargument to each argument with claim $CP < NT$ and vice versa. This is represented by the following directed graph.

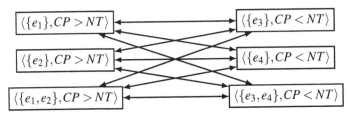

20.4.3   Identification of Preferences over Structured Arguments (Step 3)

Not all structured arguments are of the same weight. They vary in terms of the benefits that they offer, so for instance one argument may have the claim that τ_1 is superior τ_2 because of a substantial improvement in life expectancy, and another argument may have the claim that τ_2 is superior to τ_1 because the former has no side-effects, and the latter has some minor side-effects. To capture this, we use a preference relation over structured arguments that takes into account the nature and magnitude of the outcomes presented in the evidence (as we suggested in the introduction). This allows for a simple and intuitive approach to capturing subjective criteria.

Example 20.4. Continuing Example 20.1, given the outcome indicators presented in the evidence table, a clinician or patient may express the following preferences over them as following.

- (Preference 1) Substantial reduction in pregnancy is *more preferred* to modest reduction in risk of either breast cancer or DVT.
- (Preference 2) Modest reduction in risk of ovarian cancer is *equally preferred* to modest reduction in risk of either breast cancer or DVT.
- (Preference 3) Modest reduction in risk of ovarian cancer is *less preferred* to modest reduction in ower risk in both DVT and breast cancer.

In our framework, preferences over outcomes are used to refine the symmetrical (bidirectional) attacks between structured arguments. For each pair of structured arguments A and B, if the outcome indicators and their magnitude in the evidence in A are preferred to the outcome indicators and their magnitude in the evidence in B, then A attacks B and B does not attack A.

Example 20.5. The preferences in Example 20.4 can be used to refine the directed graph in Example 20.3 to give the following directed graph.

- Preference 1 is used to prefer arguments involving evidence e_1 over arguments involving evidence e_3 or e_4, and so the top and bottom arguments on the left attack each of the arguments on the right (but not vice versa).
- Preference 2 is used to identify that an argument involving just evidence e_2 is equally preferred to an argument involving just evidence e_3 and that an argument involving just evidence e_2 is equally preferred to an argument involving just evidence e_4, and so the middle argument on the left attacks the top and middle arguments on the right, and top and middle arguments on the right each attack the middle argument on the left.
- Preference 3 is used to prefer an argument involving both evidence e_3 and e_4 over an argument involving just evidence e_2, and so the bottom argument on the right attacks the middle argument on the left (but not vice versa).

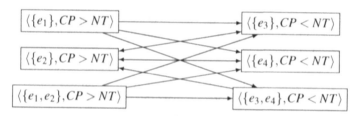

20.4.4 Generation of Meta-arguments (Step 4)

Structured arguments may vary also in terms of the quality of the evidence. For instance, one argument may be based on one small randomized clinical trial, and another may be based on a number of large randomized clinical trials. To address this, we use meta-arguments.

Each meta-argument is a counterargument to an structured argument that is generated because there is a weakness in the evidence of the structured argument. For example, if an structured argument is based entirely on evidence that is not statistically significant, then a meta-argument could be a counterargument to it.

Example 20.6. Continuing Example 20.1, we may choose the meta-argument $M =$ "Not statistically significant" to attack each structured argument that has evidence that has a p value above 0.05. So M attacks each of the following arguments.

$$\langle \{e_2\}, CP > NT \rangle$$
$$\langle \{e_1, e_2\}, CP > NT \rangle$$

There is a wide range of possible meta-arguments that can be used, and more than one meta-argument can be used at any one time. Each meta-argument attacks the evidence in a structured argument, and examples include

- The evidence contains flawed RCTs.
- The evidence contains results that are not statistically significant.
- The evidence is from trials that are for a very narrow patient class.
- The evidence has outcomes that are not consistent.

There are various ways we can formalize each of these as criteria as meta-argument (e.g. the meta-argument "Not statistically significant" could be defined as $p < 0.1$, or $p < 0.05$, or $p < 0.01$, or indeed any appropriate value for p).

Furthermore, various refinements of a meta-argument can be considered. For example, we could have a meta-argument "Not statistically significant for the intended outcome". So for instance, this would attack an structured argument that contained evidence that was not statistically significant for the outcome indicator that we want to treat, but it would not attack an structured argument only because it contained evidence that was not statistically significant for a side-effect. The rationale behind such a refinement would be that the majority of trials are set up to determine the efficacy of treatments, rather than for side-effects, and so it is normal for outcomes concerning side-effects to not be statistically significant and yet they are important in aggregating evidence about a treatment.

Obviously, using meta-arguments can have various kinds of ramification in the aggregation process, but the aim is to reflect the choices that clinicians and researchers have for attacking evidence, and moreover make this an explicit and auditable process. So if an aggregation of the evidence involves specific meta-arguments, then these are documented precisely and clearly with the outcome of the aggregation so that we have a reproducible and transparent process.

20.4.5 Generation of Evidential Argument Graph (Step 5)

An argument graph is a directed graph where each node denotes an argument, and each arc denotes an attack by one argument on another. So when one argument is a counterargument to another argument, this is represented by an arc. For each pair of treatments of interest, we construct an argument graph containing the structured arguments concerning these treatments, together with the meta-arguments that raise concerns with regard to the quality of the evidence in those structured arguments. In other words, this is the graph generated in Step 3 augmented with the meta-arguments generated in Step 4. We call this an evidential argument graph.

Example 20.7. Continuing Example 20.1, we have the following evidential argument graph. The structured arguments and the attacks between then come from Example 20.5, and the meta-argument and the attacks by the meta-argument come from Example 20.6.

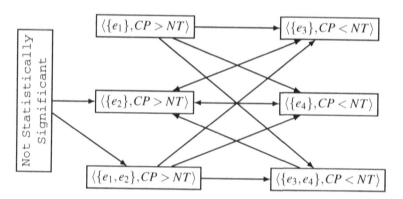

An evidential argument graph provides a clear and useful summary of the evidence in terms of the claims that can be made, the preferences over the outcomes suggested by the evidence, and the weaknesses in the evidence.

20.4.6   Evaluating the Argument Graph (Step 6)

We then evaluate the evidential argument graph to determine which arguments are warranted (i.e. which arguments "win" in the argumentation) and which arguments are unwarranted (i.e. which arguments "loose" in the argumentation). Given the graph, any argument (structured or meta) that is unattacked is warranted. For each of the remaining arguments,

- if it is attacked by a warranted argument, then it is unwarranted
- if all the arguments that attack it are unwarranted, then it is warranted
- if it is attacked by an argument that is neither warranted nor unwarranted, then it is undecided

Using this argumentation process, an argument is undecided unless there are assignments to its attacking arguments to make it either warranted or unwarranted.

Example 20.8. Continuing Example 20.7, the meta-argument is unattacked, and the structured argument $\langle \{e_1\}, CP > NT \rangle$ is unattacked, and so both are warranted. Each of $\langle \{e_2\}, CP > NT \rangle$ and $\langle \{e_1, e_2\}, CP > NT \rangle$ are attacked by the meta-argument, and so both are unwarranted. Finally, all the arguments on the right are attacked by $\langle \{e_1\}, CP > NT \rangle$, and so they are unwarranted.

Example 20.9. Returning to Example 20.3, suppose we have no preferences over the arguments, and we have no meta-arguments, then the evidential argument graph would be the graph given in Example 20.3. So every argument is unattacked, and so we cannot identify any warranted arguments or any unwarranted arguments. Therefore, all the arguments are undecided.

Note, our framework is defined so that it is not possible to have an evidential argument graph with a warranted argument with claim $\tau_1 > \tau_2$ and a warranted argument with claim $\tau_1 < \tau_2$. It is a property of our framework that we have warranted arguments with one of the claims, or we have all the structured arguments being either unwarranted or undecided.

20.4.7 Generation of Superiority Graph (Step 7)

So far, we have only considered pairs of treatments, and for each pair of treatments τ_1 and τ_2 we have an argument graph. We summarise the result of the argument graph as a superiority graph. If the winning arguments have the claim that τ_1 is superior to τ_2, then this is represented in the superiority graph by an arc from τ_1 to τ_2. For each arc in the superiority there is an associated argument graph which has been used to determine the direction of the arc. This argument graph is available to the user as an explanation for the direction of the arc.

Example 20.10. Continuing Example 20.8, there is an argument with the claim $CP > NT$ that is warranted, and all the arguments with the claim $CP < NT$ are unwarranted. So from the evidence table given in Example 20.1, we obtain the following superiority graph.

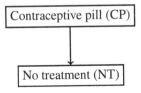

If an evidence table considers more than two treatments, as for example in Table 20.1, then an evidential argument graph needs to be generated for each pairs of treatments. So for the glaucoma evidence table, six evidential argument graphs were constructed, and the outcome from each of these gives one of the arcs in the superiority graph in Fig. 20.1.

20.4.8 Summary of Our Approach

Our framework allows for the construction of arguments on the basis of evidence as well as their syntheses. The evidence available is then presented and organized

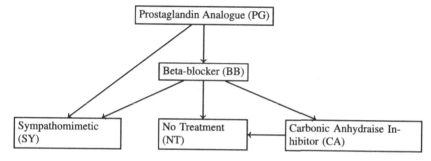

Fig. 20.1 Example of a superiority graph. This concerns treatments for glaucoma and it has been generated by our approach using the evidence table given in Table 20.1. There is an arc for each pair of treatments that we compared in one or more trials. If a pair of treatments were not compared in any trial, then there is no arc between them. When there is an arrow from treatment τ_1 to τ_2, then it means that our study found τ_1 to be superior to τ_2.

according to the agreement and conflict inherent. In addition, users can encode preferences for automatically ruling in favour of the preferred arguments in a conflict.

The **input to our framework** is a table of evidence comparing pairs of treatments. Each row in the table concerns a specific item of evidence such as a randomized clinical trial, and it gives the pair of treatments, the outcome indicator (e.g. disease-free survival, or overall survival), the outcome value, and optionally further details such as the kind of comparison (e.g. randomized clinical trial, meta-analysis, or network analysis), the statistical significance, etc. For any treatments τ_1 and τ_2 occurring in the evidence table, our framework would attempt to determine whether τ_1 is superior to τ_2, or τ_1 is equivalent to τ_2, or τ_1 is inferior to τ_2. This assessment would be justified by the arguments and counterarguments used to reach this conclusion.

The **output from our framework** is a **superiority graph** which is a directed graph where each node denotes a treatment (appearing in the input evidence table), each unidirectional arc from τ_1 to τ_2 denotes that τ_1 is superior to τ_2, and each bidirectional arc between τ_1 and τ_2 denotes that τ_1 is equivalent to τ_2.

So by determining in general whether one treatment is superior to another based on comparisons involving specific outcome indicators, we are using the items of evidence (concerning comparisons involving specific outcome indicators) as proxies for the general statement that in clinical and statistical terms one treatment is superior (or equivalent) to another. Furthermore, the items of evidence are normally incomplete and also disagree with each other as to which treatment is superior (for instance a treatment τ_1 may be superior to another τ_2 in suppressing the risk of mortality due to a particular disease, but τ_1 may be inferior to τ_2 because τ_1 has a substantial risk of a fatal side-effect and τ_2 has no risk of this side-effect). So to deal with the incomplete and inconsistent nature of the evidence, we have developed an approach that is based on a computational model of argumentation that takes into account the logical structure of individual arguments, and the dialectical structure of sets of arguments. We summarize our approach in Fig. 20.2.

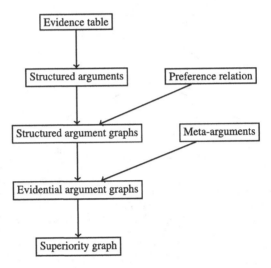

Fig. 20.2 Summary of our framework for evidence aggregation. The input is the evidence table and the output is the superiority graph. For each pair of treatments in the evidence table where there is a least one item of evidence comparing them, an evidential argument graph is produced. The evidential argument graph contains the structured arguments each of which takes a subset of the evidence to claim that one treatment is better (or equivalent) and meta-arguments that are counterarguments to structured arguments. One structured argument attacks another if their claims conflict, and the benefits of the first argument are preferred to the second. Each meta-argument attacks an structured argument when there is a weakness in the quality of the evidence used in the structured argument. If "winners" of the evidential argument graph, are all arguments for one treatment being superior to another, then this is reflected in the superiority graph.

20.5 Managing Subjectivity in Aggregation Criteria

So far in this paper we have explained how the evidence table is the input to the system, each pair of treatments is evaluated using an argument graph, and then a summary is produced in the form of a superiority graph. For this, we have assumed a single preference relation over the arguments (obtained from the preference relation), and a specific set of meta-arguments.

However, in practice it is normally not obvious that there is a single preference relation or a single set of meta-arguments. This is because, in general, the selection of a preference relation, and the selection of meta-arguments, are subjective criteria. Different clinicians, or their patients, may have different preference relations. This is an intrinsic and unavoidable feature of dealing with preferences over outcome indicators and their magnitude. Specification of the meta-arguments is also subjective because different experts judge evidence differently.

So irrespective of whether our proposal is used, aggregating clinical evidence involves subjective information. But the following are two key advantages of our approach for dealing with this subjective information:

Reproducibility. The preference relation and the set of meta-arguments are presented explicitly with the superiority graph. This means that any aggregation of the evidence is reproducible. The evidence, the preference relation, and the meta-arguments, can all be made available so that anyone can check exactly how the argument graphs and the superiority graph has been produced. This means the process is transparent and auditable.

Sensitivity analysis. Since there is not a preference relation or a set of meta-arguments that is always the right choice, different combinations of preference relation and/or meta-arguments can be used. In this way, a form of sensitivity analysis can be undertaken and so a treatment can be identified as superior for a range of preference relations and/or sets of meta-arguments. Furthermore, if the superiority graph changes little over a wide range of sensible preference relation and meta-arguments, then the superiority graph could be regarded as robust. Such sensitivity analyses may allow researchers and clinicians to categorize their findings according to robustness, and it may allow them to focus their discussions on evidence that is sensitive to the choice of preference relation or meta-arguments.

In general, we believe that a preference relation and a set of meta-arguments should be justifiable in some sense. Therefore there should be some clinical or ethical reason for adopting a particular preference relation, and there should be some methodological or clinical reason for adopting a particular set of meta-arguments.

But it may also be worthwhile to go backwards from a particular superiority graph to identify a preference relation and a set of meta-arguments that would give that superiority graph. For instance, suppose we have some evidence concerning treatments τ_1 and τ_2, and we consider τ_1 superior to τ_2. Suppose we cannot find any combination of preference relation and set of meta-arguments that is justifiable, then we have a stronger case for saying that τ_1 is not superior to τ_2.

In conclusion, using our framework, we can investigate the sensitivity of aggregations of evidence according to different subjective choices concerning the evidence table (i.e. when deciding whether two trials concern the same treatment or the same patient class is a subjective decision), and in the aggregation process (i.e. when deciding which preference relation and which meta-arguments to use). This leads to investigation of the sensitivity of a superiority graph to these subjective choices, and the identification of treatments are superior for a wide range of subjective choices (for the evidence table and the aggregation process).

20.6 Managing Subjectivity in Representing Evidence

Another kind of subjectivity in the aggregation process, concerns the way in which we group evidence. In many domains, the precise specification of the patient groups and treatments may vary across different trials. However, in order to make sense of the evidence, we accept that some treatments or patients can be grouped. This approach is common in existing systematic reviews, and also applies to our framework.

Patient class. When aggregating a set of trial results, we need to assume that the patient group is the same, and that the same treatments are being used. Normally, this is not the case. There may be small differences in the inclusion and exclusion criteria, and therefore the specification of the patient class needs to be relaxed to allow the trials to be regarded as concerning the same patient class. For example, if trial A considers male patients over 21 and trial B considers male patients over 23, then it would be reasonable to relax the patient class to being male adults and so both trials concern the same patient class.

Treatments. Similarly, the exact drug, the dosage, and the frequency of treatment might be slightly different, but for aggregation, they can be regarded as the same (e.g. for a particular drug 10% and 15% concentration may be regarded as the same treatment). Again this involves relaxation. As another example, many drugs for cancer are given in a cocktail (i.e. a mixture of therapies), and it is often difficult to find exactly the same cocktail used in more than a small number of trials. So again, the specification of the cocktail needs to be relaxed in order to aggregate the results.

Grouping of patients and treatments (relaxation) offers a valuable tool for analyzing clinical evidence in order to make more insightful and robust recommendations. To address this, we can couple the construction of arguments with an computer-readable model of the world, which contains accepted groupings of patients and treatments (an ontology), in order to automate the grouping of evidence according to patient class and/or treatment. By using the ontology to determine that two or more trials concern the same patient class and treatment, means that we have more evidence to consider for our arguments to any particular argument graph. We illustrate this idea in the next example.

Example 20.11. Suppose we have the following evidence table that is the same as the evidence table given in Example 20.1 except we have specific brands CP1 or CP2 instead of CP, where CP1 and CP2 are similar second generation low dose contraceptive pills.

ID	Left	Right	Outcome indicator	Outcome value	Net outcome	p
e1	CP1	NT	pregnancy	0.05	superior	0.01
e2	CP2	NT	ovarian cancer	0.99	superior	0.07
e3	CP1	NT	breast cancer	1.04	inferior	0.01
e4	CP2	NT	DVT	1.02	inferior	0.05

By using the ontological knowledge that CP1 and CP2 are similar, the above evidence table can be relaxed to the evidence table given in Example 20.1. In other words, by using this ontological knowledge, we can automatically replace CP1 and CP2 by CP in each entry in the Left column.

We have undertaken a theoretical analysis of how this may be done [4], and we can harness this for developing our sensitivity analysis of superiority graphs (whether by hand or by automated computer-readable ontologies).

20.7 Relationship of Our Approach with GRADE

One of the key questions when aggregating evidence is to what extent we can trust the evidence we have. There have been several approaches to considering the quality of evidence, including SIGN [18], and MERGE [12]. See [15] for a discussion. However, more recent work has aimed to achieve consensus via the GRADE guidelines [5].

We see our approach as being consistent with the GRADE approach. GRADE is a paper-based approach for making clinical recommendations based on evidence. It is an important tool for guideline development organizations such as NICE. In the approach, assignment of strength is made to each recommendation. Strong recommendations are made when the desirable effects of an intervention outweigh the undesirable effects, and weak recommendations are made when the trade-offs are less certain. Outcomes are graded according to their importance using a scale from 1 to 9. For instance, in considering phosphate lowering drugs in patients with renal failure, flatulence has grade 2, pain due to soft tissue calcification has grade 6, fractures has grade 7, myocardial infarction has grade 8, and mortality has grade 9 [6]. Allowing desirable and undesirable outcomes to be weighed. Furthermore, recommendations can be downgraded when the evidence is not of a sufficiently high quality. Items of evidence that are based on randomized clinical trials are *a priori* regarded as high quality evidence. But this assignment may be decreased for various reasons such as study limitations, inconsistency of results, indirectness of evidence, imprecisions, reporting bias, etc.

We can capture the GRADE approach in our framework using the preference relations, and the meta-arguments, in the argumentation. This means GRADE can benefit from a number of substantial advantages that come with our approach:

1. The way that the evidence is being aggregated is made explicit, with the preference relation and meta-arguments being made explicit, meaning that it is easier for third parties to inspect how the aggregation has been derived;
2. The same criteria (i.e. the same preference relations and meta-arguments) can be used systematically with new evidence tables, and so the aggregation process is consistent;
3. Different criteria (i.e. different combination of preference relation and meta-arguments) can be used in order to determine the sensitivity of ranking of treatments in a superiority graph;
4. Different strength of recommendation can be made by different choices of preference relation and meta-argument;
5. The process of generating superiority graphs can be automated.

Whilst, we have not considered diagnostic tests and strategies in our framework yet, we believe we can also capture the GRADE approach for diagnostic tests and strategies in our approach [17].

20.8 Discussion

For evidence-based decision making in healthcare, there is a need to abstract away from the details of individual items of evidence, and to aggregate the evidence in a way that reduces the volume, complexity, inconsistency and incompleteness of the information. Moreover, it would be helpful to have a method for automatically analyzing and presenting the clinical trial results and the possible ways to aggregate them in an intuitive form, highlighting agreement and conflict present within the literature.

We believe that our framework for aggregation of clinical evidence using argumentation addresses these needs. The output from our framework is a superiority graph. This is a useful summary of the aggregation of evidence for researchers and clinicians who need to aggregate evidence. Each arc connecting a pair of treatments in the graph is generated by an argumentation process that involves constructing an argument graph using the evidence concerning those two treatments, and this argument graph is available to the users of the superiority graph. They can look at the argument graph to inspect what arguments were considered and what preference criteria and meta-arguments were used. This means that it is explicit how the superiority graph was obtained, and thereby provides an audit trail of the aggregation process. Furthermore, different combinations of preference criteria and meta-arguments can be used to investigate the robustness of any superiority graphs produced.

We have already shown how clinicians use preferences in evaluating evidence [9], and it is straightforward to use our framework to represent these preferences. The advantage of allowing the user to define their own preference relations and their own meta-arguments is that they can systematically use the evidence in the context of their working environment.

We have evaluated our framework with three case studies involving 56 items of evidence, and 16 treatment options. The items of evidence come from three NICE Guidelines, and we have compared the results of our aggregation process with the recommendations made by NICE. In Table 20.1, we give one of the evidence tables used and in Fig. 20.1, we give the resulting superiority graph. The results using our framework are consistent with the NICE recommendations, though in some cases, it is apparent that they bring extra knowledge (beyond the evidence) into the process such as health economics modelling, or experiential knowledge, and so in some cases their recommendations are more refined than ours. We made simple choices for the preference relations over sets of benefits, and we believe that they are robust in the sense that they could be changed quite considerably and still we would get the same results from our aggregation process. For more details on this evaluation of our approach, please see [8].

In another case study, on lung cancer chemo-radiotherapy, we have investigated a number of different benefits preference relation and kinds of meta-argument. For this, we constructed an evidence table with 283 items of evidence (where each item of evidence concerns a pairwise comparison according to a single outcome indicator). The primary evidence on which the evidence table was based was a superset for that

Table 20.1 An evidence table concerning treatments for glaucoma. Each row is a meta-analysis from the NICE Glaucoma Guideline [14] (Appendix pages 213–223) for the class of patients who have raised intraocular pressure (i.e. raised pressure in the eye) and are therefore at risk of glaucoma with resulting irreversible damage to the optic nerve and retina. Each item is a meta-analysis (MA) generated by the guideline authors as presented in the appendix of the guideline. The medications considered are no treatment (NT), beta-blocker (BB), prostaglandin analogue (PG), sympathomimetic (SY), and carbonic anhydrase inhibitor (CA). The Net outcome column gives an interpretation of the value with respect to the type of outcome indicator: For the outcome indicator "change in IOP", if the value is negative, the left arm is superior, otherwise it is inferior. For the outcome indicator "acceptable IOP", which is a desirable outcome for the patient, if the value is greater than 1, the left arm is superior, otherwise it is inferior. For each of the remaining outcome indicators (i.e. for "respiratory problems", "cardiovascular problems", "allergy problems", "hyperaemia", "convert to COAG", "visual field progression", "IOP > 35mmHg", and "drowsiness"), which are undesirable for the patient, if the value is less than 1, then the left arm is superior, otherwise it is inferior. Note, "hyperaemia" means redness of eyes, "convert to COAG" means the patient develops chronic open angle glaucoma, "visual field progression" means that there is damage to the retina and/or optic nerve resulting in loss of the visual field and "IOP > 35mmHg" means that the intraocular pressure is above 35mmHg (which is very high).

ID	Left	Right	Outcome indicator	Outcome value	Net outcome	Sig	Type
e_{01}	BB	NT	visual field prog	0.77	superior	no	MA
e_{02}	BB	NT	change in IOP	-2.88	superior	yes	MA
e_{03}	BB	NT	respiratory prob	3.06	inferior	no	MA
e_{04}	BB	NT	cardio prob	9.17	inferior	no	MA
e_{05}	PG	BB	change in IOP	-1.32	superior	yes	MA
e_{06}	PG	BB	acceptable IOP	1.54	superior	yes	MA
e_{07}	PG	BB	respiratory prob	0.59	superior	yes	MA
e_{08}	PG	BB	cardio prob	0.87	superior	no	MA
e_{09}	PG	BB	allergy prob	1.25	inferior	no	MA
e_{10}	PG	BB	hyperaemia	3.59	inferior	yes	MA
e_{11}	PG	SY	change in IOP	-2.21	superior	yes	MA
e_{12}	PG	SY	allergic prob	0.03	superior	yes	MA
e_{13}	PG	SY	hyperaemia	1.01	inferior	no	MA
e_{14}	CA	NT	convert to COAG	0.77	superior	no	MA
e_{15}	CA	NT	visual field prog	0.69	superior	no	MA
e_{16}	CA	NT	IOP > 35mmHg	0.08	superior	yes	MA
e_{17}	CA	BB	hyperaemia	6.42	inferior	no	MA
e_{18}	SY	BB	visual field prog	0.92	superior	no	MA
e_{19}	SY	BB	change in IOP	-0.25	superior	no	MA
e_{20}	SY	BB	allergic prob	41.00	inferior	yes	MA
e_{21}	SY	BB	drowsiness	1.21	inferior	no	MA

used in a Cochrane Review on this topic [16]. For the systematic review that has resulted from our case study, the different ways of aggregating the evidence gave various insights into the evidence, such as the identification of weaknesses in the evidence base, and suggestions being made for future clinical trials to better determine which of the available treatments is superior. By exploring various relaxations of the evidence, we were able to make more refined recommendations than obtained with the original Cochrane review.

As we explained in Sect. 20.7, our approach is consistent with GRADE, and the GRADE approach for interventions can be formalized and automated in our approach giving a number of benefits. By using GRADE in our approach, any assumptions are made explicit, and the aggregation process is reproducible.

Our approach is also consistent with standard techniques such as meta-analyses. If there are multiple trials with the same outcome indicator, then standard techniques such as taking the weighted average offer substantial advantages. However, standard meta-analysis techniques do not handle multiple outcome indicators [7, 10]. So if there are multiple trials with the same outcome indicator, then standard techniques can be applied, and the result of the standard techniques used as the input to our approach. In other words, for the evidence table, a row can be based on a meta-analysis. So our approach can harness the output of standard meta-analysis techniques, but our approach can address problems that cannot be addressed by standard meta-analysis techniques

Network analysis is an increasingly popular method for systematic reviews with over 30 published in 2011, and an estimate of over 50 in 2012 [1]. In network analysis, the pairwise superiority of interventions is considered transitively. For example, if τ_1 is superior to τ_2 and τ_2 is superior to τ_3, then by transitivity τ_1 is superior to τ_3. In general, such an inference can be error-prone (for a discussion of this, see [2]). But with further information about the trials (such as details about the populations, results, etc.), then there are network analysis techniques that can qualify the transitive inference [13]. Also, see [11] for a discussion of network analysis. However, as with meta-analysis techniques, network analysis techniques assume a common outcome indicator. So again, we believe that our approach is consistent with network analysis techniques. Our approach can harness the output of network analysis techniques, but our approach can address problems that cannot be addressed by network analysis techniques.

Acknowledgements The authors would like to thank Jiri Chard and Cristina Visintin for valuable feedback on this tutorial.

References

1. Bafeta, A., et al.: Analysis of the systematic reviews process in reports of network meta-analyses: methodological systematic review. Br. Med. J. **347**, f3675 (2013)
2. Baker, S., Kramer, B.: The transitive fallacy for randomized trials: If A beats B and B beats C in separate trials, is A better than C? BMC Med. Res. Methodol. **2**, 13 (2002)
3. Besnard, P., Hunter, A.: Elements of Argumentation. MIT Press, Cambridge (2008)
4. Gorogiannis, N., Hunter, A., Williams, M.: An argument-based approach to reasoning with clinical knowledge. Int. J. Approximate Reasoning **51**(1), 1–22 (2009)

5. Guyatt, G., et al.: GRADE: an emerging consensus on rating quality of evidence and strength of recommendations. Br. Med. J. **336**, 924–926 (2008)
6. Guyatt, G., et al.: GRADE: what is quality of evidence and why is it important to clinicians. Br. Med. J. **336**, 995–998 (2008)
7. Hackshaw, A.: A Concise Guide to Clinical Trials. Wiley Blackwell, London (2009)
8. Hunter, A., Williams, M.: Aggregating evidence about the positive and negative effects of treatments. Artif. Intell. Med. **56**, 173–190 (2012). Edited by Baroni, P., et al
9. Hunter, A., Williams, M.: Using clinical preferences in argumentation about evidence from clinical trials. In: Veinot, T., et al. (eds.) Proceedings of the First ACM International Health Informatics Symposium, pp. 118–129. ACM Press (2010)
10. Kirkwood, B., Sterne, J.: Essential Medical Statistics. Blackwell, Oxford (2003)
11. Li, T., et al.: Network meta-analysis-highly attractive but more methodological research is needed. BMC Med. **9**(1), 79 (2011)
12. Liddle, J., Williamson, M., Irwig, L.: Method for Evaluating Research and Guideline Evidence. New South Wales Health Department, Sydney (1996)
13. Lumley, T.: Network meta-analysis for indirect treatment comparison. Stat. Med. **21**, 2313–2324 (2002)
14. NICE. Glaucoma: Clinical Guidelines CG85. London, UK: National Institute for Health and Clinical Excellence (2009). www.nice.org.uk. Accessed 1 April 2012
15. NICE. The Guidelines Manual. National Institute for Health and Clinical Excellence (2009)
16. N. O'Rourke et al. "Concurrent chemoradiotherapy in non-small cell lung cancer". In: Cochrane Database of Systematic Reviews. Article. No.: CD002140. 6 (2010). doi:10.1002/14651858
17. Schnemann, H., et al.: GRADE: grading quality of evidence and strength of recommendations for diagnostic tests and strategies. Br. Med. J. **336**, 1106–1110 (2008)
18. SIGN. SIGN 50: A Guideline Developers Handbook. Scottish Intercollegiate Guidelines Network (2011)

Author Index

Printed in the United States
By Bookmasters